Practical Infection Control in Dentistry

Practical Infection Control in Dentistry

JAMES A. COTTONE, DMD, MS

Professor and Director
Division of Oral Diagnosis and Oral Medicine
Department of Dental Diagnostic Science
The University of Texas Health Science Center at San Antonio Dental School
San Antonio, TX

GEZA T. TEREZHALMY, DDS, MA

Dean
School of Dentistry
Case-Western Reserve University
Cleveland, OH

JOHN A. MOLINARI, PhD

Professor and Chairman
Department of Biomedical Sciences
University of Detroit Mercy School of Dentistry
Detroit, MI

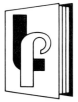

Lea & Febiger • Philadelphia • London

Lea & Febiger
200 Chester Field Parkway
Malvern, Pennsylvania   19355-9725
U.S.A.
(215) 251-2230

Library of Congress Cataloging-in-Publication Data

Practical infection control in dentistry / edited by James A. Cottone,
   Geza T. Terezhalmy, John A. Molinari.
        p.   cm.
     ISBN 0-8121-1326-8
     1. Dental offices—Sanitation.   2. Communicable diseases—
Prevention.   3. Asepsis and antisepsis.   I. Cottone, James A.
II. Terezhalmy, Geza T.   III. Molinari, John A.
     [DNLM: 1. Communicable Disease Control—methods.   2. Dentistry.
WA 110 P895]
RK52.P73   1991
617.6'01—dc20
DNLM/DLC
for Library of Congress   90-5643
                                                                          CIP

PRINTED IN THE UNITED STATES OF AMERICA

Print number: 5

Reprints of chapters may be purchased from Lea & Febiger in quantities of 100 or more.
Contact Sally Grande in the Sales Department

Preface

Until recently the basic sources for infection control information for the dental practitioner were:
1. Advice from older practitioners whose knowledge was usually minimal or outdated.
2. Dental supply personnel who lacked formal education in this area and could be biased towards their own products.
3. A trained assistant whose knowledge was variable depending on his or her experience.
4. A trained hygienist, who usually was the most knowledgeable but was discouraged once out in practice with statements such as "we don't do it that way here."
5. Miscellaneous articles and research reports in the literature, many of which perpetuate myths or sometimes are even misleading or wrong in their results and advice as they may have been authored by individuals who thought they knew the basics of something as "simple" as infection control.

In the past, few dental education institutions included sufficient classroom and clinical teaching of infection control. The basic information was usually discussed in microbiology or in a clinical introduction. Most schools prepared and sterilized the students' instruments for them, resulting in students graduating with little real experience in sterilization or other infection control procedures. The new graduate then embarked on a "do-it-yourself" project to develop some type of infection control system for their office. This system consisted of a blend of instrument disinfection, instrument sterilization, and household cleaning procedures adapted for the dental office, again depending on the quality of his or her staff.

Recent information regarding the transmission of hepatitis and herpes, and the emergence of Human Immunodeficiency Virus (HIV) infection and AIDS, along with the impact of standards from governmental agencies such as the Occupational Safety and Health Administration (OSHA) and the Environmental Protection Agency (EPA), have led to an increased interest in infection control in general and as it relates to dentistry in particular. This interest is warranted because of the lack of traditional infection control procedures in dentistry over the years. In some instances, these events have led to the development of infection control protocols that are overly detailed and elaborate, incorporating every conceivable barrier, product, and procedure. Infection control procedures have gone too far in many facilities. There are some basic procedures that need to be followed.

The *GOAL* of good infection control in dentistry is to treat *every* patient as though he or she is infected with an incurable disease (universal precautions). The method to implement this goal is to develop *one* infection control protocol for use in the dental operatory that is simple and effective for use with *all* patients, including hepatitis B carriers, HIV antibody positive, and diagnosed AIDS patients. If appropriate measures are taken, infection control will then occur as a routine component of dental practice.

In order to assist in the development of one infection control protocol for all patients, this textbook has been divided into the following major areas:
1. Patient Assessment
2. Personal Protection
3. Sterilization and Chemical Disinfection
4. Environmental Surface and Equipment Disinfection
5. Aseptic Technique

Each of these areas is explored thoroughly in the chapters that follow, with a discussion of medical and legal considerations and today's minimum requirements in infection control at the end of the text.

This volume contains much information about infection control protocols and procedures. Although the authors, contributors and publisher have taken meticulous care to ensure the accuracy of the product formulations and manufacturer recommendations, the law requires the reader to consult information about changes in formulation and methods of product use printed in the package insert before using any product. The reader then can be certain that new data has not led to altered instructions.

Additionally, the area of infection control is changing daily with new products and techniques. The reader will need to become an evaluator of these advances. The use of this text as part of the reader's infection control education and training programs is encouraged because good infection control is a *philosophy*, not a series of "cookbook" steps. Practical infection control in dentistry is making a needed permanent change in the dental profession as we know it.

J.A. Cottone, San Antonio
G.T. Terezhalmy, Cleveland
J.A. Molinari, Detroit

Contributors

A special note of thanks to the following contributors for adding their expertise to that of the authors:

Bill R. Baker, DDS, MSD

Department of Dental Diagnostic Science
The University of Texas Health Science Center
at San Antonio Dental School
San Antonio, TX (Chapter 5)

Constance Baker, JD

Venable, Baetjer and Howard
Baltimore, MD (Chapter 16)

James J. Crawford, PhD

Department of Endodontics
University of North Carolina School of Dentistry
Chapel Hill, NC (Chapter 12)

Birgit Junfin Glass, DDS, MS

Department of Dental Diagnostic Science
The University of Texas Health Science Center
at San Antonio Dental School
San Antonio, TX (Chapter 13)

Chris H. Miller, PhD

Department of Oral Microbiology
Indiana University School of Dentistry
Indianapolis, IN (Chapter 7)

Risa Pollock, CDA, RDA

Teamwork Concepts
Burlingame, CA (Chapter 14)

Sam Rosen, PhD

College of Dentistry
Section of Oral Biology
Ohio State University
Columbus, OH (Chapter 8)

Robert R. Runnells, DDS

University of Utah Medical School
Salt Lake City, UT (Chapter 1)

Bernard M. Sabatini, CDT

Wolverine Dental Laboratory
Hazel Park, MI (Chapter 15)

Linda Stokes, CDA

c/o Cottrell Ltd.
Englewood, CO (Chapters 12 and 14)

John M. Young, DDS, MSc

Department of General Practice
The University of Texas
Health Science Center at San Antonio
San Antonio, TX (Chapters 11, 12, 14, and 15)

The authors also wish to thank Deborah Willoughby, Peggy Campbell, Carol Grennan, Marion Mora, and the Office Sterilization and Asepsis Procedures (OSAP) Research Foundation for their assistance in the preparation of the manuscript.

This text represents the consensus of the authors and contributors and not necessarily the private views of any one individual.

Contents

section one

Patient Assessment

Chapter 1

Infectious Diseases Important in Dentistry

Infections present a significant hazard in the dental environment. For this reason, the essence of basic asepsis in dental practice cannot be overemphasized. Although protection of the patient is an obvious priority, oral health care personnel are also vulnerable to cross-infections. Much of this awareness is in response to problems associated with patients and dental personnel who contract hepatitis or who are carriers of the virus. Although hepatitis may have generated the initial concern about cross-infection, practitioners have grown aware of the threat posed by other infectious diseases. The incidence of certain microbial cross-infections in the dental environment has been well documented. However, the transmission of other pathogens, while highly probable, has not been definitely established. Consequently, dental personnel may not take the problem of cross-infection as seriously as they should, and they may transmit or contract more infections than they realize.

HISTORICAL PERSPECTIVE

In 2700 B.C., Huang-Ti wrote the *Canon of Medicine*, the oldest medical manuscript to refer to dental and gingival diseases, and the Egyptians, who had rudimentary knowledge of oral surgery, treated dental diseases as early as the sixth century B.C. However, microorganisms were not discovered in the mouth until 1685, when van Leeuwenhoek, using a microscope he had constructed, examined dental plaque.

In 1881, Miller recommended that microbiology be made an integral part of dental curricula and, in 1884, Koch demonstrated that tuberculosis could be transmitted by airborne droplets from the mouth and respiratory tract. In 1911, a paper by William Hunter, an English physician, claimed that the causes of many ailments could be traced to infections in the oral cavity. The electric dental engine, introduced in the 1920's, was shown to have produced aerosols that exposed dental personnel to more diseases than did the foot-driven engine and, in 1931, a report confirmed that the incidence of airborne infections was greater for dentists than for other professionals.

The introduction of the high-speed turbine engine and ultrasonic scalers in the late 1950's significantly contributed to bacteria-laden aerosol contamination of the dental operatory. In a study conducted in 1962, tracer organisms, *Serratia marcescens*, were recovered as far as 6 feet from the handpiece when the turbine was used with a water spray. Despite the evidence, it was not until the early 1970's that the dental profession began to realize the potential for cross-infection in the dental environment.

RESPIRATORY INFECTIONS

The Common Cold. This is a brief, self-limiting respiratory illness most frequently caused by a group of viral agents that include influenza, parainfluenza, respiratory syncytial virus, coronavirus, rhinovirus, echovirus, adenovirus, Coxsackie A and B, and other viruses. Some of these viruses have been isolated in dental aerosols and a positive correlation has been shown between the incidence of common cold epidemics in patients and in the oral health care personnel who treated them. In another study, dental students experienced a consistently higher incidence of respiratory diseases than their counterparts in medical and pharmacy schools.

A survey of the incidence of respiratory diseases in dental hygienists and dieticians during a 1-year period revealed that hygienists experienced significantly more colds than did the dieticians. Dental hygienists, however, did not miss significantly more work days, suggesting the potential for transmission of their infection to others.

Acute or Chronic Sinusitis. The initial viral infection of the common cold may be followed by a secondary bacterial infection that may go on for weeks. Sinusitis is more common in individuals with nasal polyps and allergic rhinitis, and among heavy smokers. Pneumococci, *Haemophilus influenzae*, and anaerobes identified in dental aerosols and contaminated water lines are common isolates in chronic sinusitis.

Acute Pharyngitis. Acute pharyngitis may be of viral or streptococcal etiology. Adenovirus pharyngitis is common in military populations. *Herpesvirus hominis* may cause ulcerative pharyngitis and subsequent recurrent herpetic infections. The Coxsackie viruses may cause herpangina, especially in children, and infectious mononucleosis (Epstein-Barr virus) in adolescence may present with similar clinical manifestations. Infection with *Streptococcus pyogenes*, isolated from dental aerosols, may produce classical bacterial pharyngitis. Gonococcal pharyngitis is commonly asymptomatic but may resemble either viral or streptococcal disease.

Pneumonia. Defective leukocyte activity predisposes to infections with pneumococci, streptococci, *Haemophilus influenzae*, and *Pneumocystis carinii*. Pneumococci are responsible for 98%, staphylococci for 1%, *Klebsiella pneumoniae* for 0.6%, and *H. influenzae* for 0.3% of the bacterial pneumonias. Friedlander's pneumonia (*Klebsiella pneumoniae*) is most common among alcoholic males between the age of 40 and 60 with mortality rates of 40 to 60% compared to 5% for pneumococcal infections. Staphylococcal pneumonia occurs primarily in children, patients with altered pulmonary function, and hospitalized patients. It is frequent during influenza epidemics and is associated with an overall mortality rate ranging from 25 to 60%. *H. influenzae* pneumonia is also most common in alcoholic males and the condition may be on the rise because the treatment of childhood infections with this organism may reduce protective antibody response.

Tuberculosis. Although morbidity and mortality from tuberculosis have declined steadily for several decades, this disease persists as an important health problem in the United States. The infection and disease are caused by *Mycobacterium* *tuberculosis.* The inhalation of a small number of bacilli may lead to bacterial multiplication in the respiratory bronchioles, alveolar ducts, or alveoli.

Tuberculous Infection. This is a state in which the tubercle bacillus has become established in the body but there are no symptoms, no radiographic abnormalities compatible with tuberculosis, and bacteriologic studies are negative. Infection in a person who is otherwise well can usually be diagnosed by demonstrating that the tuberculin test is positive. *Tuberculosis,* however, indicates a state in which an infected person has a disease process involving one or more of the organs of the body. Bacteriologic studies will usually confirm the presence of disease. Only about 5 to 15% of those infected ever become ill with tuberculosis, and the risk of developing tuberculosis for newly infected individuals is about 4% per year for the first 1 or 2 years following infection.

The diagnosis of tuberculous infection is important both clinically and epidemiologically. Such a diagnosis may be the first hint to the clinician that tuberculosis is present. Other infected persons may be candidates for preventive therapy with isoniazid. The tuberculin skin test has been the traditional method of diagnosing tuberculous infection, and the intradermal (Mantoux) test using five tuberculin units (TU) of Tween-stabilized PPD- tuberculin is the test of choice because of its relative specificity.

A study of English medical and dental students revealed that tuberculosis was more prevalent in dental students. Another study confirmed that by the end of their senior year, 33% of the dental students were PPD converters in contrast to only 5% at the beginning of their junior or first clinical year.

CHILDHOOD DISEASES

Childhood diseases are another potential source of cross-infections in the dental environment. The past low incidence of these conditions contributed to apathy both among physicians and parents and the immunization status of many oral health care professionals and their patients may be deficient.

Chickenpox. Primary infections by the *Varicella-Zoster* virus usually occurs in childhood. It is highly contagious and transmitted commonly by droplet inhalation or by direct skin contact. Dissemination of the virus within the body is probably hematogenous, and the typical rash develops after an incubation period of about 2 weeks. Oral lesions, affecting the tongue and oral mucosa, are a fairly common feature of this infection and may precede the skin lesions.

Herpangina. This is a common viral disease of the oral cavity and oropharynx of children and young adults caused by a *Coxsackie* virus. The typical course begins with fever and malaise followed in 24 to 48 hours by acute inflammation of the soft palate and oropharynx. The rest of the mouth is characteristically unaffected. Duration is 7 to 10 days and resolution is uneventful.

Hand-Foot-and-Mouth Disease. This is an infection of children and young adults also attributed to a *Coxsackie* virus. The pattern of vesicle formation, rupture, and ulceration of the oral mucosa is differentiated from that of herpangina by the involvement of any part of the oral cavity and from herpetic gingivostomatitis by the presence of the lesions on the hands and feet.

Rubella (German Measles). This is a mild respiratory infection associated with an exanthem and occurs predominantly in the spring and summer. The incubation period is 14 to 21 days. A typical rash appears as a maculopapular eruption on the face and neck and is preceded by or associated with posterior cervical lymphad-enopathy. The rash descends from head to foot over 2 to 3 days. An exanthem may develop simultaneously with the rash and consists chiefly of petechial lesions of the soft palate (Forscheimer spots). Fever is present for 1 to 2 days at the onset of the rash. The manifestations of rubella may be sufficiently mild that many cases go undiagnosed although 30 to 40% of adult women with rubella may develop arthritis, or arthralgia of the fingers, wrists, and knees. Of major importance is the fetal damage that follows transplacental infection occurring during the first 12 weeks of gestation resulting in severe birth defects, cardiac anomalies, or spon-taneous abortions. Later infections during pregnancy may lead to hepatitis, jaun-dice, thrombocytopenia, lymphadenopathy, pneumonitis, and progressive mental retardation of the child. Postnatally acquired rubella is generally a benign disease of children and adults.

Rubeola (Measles). Measles is also an acute respiratory infection characterized by a maculopapular rash on the face and neck. It spreads in a descending pattern to reach the hands and feet and lasts 5 to 7 days. It occurs in young school-age children worldwide. The incubation period is 10 to 14 days in children but may be as long as 21 days in adults. A prodroma of increasing severity is associated with cough, conjunctivitis, fever, malaise, loss of appetite, coryza, and Koplik's spots (multiple 0.25 to 1 mm whitish-blue spots on a red base found in clusters on the buccal mucosa usually opposite the second molars). Rubeola may ultimately lead to croup and bronchopneumonia.

Mumps. This infection is characterized by an incubation period of 14 to 21 days followed by fever, swelling, and tenderness of the parotids. It occurs primarily between 5 and 15 years of age. Transmission of the virus is by direct contact with droplets of saliva that contain the virus several days before and up to 1 week after swelling of the parotid is noted. In addition to the parotids, the condition may involve the pancreas, testes, and the CNS.

Cytomegalovirus (CMV). CMV infection, an apparently endemic disease that can be transmitted through saliva and is usually asymptomatic, has been shown to be common among children attending day-care centers. CMV infection can cause a form of lymphatic disease resembling mononucleosis in older children and adults. CMV infection is of greatest concern when infection occurs in utero, and it may account for approximately 0.1% of deaths among newborn infants. Because of this finding, oral health care professionals are being urged to carefully follow proper aseptic procedures to avoid transmitting the infection.

SEXUALLY TRANSMITTED DISEASES

Venereologists recognize an increasing number of sexually transmissible dis-eases, many of which have reached epidemic proportions. When we discuss sexual activity and disease, we must take into account the possibility of persons having multiple sexual partners and engaging in a greater variety of sexual acts than in the past. Increases in orogenital activity can be expected to be accompanied by corresponding increases in the oral manifestations of sexually related diseases. Clinicians must have an acute awareness of these infections to minimize the po-tential for cross-infection.

A striking characteristic of many of the sexually transmissible diseases is that their most severe consequences, with the notable exception of AIDS, are seen in women and young children.

Herpetic Infections. These infections have evoked increasing interest over the past several years because they are a common venereal disease. Both antigenically distinct types of *Herpesvirus hominis* (HVH-1 and HVH-2) can produce local skin, oropharyngeal, genital, and CNS infections, as well as disseminated visceral viremia. Cases of HVH-1 and HVH-2 infections of oropharyngeal and genital sites of sexual partners have been observed and autoinoculation from oropharynx to genitalia, genitalia to oropharynx, or other body sites with either virus type can occur.

The clinical manifestations of herpetic infections have been clearly described for the last 250 years. Despite this, the causative agent was not identified as a herpes virus until the 20th century. Seroepidemiologic studies indicate that 80 to 90% of the adult population has been exposed to the herpes virus and 40% of those individuals with serologic evidence of primary infection experience recurrent lesions. Because of this widespread occurrence, localized herpetic infections constitute a significant problem for the dental profession.

Acute Herpetic Gingivostomatitis. This is the most common form of primary invasion by HVH-1. In young children, the infection may only be transient or subclinical. In adults, however, it is often more dramatic. Following an incubation period of 4 to 5 days, the patient complains of malaise, irritability, headache, fever, lymphadenopathy, and within 1 or 2 days, the mouth becomes uncomfortable. Examination shows widespread inflammation of the marginal and attached gingivae characterized by erythema, edema, and capillary proliferation. Numerous small vesicles may develop anywhere on the oral mucosa and lips. The vesicles soon ulcerate and may become secondarily infected. The ulcers on the lips become crusted and if saliva dribbles from the mouth, similar lesions may develop on the face. The symptoms begin to subside about the sixth day of fever, and the oral lesions and lymphadenopathy take 10 to 14 days to resolve.

Primary HVH infection is a frequent cause of pharyngitis in young adults, and HVH-1 and HVH-2 have been isolated from the oropharynx of patients with primary and recurrent genital herpes. Clinical signs of herpetic pharyngitis range from mild erythema to severe diffuse ulcerative or exudative pharyngitis of the posterior pharynx. Occasionally, the lesions extend into other areas of the oral cavity. Fever, malaise, myalgia, headache, and tender anterior cervical lymphadenopathy are usually present. Severe herpetic pharyngitis may lead to laryngeal edema and obstruction.

Herpes Labialis. This is the most frequent type of recurrent herpetic infection. It is characterized by marked local symptoms unaccompanied by systemic illness. There is an apparent increased prevalence with age and the lesions tend to recur in a similar site in any one individual, most commonly on or adjacent to the vermilion border of the lip. The clinical course is marked by a prodromal period of hyperesthesia or altered sensation, and erythema and edema at the site of involvement. Prodromata is followed by the eruption of clusters of vesicles that coalesce and crust.

Recurrent Intraoral Infections. The typical features of recurrent intraoral herpetic infections include single or small clusters of vesicles that rapidly break down into ulcers. These lesions occur on the keratinized mucosa of the hard palate or gingivae and may occasionally be associated with herpes labialis.

Herpetic Whitlow. A particular problem to dental and medical personnel, herpetic whitlow is a type of primary HVH-1 infection that affects one or several fingers, characteristically presenting with an extremely painful finger and vesicles that initially contain a clear fluid. Local adenitis and, frequently, a marked constitutional disturbance, are noted.

In a study of Michigan dentists, it was found that more dentists experience *Herpesvirus hominis* infections of the finger or hand than their age and sex-matched controls, and an increased incidence of herpetic keratoconjunctivitis from autoinoculation has been reported in association with herpetic whitlow.

There is also documented evidence of *Herpesvirus hominis* transmission from an oral health care professional to patients. Twenty of 46 patients seen by a dental hygienist in a 4-day period developed gingivostomatitis. The week before this 4-day period, the hygienist cleaned the teeth of a patient with a "cold sore" on the lower lip and did not wear gloves. Four days after exposure, the hygienist noticed a worsening of her chronic dermatitis and later developed vesicles. After she started wearing gloves, no new cases of herpetic gingivostomatitis developed. The area of chronic dermatitis was probably the portal of entry for the hygienist, and the mucosal trauma produced by the various cleaning procedures facilitated transmission of infection to her patients. All cases occurred before the hygienist noted the formation of vesicles. Thus, at the time she transmitted the virus to her patients, the hygienist was unaware of the fact that her dermatitis was complicated by a herpetic infection.

HVH may be identified by tissue culture methods in 1 to 3 days. The Leibovitz-Emory or Stuart's transport mediums allow storage and transport of the specimens at room temperature. A variety of serologic tests have also been developed to measure HVH antibodies, including radioimmunoassays that permit the detection of IgM, IgG, and IgA antibodies specific to HVH. However, most clinicians have greater access to cytologic rather than virologic laboratory aids. The major cytologic features of HVH infections are multinucleated giant cells with eosinophilic intranuclear inclusion bodies. These can be readily appreciated with the fixative and stains used for Papanicolau smears, but the technique will not differentiate HVH-1 from HVH-2.

Gonococcal Infections. Infection caused by *Neisseria gonorrhoeae* has the distinction of being not only one of the most prevalent, but also the oldest of the venereal diseases. Oral gonorrheal lesions are infrequently recognized but not uncommon signs of this disease. Although almost any oral soft tissue can be affected in gonococcal infection, most clinicians agree that gonococcal pharyngitis from orogenital exposure is the most frequent. Clinically, three variations may be observed: a strep-like throat with diffuse erythema and edema, with or without small punctate pustules in the tonsillar area; a viral throat with patchy erythema and edema of the tonsillar area and uvula, and the normal-appearing throat of the gonococcal carrier. The intensity of inflammation may be mild, moderate, or severe, with or without lymphadenopathy. Initial symptoms may include burning or itching, alterations in salivary flow, and halitosis. Although asymptomatic carriers are usually afebrile, fever may accompany the more severe cases.

Other oral manifestations of gonococcal infection include painful ulcerations of the lips; tender, edematous inflammation of the gingivae with or without punched-out interdental papillae; glossodynia with ulcerations and edema, as well as diffuse inflammation and ulcerative mucosal lesions covered with white, yellow, or gray pseudomembranes. In some instances, the condition may be so severe that it interferes with normal deglutition and phonation. The significance or persistent oropharyngeal carriage of *Neisseria gonorrhoeae* in asymptomatic persons is not clear, but the oropharynx may be a site from which disseminated gonococcal disease develops.

Because of the diverse clinical manifestations of this infectious process, the diagnosis of oral gonorrhea can be difficult to make; thus a high index of suspicion is a primary prerequisite. Confirmation of the diagnosis is obtained by culture on chocolate agar with gram staining and fluorescent antibody studies. Pharyngeal cultures should be obtained from homosexual men and from women practicing fellatio. Gonococci die within hours if allowed to dry; therefore, the exudates must be inoculated as soon as possible on Thayer-Martin medium or placed in a suitable transport medium. With the use of fluorescent antibody, it is possible to make a definite identification of *Neisseria gonorrhaoeae* in exudate within an hour of obtaining a specimen.

Chlamydial Infections. Infections caused by *Chlamydia trachomatis* are now recognized as the most prevalent of all sexually transmitted diseases. Chlamydiae are unique microorganisms with cell walls similar to those of gram-negative bacteria, but like viruses, they grow only intracellularly. The morbidity caused by chlamydial infections probably exceeds that of gonorrhea. This infection may be spread through contact with hands contaminated by genital secretions or secretions from the eyes. *Chlamydia trachomatis* also has been recovered from throat swabs collected from patients with inclusion conjunctivitis and concurrent pharyngitis. In these instances, positive cultures may have been the result of drainage of the infected eye. However, pharyngeal infection from apparent direct inoculation has been reported.

Because chlamydiae are the most common pathogens in the genital tract responsible for nongonococcal urethritis and cervicitis, perhaps chlamydial infection should also be included in the differential diagnosis of pharyngitis. Chlamydial pharyngitis may be associated with the complaint of a sore, "lumpy" throat or mild pharyngitis and the finding of small pustular lesions in the tonsillar area.

Although cell culture isolation, direct chlamydia enzyme immunoassay, and fluorescent fluorescein-conjugated monoclonal antibody tests are more sensitive, Giemsa staining is the most widely used laboratory test for detecting chlamydial inclusions in epithelial cells. Giemsa staining shows typical intracytoplasmic inclusions in epithelial cells often associated with prominent polymorphonuclear leukocytes. In the differential diagnosis, adenovirus and herpetic infections, reactions to allergens and irritating chemicals, and certain bacterial infections must be considered.

Trichomonal Infections. *Trichomonas vaginalis* has been recovered from throat swabs collected from patients exposed to sexual partners with trichomonal vaginitis or urethritis. Mucosal involvement is characterized by strawberry-like inflammation from vasodilitation. The surfaces of the lesions are covered with an exudate containing polymorphonuclear leukocytes and mononuclear cells. Diagnosis is made by observing motile organisms in fresh specimens. A drop of warm saline solution containing methylene blue is mixed with the exudate and examined immediately with low-power microscopy. It must be remembered, however, that of the three site-specific trichomonads affecting man (*T. tenax* in the oral cavity; *T. hominis* in the gastrointestinal tract; and *T. vaginalis* in the genitourinary tract), *T. vaginalis* and *T. hominis* show striking similarities. *Trichomonas vaginalis* is a pear-shaped, colorless, unicellular organism with two pairs of anterior flagella, an eccentrically located nucleus, an undulating membrane, and a structure termed an axostyle leading to a posterior flagellum. *Trichomonas vaginalis* can also be identified by means of cultures.

Condyloma Acuminatum. This transmissible and autoinoculable papillomatous growth caused by the papova virus, occurs most frequently on anogenital skin and mucosa. It may involve other warm, moist, intertriginous areas, however, and is increasingly recognized in the oral cavity. Although of low infectivity, after repeated exposure and trauma the lesions start as multiple, small, pink, nodular areas or flat acuminate condylomas following a 1-to-3 months incubation period. The nodules proliferate and coalesce to form soft, red or dirty-gray, sessile or pedunculated papillary growths. The lesions develop rapidly to form discrete singular or, more often, extensive clusters of granular or cauliflower-like neoplasms.

The digitating, verrucous lesions may affect all oral tissues and appear as fleshy, fibroma-like lesions of the oral mucosa, lips, and tongue. Extensive involvement of the attached gingivae and hard palate may occur as firm, irregularly shaped, but well-demarcated enlargements with multiple satellite lesions. In differential diagnosis, hereditary fibromatosis, Dilantin hyperplasia, papillary hyperplasia, focal epithelial hyperplasia, verruca vulgaris, verruca planus, and verrucous carcinoma must be considered.

Primary Syphilis. Although most chancres appear on the genitals, and the chance of primary syphilis occurring in the oral cavity is relatively low, increases in orogenital activity should alert the practitioner to this clinical entity. Chancres may affect all tissues of the oral cavity, but the lips represent the most common site of involvement, followed by the tongue and tonsillar areas.

A distinct characteristic of oral syphilis is the painless lesion, although this growth must be differentiated from malignancy. The patient may complain of a "lump" in the throat that does not appear to interfere with normal deglutition. After an average incubation period of 3 weeks, a papule develops; it soon erodes and becomes ulcerated.

The clinical appearance of palatal involvement, characterized by edema and erythema, is not unlike that associated with the fellatio syndrome. The presence of a punched-out intraoral erosion or ulceration associated with a yellow serous discharge and nontender anterior cervical lymphadenopathy should elicit a high degree of suspicion. Similarly, a hard, nontender lingual ulcer with induration and enlargement of the foliate papillae or displacement of uvula and anterior tonsillar pillar should be ominous signs.

The oral lesions of primary syphilis are teeming with spirochetes, although the lip represents the only meaningful area from which specimens can be collected for darkfield examination. *Treponema microdentium,* a common inhabitant of the oral cavity, may be most difficult to distinguish with certainty from *Treponema pallidum,* which causes syphilis. Therefore, confirmation of the clinical diagnosis must be based on nonspecific and specific treponemal antibody tests.

The differential diagnosis of primary syphilis should include herpesvirus hominis type I and type II infection. These infections are painful, may be recurrent, and have a positive Tznack test. Other conditions that must be distinguished include trauma, squamous cell carcinoma, erosive lichen planus, and fungal infections.

Secondary Syphilis. After a latent period, the secondary stage of syphilis appears within 6 months of exposure. Protean signs and symptoms are primarily systemic.

Patients may complain of a grippe-like syndrome characterized by headaches, lacrimation, nasal discharge, sore throat, and generalized arthralgia. Hard, nontender, generalized lymphadenopathy may be associated with a slight elevation of temperature, severe loss of weight, and anemia.

The lymphadenopathy may be followed by a painless, nonpruritic maculo-papular cutaneous rash with notable palmar-plantar eruptions. The oral lesions of secondary syphilis appear concurrently with the cutaneous lesions. Although associated with systemic findings, the oral lesions may represent the only evidence of undiagnosed syphilis. The typical oval red macules or maculopapules and mucous patches may affect all tissues of the oral cavity or appear as split papules of condyloma lata at the commissures. The papules usually are nodular and firm, whereas the mucous patches are slightly raised erosions or shallow ulcerations covered by a grayish-white pseudomembrane.

The differential diagnosis of secondary syphilis should include oral candidiasis, herpetiform ulcerations, and infectious mononucleosis. In some cases, a high degree of suspicion is needed to request specific serologic tests for syphilis to establish the diagnosis.

Late Syphilis. Delayed manifestations of syphilis may occur 10 or more years after the initial infection. Late syphilis is most often associated with the presence of a large lobulated, irregularly shaped tongue, with areas of leukoplakia. A solitary gumma may occasionally be seen; more common, however, is a diffuse gummatous infiltration, which produces initial vasculitis and subsequent obliterative endarteritis. Chronic interstitial glossitis may be characterized by marked papillary atrophy and irregular deep fissuring. These lesions do not respond to treatment, are considered to be premalignant, and therefore, regular followup every 3 to 6 months is indicated. Late syphilis of the hard palate consists of gummatous infiltration and subsequent perforation of the palate. Initial signs include a voice of distinctive nasal quality, followed by complaints of oronasal communication that makes drinking difficult.

Congenital Syphilis. At the present time, congenital syphilis is a preventable disease, and occurs when the fetus is infected in utero by the mother. Early adequate prenatal care, including a blood test for syphilis at the first prenatal visit, should detect almost all infected pregnant women. During the first 16 weeks of pregnancy, the fetus is protected from infection because spirochetes from the maternal circulation are unable to penetrate the placenta. The fetus becomes vulnerable to infection after week 16, with most infections occuring after the sixth month.

The possibility of fetal infection depends on the stage of the disease in the mother. Early syphilis almost always produces miscarriage, stillbirth, or an infant with congenital syphilis. The longer a mother has had the disease, the less chance for fetal infection; however, the possibility is never eliminated. Congenital syphilis has 14 common stigmata associated with it, most affecting the oral cavity, head, and neck.

Frontal bossae of Parrot, the most commonly observed stigma (86.7%), represents the manifestation of localized periostitis of the frontal and parietal bones. It is characterized by rounded, lens-shaped exostoses; if the supraorbital area is involved, the overhanging forehead creates the appearance of the "Olympian brow."

Because frontal bossae may also be associated with rickets and acromegaly, they are not in themselves pathognomonic of congenital syphilis.

Syphilitic rhinitis is usually the first manifestation of congenital syphilis in the neonatal period. Inflammation of the nasal mucosa may destroy the underlying bone and cartilage, perforate the nasal septum, interfere with normal development, and manifest as a *saddle nose* in a sizable number (73.4%) of patients; however, the condition may simply be the result of broad depression of the lower or cartilaginous portion of the nose, a nonsyphilitic infection, or trauma.

A *short maxilla* (83.8%) may also be the sequela to syphilitic rhinitis. When the rhinitis extends to the maxilla, it interferes with normal development, causing a concave or shallow-dish configuration in the middle section of the face. Failure of the maxilla to develop fully is further characterized by a *high palatal arch* (76.4%) and a *relative protuberance of the mandible* (25.8%) that produces a "bulldog" jaw; however, these clinical manifestations in themselves are not diagnostic of congenital syphilis.

Hutchinson's triad (Hutchinson's teeth, interstitial keratitis, and eight-nerve deafness) is pathognomonic of congenital syphilis. Short, barrel-shaped or peg-shaped, widely spaced central incisors characterize Hutchinson's teeth (63.1%). The middle gemma fails to form, and the consequent defective enamel in the middle third of the incisal edge contributes to the formation of a notch. The first molars may be similarly affected because they develop at the same time as the incisors. Mulberry molars (64.9%) are recognized by narrowing of the occlusal table, and poorly developed cusps that appear dome-shaped. Hypocalcification of the enamel predisposes these teeth to extensive caries.

Between the ages of 5 and 25 years, the victim may develop interstitial keratitis (8.8%) associated with symptoms of acute iritis, pain, lacrimation, and photophobia. The latter is followed by clouding of the cornea as a result of vascular proliferation on the inner surface and stroma. The keratitis may reflect local antigen-antibody reaction in tissue sensitized by transient spirochetal invasion in fetal life. A similar condition may be caused by tuberculosis. Interstitial keratitis can be suppressed with corticosteroids, and permanent damage may require keratoplasty.

Eight-nerve deafness occurs infrequently in clinical practice today (3.3%), and is never the only sign of infection. It usually is seen in the early teens, and is considered to be secondary to syphilitic labyrinthitis. The onset is heralded by vertigo and loss of high-frequency hearing. Ultimately, the person loses the ability to hear conventional tones.

Rhagades (7.6%) or linear scars extend like the spokes of a wheel from the angle of the eyes, nose, mouth, and anus; confluent macular, papular, and maculopapular lesions may be seen in some newborn patients. Skin movement that produces linear fissures, ulcerations, and eventual scarring is responsible for rhagades.

Higoumenakis' sign (39.4%) or irregular thickening of the sternoclavicular portion of the clavicle may be the result of unilateral periostitis. Periostitis of the anterior and middle portions of the tibia may cause thickening and anterior bowing, *saber skin* (4.1%), and *scaphoid scapulae* (0.7%), producing concavity of the vertebral border of the scapula. A history of rickets, fracture, or nonsyphilitic infection must be considered in the differential diagnoses. About the age of puberty, a painless synovitis associated with doughy swelling of the joint without bony involvement suggests *Clutton's joint* (0.3%). The joint fluid is positive for syphilis and the condition appears to respond to intrajoint or systemic steroid therapy.

Infectious Mononucleosis. This is the best-known syndrome associated with primary infection by the Epstein-Barr virus (EBV) and a variety of cutaneous and mucosal manifestations are recognized. The recovery in culture of EBV from patients with genital ulcerations suggests the potential for transmission by a venereal route.

Cytohybridization studies have demonstrated the EBV genome within oropharyngeal squamous cells during infectious mononucleosis. Cell-free virus has also been found in parotid secretions and the shedding of EBV in the saliva of persons convalescing from infectious mononucleosis may persist for many months. Lymphocytes carrying the EBV genome are also present in the peripheral circulation. Similarly, the EBV may also be present in semen and cervical secretions. Viral shedding can be associated with cytolysis, as is clearly the case in the pathogenesis of HVH infections, or transmitted percutaneously by B lymphocytes following orogenital activity.

Cutaneous manifestations of infectious mononucleosis may include a maculopapular rash, urticaria, and petechiae. Evidence of localized, small vessel vasculitis and thrombosis, seen on skin biopsy, may be explained on the basis of immune-complex deposition. Subsequent to orogenital activity, patients will complain of severe fatigue followed by vulvar pain, burning dysuria, bluish-black irregular lesions of the labia, eye pain, swelling of the eyelids, and a low-grade fever. As the genital lesions persist, the patient will report a sore throat at times with exudate and cervical lymphadenopathy. Oral manifestations may include acute gingivitis, stomatitis, and palatal petechiae that are early clinical signs of infectious mononucleosis. Recovery may take up to 30 days.

The diagnosis of infectious mononucleosis may be confirmed by Monospot (Horner) or Monosticon (Organon) rapid slide tests, or by immunofluorescent serologic test for the EBV. In the differential diagnosis, the clinician should consider HVH infections, chancroids, and syphilis.

Hepatitis. Studies have shown that dentists have a greater incidence of hepatitis B than the general population. The hepatitis B virus may be transmitted both percutaneously and nonpercutaneously. To date, no other health care provider transmitted more cases of hepatitis B to patients than a dentist, primarily because of inadequate barrier techniques. A complete treatment of the subject can be found in Chapter 2.

Acquired Immunodeficiency Syndrome (AIDS). To date, there are only a few reported cases of AIDS among health care workers (HCWs) in the United States that can be linked to a specific occupational exposure. Most HCWs who have been diagnosed as having AIDS have been shown to belong to known AIDS risk groups and epidemiologic investigations suggest that nonoccupational exposures were the most likely sources of infection. A complete treatment of the subject can be found in Chapter 3.

SUMMARY

The incidence of certain microbial cross-infections occurring in the dental environment is well documented, but the transmission of other pathogens, while highly probable, has not been established with certainty. However, considerable recent interest in the incubation period of various infections and improved community surveillance programs combine to ascribe infection to specific incidents. It would seem prudent for oral health care personnel to acknowledge the potential for the transmission of infectious diseases in the dental environment and institute aseptic office procedures as a matter of normal course.

REFERENCES

Traumatic Lesions of the Lingual Frenum

Fiumara, N.J.: Venereal diseases of the oral cavity. Journal of Oral Medicine, *31*:36–40,55, 1976.
Mader, C.L.: Lingual frenum ulcer resulting from orogenital sex. Journal of the American Dental Association, *103*:888–890, 1981.

Fellatio Syndrome

Belizzi, R., Krakow, A.M., and Plack, W.: Soft palate trauma associated with fellatio: Case report. Military Medicine, *145*:787–788, 1980.
Ginasanti, J.S., Cramer, J.R., and Weathers, D.R.: Palatal erythema: Another etiologic factor. Oral Surgery, *40*:379–381, 1975.
Rattner, H.: A strange case of palatitis. Archives of Dermatology, *60*:624, 1949.
Schlesinger, S.L., Borbotsina, J., and O'Neill, L.: Petechial hemorrhages of the soft palate secondary to fellatio. Oral Surgery, *40*:376–378, 1975.

Herpetic Infections

Bryson, Y.J., et al.: Treatment of first episodes of genital herpes simplex virus infection with oral acyclovir. New England Journal of Medicine, *308*:916–921, 1983.
Corey, L., et al.: Genital herpes simplex virus infections: Clinical manifestations, course, and complication. Annals of Internal Medicine, *98*:958–972, 1983.
Corey, L., et al.: Intravenous acyclovir for the treatment of primary genital herpes. Annals of Internal Medicine, *98*:914–921, 1983.
Corey, L., et al.: A trial of topical acyclovir in genital herpes simplex virus infections. New England Journal of Medicine, *306*:1313–1319, 1982.
Douglas, J.M., et al.: A double-blind study of oral acyclovir for suppression of recurrences of genital herpes simplex virus infection. New England Journal of Medicine, *310*:1551–1556, 1984.
Nahmias, A.J., et al.: Genital herpetic infection: The old and the new. *In*: Sexually Transmitted Diseases, R.D. Cattaroll and C.S. Nicol, editors, London: Academic Press, 1976, pp. 135–151.
Straus, S.E., et al.: Suppression of frequently recurring genital herpes. New England Journal of Medicine, *310*:1545–1550, 1984.

Gonococcal Infections

Ashford, W.A., Adams, H.J.U., Johnson, S.R., et al.: Spectinomycin-resistant penicillinase-producing Neisseria gonorrhoeae. Lancet, *2*:1035–1037, 1981.
Bro-Jorgensen, A., and Jensen, T.: Gonococcal pharyngeal infections. British Journal of Venereal Disease, *49*:491–499, 1973.
Bro-Jorgensen, A., and Jensen, T.: Gonococcal tonsilar infections. British Medical Journal, *4*:660–661, 1971.
Bronson, F.R.: Gonorrhea buccalis. American Journal of Urology and Sexology, *15*:59–69, 1919.
Bruusgaard, E. and Thjotta, T.: A case of meningitis and purpura gonorrhoica. Acta Dermato-Venereologica, *26*:262–274, 1925.
Center for Disease Control: Gonorrhea. CDC recommended treatment schedules. Morbidity Mortality Weekly Report, *28*:13–24, 1979.
Chue, P.W.J.: Gonorrhea—its natural history, oral manifestations, diagnosis, treatment, and prevention. Journal of the American Dental Association, *4*:567, 1954.

Copping, A.A.: Stomatitis caused by gonococcus. Journal of the American Dental Association, 49:567, 1954.

Cowan, L.: Gonococcal ulceration of the tongue in gonococcal dermatitis syndrome. British Journal of Venereal Disease, 45:228–231, 1969.

Diefenbach, W.C.I.: Gonorrheal parotitis. Oral Surgery, 6:974–975, 1953.

Fiumara, N.J., Wise, H.M. Jr., and Many, M.: Gonorrheal pharyngitis. New England Journal of Medicine, 276:1248–1250, 1967.

Handsfield, H.H., and Holmes, K.K.: Treatment of uncomplicated gonorrhea with cefotaxime. Sexually Transmitted Diseases, 8:187–191, 1981.

Holmes, K.K.: Pharyngeal gonorrhea in Internal Venereal Disease Symposium, second edition, New York: Laboratories Division of Pfizer, Inc., 1973, pp. 27–29.

Iqbal, Y.: Gonococcal tonsillitis. British Journal of Venereal Disease, 47:144–145, 1971.

Jaffe, W.H., Biddle, J.W., Johnson, S.R., et al.: Infections due to penicillinase-producing Neisseria gonorrhoeae in the United States: 1976– 1980. Journal of Infectious Diseases, 144–191, 197, 1981.

Jones, R.B., Stimson, J., Counts, J.W., et al.: Cefoxitin in the treatment of gonorrhea. Sexually Transmitted Diseases, 6:239–242, 1979.

Keil, H.: A type of gonococcal bacteraemia with characteristic haemorrhagic vesiculopustular and bullous skin lesion. Quarterly Journal of Medicine, 7:1–15, 1938.

Kohn, S.R., Shaffer, J.F., and Chomenko, A.G.: Primary gonococcal stomatitis. Journal of the American Medical Association, 219:86, 1972.

Metzger, A.L.: Gonococcal arthritis complicating gonorrheal pharyngitis. Annals of Internal Medicine, 73:267–269, 1970.

Ratnatunga, C.S.: Gonococcal pharyngitis. British Journal of Venereal Disease, 48:184–186, 1972.

Rodin, P., Monteiro, G.E., and Scrimgeour, G.: Gonococcal pharyngitis. British Journal of Venereal Disease, 48:182–183, 1972.

Schmidt, H., Hjorting-Hansen, E., and Philpsen, H.P.: Gonococcal stomatitis. Acta Dermato-Venerologica (Stock), 41:324–327, 1961.

Stamm, W.E., et al.: Effect of treatment regimens for Neisseria Gonorrhoeae on simultaneous infection with Trachomatis Chlamydia. New England Journal of Medicine, 310:545–549, 1984.

Thatcher, R.W., McCraney, W.T., Kellogg, D.S., et al.: Asymptomatic gonorrhea. Journal of the American Medical Association, 210:315–321, 1969.

Thompson, S.E., III., Jacob, N.F., Zakarias, F., et al.: Gonococcal tenosynovitis-dermatitis and septic arthritis. Journal of the American Medical Association, 244:1101–1102, 1980.

Wallin, J., and Siegel, M.S.: Pharyngeal neisseria gonorrhoeae: Colonizer of pathogen? British Medical Journal, 1:1462–1463.

Weisner, P.M., Tronca, E., Bonin, P., et al.: Clinical spectrum of pharyngeal gonococcal infection. New England Journal of Medicine, 288:181–185, 1973.

Chlamydial Infections

Center for Disease Control: Chlamydia Trachomatis infections. Morbidity Mortality Weekly Report, 34(35):535–745, 1985.

Dawson, C., and Schachter, J.: TRIC agent infections of the eye and genital tract. American Journal of Ophthalmology, 263:1288–1298, 1967.

Hammerschiag, M.R., Chandler, J.W., Alexander, E.R., et al.: Erythromycin ointment for ocular prophylaxis of neonatal chlamydial infection. Journal of the American Medical Association, 244:2291–2293, 1980.

Harrison, R.H., English, M.G., Lee, C.K., et al.: Chlamydia trachomatis infant pneumonitis. New England Journal of Medicine, 298:702–708, 1978.

Oriel, J.D., Reeve, P., and Nichol, C.S.: Minocycline in the treatment of nongonococcal urethritis: Its effect on Chlamydia trachomatis. Journal of the American Venereal Disease Association, 2:17–19, 1975.

Quinn, T.C., Goodell, S.E., Mkrichian, E.M., et al.: Chlamydia trachomatis proctitis. New England Journal of Medicine, 305:195–200, 1981.

Schachter, J., and Atwood, G.: Chlamydial pharyngitis. Journal of the American Venereal Disease Association, 2:12, 1975.

Tam, M.R., et al.: Culture-independent diagnosis of Chlamydia Trachomatis using monoclonal antibodies. New England Journal of Medicine, 310:1146–1150, 1984.

Trichomonal Infections

Fiumara, N.J.: Venereal diseases of the oral cavity. Journal of Oral Medicine, 31:36–40,55, 1976.

Lohmeyer, H.: Treatment of candidiasis and trichomoniasis of the female genital tract. Postgraduate Medical Journal, 50(Suppl.):78–79, 1974.

Muller, M., Meingassner, J.G., Miller, W.A., et al.: Three metronidazole-resistant strains of trichomonas vaginalis from the United States. American Journal of Obstetrics and Gynecology, 138:808–812, 1980.

Rein, M.F.: Current therapy of vulvovaginitis. Sexually Transmitted Diseases, 8:316–320, 1981.

Condyloma Acuminatum

Chonkas, N.C., and Toto, P.D.: Condylomata acuminatum of the oral cavity. Oral Surgery, Oral Medicine, Oral Pathology, 54(4):480–485, 1982.

Dawson, D.F., Duckworth, J.K., Berhardt, H., et al.: Giant condyloma and verrucous carcinoma of the genital area. Archives of Pathology, 79:225–231, 1965.

Doyle, J.L., Gordjesk, J.E., Manhold, J.H.: Condyloma acuminatum occurring in the oral cavity. Oral Surgery, 26:434–440, 1968.

Frihiof, L., and Wersall, J.: Virus-like particles in human oral papilloma. Acta Otolaryngologica (Stockh), 64:263–266, 1967.

George, D.I., and Farman, A.G.: Ultrastructural features of oral condyloma acuminatum. Journal of Oral Medicine, 39(3):169–172, 1984.

Goldschwidr, H., and Gligman, A.M.: Experimental inoculation of humans with ectodermotrophic viruses. Journal of Investigative Dermatology, 31:175–182, 1958.

Haye, K.R.: Treatment of condyloma acuminata with 5 percent 5-fluorouracil (SFU) cream. British Journal of Venereal Disease, 50:466, 1974.

Knapp, M.J., and Uohara, G.I.: Oral Condyloma acuminatum. Oral Surgery, 23:538–545, 1967.

Litvak, A.S., Meinick, I.M., and Lieberman, P.R.: Giant condylomata acuminata associated with carcinoma. Journal of the Medical Society of New Jersey, 63:165–167, 1966.

Machuach, G.F., and Weakley, D.R.: Giant condyloma acuminata of Buscke and Lowenstein. Archives of Dermatology, 82:41–47, 1960.

McClatchey, K.D., Colquitt, W.N., and Robert, R.C.: Condyloma acuminatum of the lip: Report of a case. Journal of Oral Surgery, 37:751–752, 1979.

Pareek, S.: Treatment of condyloma acuminatum in 5 percent 5-fluorouracil. British Journal of Venereal Disease, 55:65–67, 1979.

Praetorius-Clausen, F.: Rare oral viral disorders (molluscum contagiosum, localized keratoacanthoma, verrucae, condyloma acuminatum, and focal epithelial hyperplasia). Oral Surgery, 34:604–618, 1972.

Seibert, J.S., Shannon, C.J., and Jacoway, J.R.: Treatment of recurrent condyloma acuminatum. Oral Surgery, 27:398–409, 1969.

Simmons, P.D.: Podophyllin 10% and 25% in the treatment of anogenital warts. British Journal of Venereal Disease, 57:208–209, 1981.

Summers, L., and Booth, D.R.: Intraoral condyloma acuminatum. Oral Surgery, 38:273–278, 1974.

Von Krogh, G.: The beneficial effect of 1% 5-fluorouracil in 70% ethanol on therapeutically refractory condylomas in the preputial cavity. Sexually Transmitted Diseases, 5:137–140, 1978.

Von Krough, G.: Topical treatment of penile condylomata acuminata with podophyllotoxin and colchicine. Acta Dermato-Venerologica (Stockh), 58:163–168, 1978.

Syphilis of the Oral Cavity

Fiumara, N.J.: A legacy of syphilis. Archives of Dermatology, 92:676–678, 1965.

Fiumara, N.J., and Berg, M.: Primary syphilis in the oral cavity. British Journal of Venereal Disease, 50:463–464, 1974.

Fiumara, N.J.: Cutaneous lesions of syphilis. Cutis, 9:184–190, 1972.

Fiumara, N.J., Grande, D.J., and Giunta, J.I.: Papillar secondary of the tongue. Oral Surgery, 45:540–542, 1978.

Fiumara, N.J., and Lesell, S.: Manifestations of late congenital syphilis. Archives of Dermatology, 102:78–83, 1970.

McCormack, W.M., George, H., Donner, A., et al.: Hepatotoxicity of erythromycin estolate during pregnancy. Antimicrobial Agents and Chemotherapy, *12*:630–635, 1977.

Robinson, R.C.V.: Congenital syphilis. Archives of Dermatology, *99*:599–610, 1969.

Treatment of sexually transmitted diseases. Medical Letter on Drugs and Therapeutics, *26*:5–10, 1984.

Hepatitis

Baker, C.H., and Hawkins, V.L.: Law in the dental workplace: Legal implications of hepatitis B for the dental profession. Journal of the American Dental Association, *110*:637–642, 1985.

Centers for Disease Control: ACIP recommendations for protection against viral hepatitis. Morbidity, Mortality Weekly Report, *34(22)*:313–335, 1985.

Cottone, J.A.: Hepatitis B virus infection in the dental profession. Journal of the American Dental Association, *110*:617–621, 1985.

Crawford, J.J.: State of the art: practical infection control in dentistry. Journal of the American Dental Association, *110*:629–633, 1985.

Gitnick, G.: Non-A non-B hepatitis: Etiology and clinical care. Lab Med, *14(11)*:721–726, 1983.

Goebel, W.M.: Reliability of the medical history in identifying patients likely to place dentists at an increased hepatitis risk. Journal of the American Dental Association, *98*:907–918, 1979.

Hollinger, F.B., Khan, N.C., Oefinger, P.E., Yawn, D.H., Schmullens, A.C., Driesman, G.R., and Melnick, J.L.: Posttransfusion hepatitis type A. Journal of the American Medical Association, *250(17)*:2313–2317, 1983.

McLean, A.A.: Hepatitis B vaccine: A review of the clinical data to date. Journal of the American Dental Association, *110*:624–628, 1985.

Nath, N., Fang, C.T., Berberian, H., Mushahwar, I.K., and Dodd, R.Y.: Antibodies to delta antigen among asymptomatic HBzsAg-positive volunteer blood donors in the U.S. The 1984 International Symposium on Viral Hepatitis, 1984, p. 23.

Rizzetto, M., Canese, M.G., Arico, S., Crivelli, O., Irepo, C., Bonino, F., and Verme, G.: Immunofluorescence detection of new antigen-antibody system (delta/anti-delta) associated to hepatitis B virus in liver and in serum of HGzsAg carriers. Gut, *18*:997–1003, 1977.

Rizzetto, M., Hoyer, B., Canese, M.G., Shih, J.W.K., Purcell, R.H., and Gerin, J.L.: Delta agent: Association of delta antigen with hepatitis B surface antigen and RNA in serum of delta-infected chimpanzees. Proceedings of the National Academy of Sciences, *77*:6124–6128, 1980.

Seto, B., Awarson, S., Colemann, W.G., Gerety, Nd R.J.: Detection of reverse transcriptase activity in association with the non-A non-B hepatitis agent(s). Lancet, *vol. II*:941–943, 1984.

Smedile, A., Lavarini, C., Farci, P., Arico, S., Marinucci, G., Dentico, P., Giuliani, G., Cargnel, A., del Vecchio Blanco, C., and Rizzetto, M.: Epidemiologic patterns of infection with the hepatitis B virus-associated delta agent in Italy. American Journal of Epidemiology, *117*:223–229, 1983.

Tullman, M.J. and Boozer, C.H.: Past infection in the dental profession. Journal of the American Dental Association, *110*:624–628, 1985.

AIDS

Centers for Disease Control: Revision of the case definition of acquired immunodeficiency syndrome. Morbidity, Mortality Weekly Report, *34(25)*:373–375, 1985.

Centers for Disease Control: Update: Evaluation of human T-lymphotropic virus type III/Lymphadenopathy-associated virus infection in health-care personnel–United States. Morbidity, Mortality Weekly Report, *34(38)*:575–578, 1985.

Centers for Disease Control: Oral viral lesion (hairy-leukoplakia) associated with acquired immunodeficiency syndrome. Morbidity Mortality Weekly Report, *34(36)*:549–550, 1985.

Klein, R.S., et al.: Oral candidiasis in high-risk patients as the initial manifestation of the acquired immunodeficiency syndrome. New England Journal of Medicine, *311*:354–358, 1984.

Wofford, D.T. and Miller, R.I.: Acquired immune deficiency syndrome (AIDS): disease characteristics and oral manifestations. Journal of the American Dental Association, *111*:258–261, 1985.

Infectious Mononucleosis

Portnoy, J., et al.: Recovery of Epstein-Barr virus from genital ulcers. New England Journal of Medicine, *311*:966–968, 1984.

Chapter 2

The Challenge of Viral Hepatitis

Dentists and dental staff members have always known that they are susceptible to many diseases in their office setting. Winters seem to bring more colds to dental staff members than to control populations. Gonorrhea and syphilis are presented to the profession as risks but most dental staffs know no one who has contracted these diseases in the dental office. Possibly a dental office staff member has contracted herpes through occupational exposure, but this too is rare. Tuberculosis is a disease that most of the dental profession thought was almost extinct until recently. Now, two other diseases have come to the forefront: hepatitis and AIDS.

Viral hepatitis is a disease that dentists and staff members learned about in school, but because there was no real way to avoid it, everyone just took their chances with little worry. In 1982, a vaccine became available against hepatitis B. Many studies were performed in preparation for the introduction of the vaccine documenting various populations at a higher risk of hepatitis B exposure. The dentist appeared near the top of the seropositive list followed by various members of the dental staff. These results were alarming to some but not alarming enough for action for the bulk of the dental profession.

Thundering right behind the introduction of the hepatitis B vaccine was Acquired Immune Deficiency Syndrome (AIDS). Now *here* was a disease that captured the attention of the dental profession along with the majority of the world. Here was a disease that, if one could contract it in the dental office, would make the practice of dentistry a potentially suicidal occupation. The profession had to fall back on knowledge of hepatitis B to initially provide safeguards as there was much uncertainty, many misconceptions, and little knowledge about AIDS. However, when all the facts are examined, AIDS is not nearly as large a problem in dentistry as hepatitis B. But, AIDS challenged dentistry—it challenged it to learn and to practice in a safer manner that would prevent transmission of ALL diseases.

The purpose of this chapter is to examine the challenge that viral hepatitis delivers to the dental profession and to put this challenge in proper perspective. Human immunodeficiency virus (HIV) infection and AIDS will be reviewed in the next chapter.

VIRAL HEPATITIS: THE REAL CHALLENGE

Hepatitis, or inflammation of the liver, can be caused by agents other than viruses such as various disease states and drug reactions. Viral hepatitis is commonly divided into hepatitis A, B, non-A non-B, and delta. Table 2–1 lists the many viruses that can cause viral hepatitis.

Table 2–1.   Viruses That May Be Involved in Human Hepatitis

RNA Viruses	DNA Viruses
Picornaviruses (enteroviruses)	Hepadnavirus
Hepatitis A virus	Hepatitis B virus
Delta hepatitis virus	Herpes viruses
Coxsackie viruses	Cytomegalovirus
Echo viruses	Epstein-Barr virus
Togaviruses	Herpes Simplex viruses
Yellow Fever virus	Varicella-Zoster virus
Rubella virus	Unclassified
Arenaviruses	Non-A Non-B Hepatitis viruses
Junin virus (Argentina)	
Machupo virus (Bolivia)	
Lassa virus (Lass fever—Africa)	
Rift Valley Fever virus (Africa)	
Rhabdoviruses	
Marburg virus (Marburg disease—Africa)	
Ebola virus (Africa)	
Paramyxovirus	
Measles virus	

Hepatitis A (formerly called infectious or short incubation hepatitis) and hepatitis B (formerly called serum or long incubation hepatitis) have been recognized as separate entities since the early 1940s. They can be diagnosed with specific serologic tests that have been readily available since 1980.

The third form of hepatitis, currently known as non-A non-B, is caused by at least two different viral agents. Additionally, there are two epidemiologically distinct types of non-A non-B hepatitis: parenterally transmitted and enterically transmitted. Non-A non-B hepatitis has been a disease diagnosed by exclusion because of the lack of specific diagnostic tests. Major advances are occurring to remedy this problem. It is an important form of acute viral hepatitis in adults and currently accounts for most of the post-transfusion hepatitis seen in the United States.

A fourth type of viral hepatitis, delta hepatitis, was recognized as an infection dependent on hepatitis B virus. It may occur as a *co-infection* with acute hepatitis B infection or as *superinfection* in a hepatitis B carrier.

HEPATITIS A

Hepatitis A (Table 2–2) is caused by the hepatitis A virus (HAV), a 27-nm ribonucleic acid (RNA) agent that is a member of the picornavirus family. It was

Table 2–2.   Comparison of Hepatitis A and B

	A	B
Virus	RNA 27 nm	DNA 42 nm + 20 nm
Former nomenclature	Infectious Short incubation	Serum Long incubation
Routes of transmission	Fecal-oral	Intimate contact with body secretions
Incubation period	2 to 6 weeks	2 to 6 months
Sequelae	Rare	Chronic hepatitis, cirrhosis, liver cancer
Carrier State	No	Yes

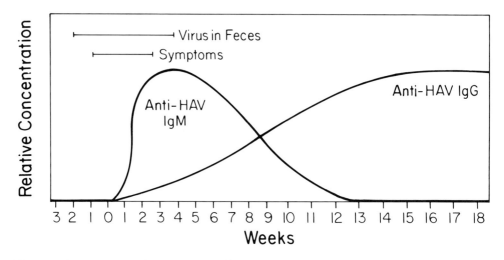

Fig. 2–1. Hepatitis A serology. (From Serodiagnostic Assessment of Acute Viral Hepatitis. Abbott Laboratories, Diagnostic Division, North Chicago, IL 60064.)

first described in 1973. The illness caused by HAV characteristically has an abrupt onset with fever, malaise, anorexia, nausea, abdominal discomfort, and jaundice. Severity is related to age. In children, most infections are asymptomatic, and illness is usually not accompanied by jaundice. Most infected adults become symptomatically ill with jaundice. Fatality among reported cases is infrequent (about 0.6%).

Hepatitis A is primarily transmitted by person-to-person contact, generally through fecal contamination. Transmission is facilitated by poor personal hygiene, poor sanitation, and intimate (intrahousehold or sexual) contact. Epidemics from contaminated food and water occur. Sharing utensils, cigarettes, or kissing are *not* believed to transmit the infection.

The incubation period of hepatitis A is 15 to 50 days (average 28 to 30). High concentrations of HAV are found in stools of infected persons. Fecal virus excretion reaches its highest concentration late in the incubation period and early in the prodromal phase of illness, and diminishes rapidly once jaundice appears. Greatest infectivity is during the 2-week period immediately before the onset of jaundice. Viremia is of short duration and virus has not been found in urine or other body fluids. A chronic carrier state with HAV has not been demonstrated. Transmission of HAV by blood transfusions has occurred but is rare.

The diagnosis of acute hepatitis A is confirmed by finding IgM-class anti-HAV in serum collected during the acute or early convalescent phase of disease. IgG-class anti-HAV, which appears in the convalescent phase of disease and remains detectable in serum thereafter, confers enduring protection against disease (Fig. 2–1). Commercial tests are available to detect IgM anti-HAV and total anti-HAV in serum.

Although the incidence of hepatitis A in the United States had decreased, increased frequency of infection has been reported in recent years, especially among intravenous drug users. HAV is still a common infection in older children and young adults. About 50% of reported hepatitis cases in this country are attributable to hepatitis A.

HAV has been successfully grown in culture and its genome has been cloned. A vaccine against hepatitis A is under development.

HEPATITIS B

Hepatitis B virus (HBV) infection is a major cause of acute and chronic hepatitis, cirrhosis, and primary hepatocellular carcinoma worldwide. The virus was first described in 1965. The frequency of HBV infection and patterns of transmission vary significantly in different parts of the world (Fig. 2–2). In the United States, Western Europe, and Australia, it is a disease of low endemicity, with only 0.2 to 0.9% of the population being virus carriers and infection occurring primarily during adulthood. However, HBV infection is highly endemic in China and Southeast Asia, much of Africa, most Pacific Islands, the Amazon Basin, and parts of the Middle East. In these areas, 8 to 15% of the population carry the virus, and most persons acquire infection at birth or during childhood.

Hepatitis B infection is caused by HBV, a 42-nm, double-shelled deoxyribonucleic acid (DNA) virus (Fig. 2–3, Table III). Several well-defined antigen-antibody systems have been associated with HBV infection. HBsAg, formerly called "Australia antigen" or "hepatitis-associated antigen," is found on the surface of the virus and on accompanying 22-nm spherical and tubular forms. The various subtypes (adr, adw, ayw, ayr) of HBsAg provide useful epidemiologic markers. Antibody against HBsAg (anti-HBs) develops during a resolved infection and is responsible for long-term immunity. Anti-HBc, the antibody to the core antigen (an internal component of the virus), develops in all HBV infections and persists indefinitely. IgM anti-HBc appears early in infection and persists for 6 or more months; it is a reliable marker of acute or recent HBV infection. The hepatitis B antigen (HBeAg) is a third antigen, the presence of which correlates with HBV replication and high infectivity. Antibody to HBeAg (anti-HBe) develops in most HBV infections and correlates with lower infectivity. Figure 2–4 shows the typical serologic pattern of a hepatitis B infection.

The onset of acute hepatitis B is generally insidious. Clinical symptoms and signs include various combinations of anorexia, malaise, nausea, vomiting, abdominal pain, and jaundice. Skin rashes, arthralgias, and arthritis can also occur. Overall fatality rates for reported cases generally do not exceed 2%. The incubation period of hepatitis B is long: 45 to 160 days (average 60 to 120). There is a variety of ultimate outcomes of this disease including a carrier state, cirrhosis, acute hepatitis, and primary liver cancer (Fig. 2–5).

Modes of Transmission

HBV is transmitted by percutaneous and nonpercutaneous modes, both of which have significance in dentistry. The delivery of dental treatment involves the use of many small, sharp instruments, which provides multiple opportunities for inadvertent percutaneous wounds to the operator. The remainder of the dental staff is also at risk, performing dental hygiene procedures, handling impressions and dental casts, and particularly while gathering contaminated instruments (often by the handful) and scrubbing them to remove debris before sterilization.

Nonpercutaneous dental transmission includes the transfer of infectious body secretions such as saliva, blood, and a mixture of both. The percutaneous route of

Geographic Pattern of Hepatitis B Prevalence

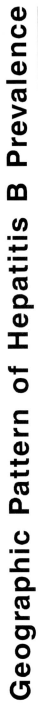
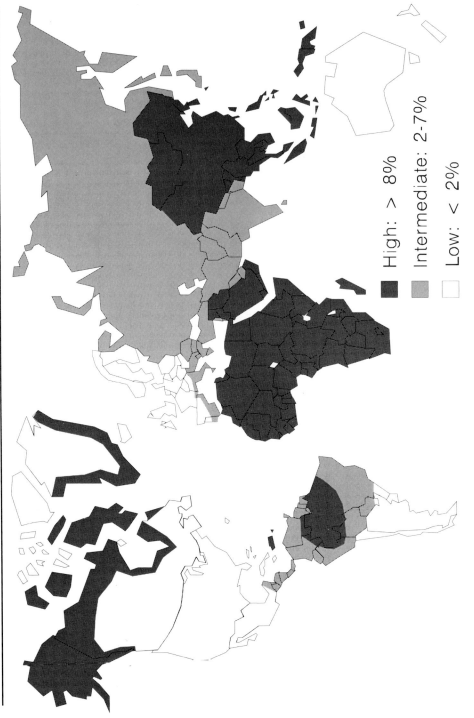

High: > 8%

Intermediate: 2-7%

Low: < 2%

Fig. 2–2. Prevalence of hepatitis B worldwide.

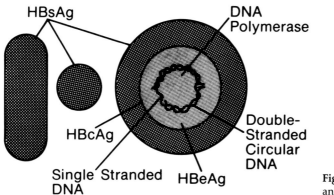

Fig. 2–3. Hepatitis B virus and antigens.

transmission is more efficient for virus transmission in that the incubation period prior to HBsAg titer elevation can be as short as 7 days, whereas oral transmission involving intact mucosa usually involves a longer incubation period (approximately 54 days). In reality, this longer incubation period is advantageous to further virus transmission as it is then more difficult to associate the source of infection with any one patient and allows the infected dental staff member a longer period of time to potentially transmit the virus to other staff members, patients, and family members.

Hepatitis B transmission in the dental operatory occurs primarily in the horizontal mode—that is among the staff, patients, and family members who associate with one another (Fig. 2–6). Studies have shown that this transmission is predominantly from patient to health care provider and less often from health care provider to patient. Nevertheless, transmission via this latter route does occur and has been documented. Vertical transmission is also possible as when an infected dentist transmits hepatitis B to his children via intimate contact.

The potential of transmission of hepatitis B at birth by a female who has developed the carrier state by infection from her husband/dentist, her own occupational exposure or personal risk behavior also exists. The development of the carrier state in the newborn infant is then possible with a resultant increase in that child's probability of ultimately developing primary hepatocellular carcinoma later in life. For this reason, it was initially recommended that all pregnant women in high-risk groups (including health care workers) be serologically tested to determine HBsAg status. This recommendation was broadened in 1988 to include screening of *all* pregnant women during an early prenatal visit. If they are hepatitis B carriers, their newborn must receive hepatitis B immune globulin (HBIG) and hepatitis B vaccine within days of birth to avert development of infection.

Frequency of Infection

Most dentists feel there are few potential hepatitis B carriers in their practice and hence little chance of infection in their office or indeed in the profession as a whole. They are not alone as the majority of the medical profession including most hospitals believed the same myth until recently. The number of patient population groups that have a significantly increased prevalence of hepatitis B infection and hence an increased prevalence of the carrier state is much larger than one would imagine (Table 2–4). Many of these patient populations are themselves unaware

Table 2–3. Hepatitis Terminology

Abbreviation	Term	Comments
	Hepatitis A	
HAV	Hepatitis A virus	Etiologic agent of "infectious" hepatitis
Anti-HAV	Antibody to HAV virus	Detectable at onset of symptoms; lifetime persistence
IgM anti-HAV	IgM class antibody to HAV virus	Indicates recent infection with hepatitis A; positive up to 4 to 6 months after infection
	Hepatitis B	
HBV	Hepatitis B virus	Etiologic agent of "serum" or "long-incubation" hepatitis; also known as Dane particle
HBsAg	Hepatitis B surface antigen	Surface antigen(s) of HBV detectable in large quantity in serum; several subtypes
HBeAg	Hepatitis B e antigen	Soluble antigen; antigen correlates with HBV replication, higher titer HBV in serum, and infectivity of serum
HBcAg	Hepatitis B core antigen	No commercial test available
Anti-HBs	Antibody to HBsAg	Indicates past infection with, and immunity to, HBV, passive antibody from HBIG, or immune response from HB vaccine
Anti-HBe	Antibody to HBeAg	Presence in serum of HBsAg carrier suggests lower titer of HBV
Anti-HBc	Antibody to HBcAg	Indicates past infection with HBV at some undefined time
IgM Anti-HBc	IgM class antibody to HBcAg	Indicates recent infection with HBV; positive for 4 to 6 months after infection
	Non-A Non-B Hepatitis	
PT-NANB	Parenterally transmitted non-A non-B hepatitis	Diagnosis of exclusion. At least two candidate viruses; epidemiology parallels that of hepatitis B
HCV	Hepatitis C virus	Proposed name for one virus associated with PT-NANB
ET-NANB	Enterically transmitted non-A non-B hepatitis	Diagnosis by exclusion. Causes large epidemics in Asia, Africa and Mexico
HEV	Hepatitis E virus	Proposed name for ET-NANB
	Delta Hepatitis	
HDV	Delta virus	Etiologic agent of delta hepatitis; only causes infection in presence of HBV
HDAg	Delta antigen	Detectable in early acute delta infection
Anti-HDV	Antibody to delta antigen	Indicates past or present infection with delta virus
	Immune Globulins	
IG	Immune globulin (previously ISG, immune serum globulin, or gamma globulin)	Contains antibodies to HAV; lower titer antibodies to HBV
HBIG	Hepatitis B immune globulin	Contains high titer antibodies to HBV

Adapted from Centers for Disease Control (ACIP): Protection against viral hepatitis. MMWR, *39*(RR-2):6–7, 1990.

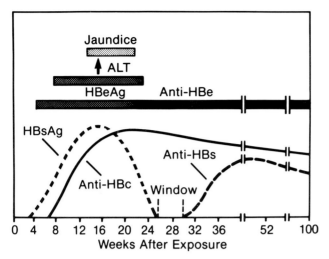

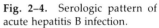

Fig. 2–4. Serologic pattern of acute hepatitis B infection.

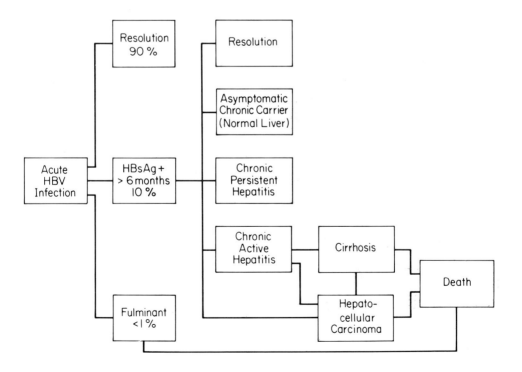

Fig. 2–5. Outcomes of hepatitis B infection.

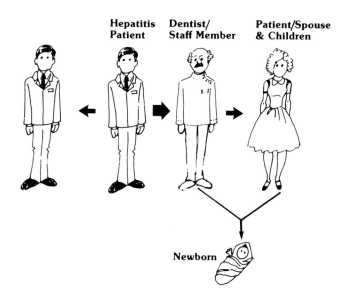

Fig. 2–6. Vertical and horizontal transmission of HBV in the dental office.

Table 2–4. Hepatitis B High-Risk Populations

Health care personnel
   Dentists and physicians
   Nurses, dental hygienists, and dental assistants
   Paramedical personnel and custodial staff who may be exposed to the virus
   Laboratory personnel handling blood, blood products, and other patient samples
   Dental, medical, and nursing students
   Dental laboratory technicians

Selected patients and patient contacts
   Patients and staff in hemodialysis units and hematology/oncology units
   Patients requiring frequent or large-volume blood transfusion or clotting-factor concentrates
      (for example, persons with hemophilia or thalassemia)
   Clients (residents) and staff of institutions for the developmentally disabled
   Classroom contacts of deinstitutionalized developmentally disabled persons with persistent hepatitis
      B antigenemia
   Household and other intimate contacts of persons with persistent hepatitis B antigenemia
   Newborns of HBsAg-carrier mothers

Populations with high incidence of the disease
   Alaskan natives and Pacific Islanders
   Refugees from Africa, Eastern Asia, Middle East and Haiti
   Adoptees from countries of high HBV endemicity

Military personnel who have been stationed outside the USA

Morticians and embalmers

Blood bank and plasma fractionation workers

Persons at increased risk of disease because of multiple sex partners
   Persons who repeatedly contract sexually transmitted diseases

Homosexually and heterosexually active individuals
   Homosexually active males
   Female prostitutes

Inmates of long-term correctional facilities

Users of illicit injectable drugs

International travelers

of their increased prevalence of hepatitis B infection. The dentist and the entire dental staff is one of these high-risk populations. Why is this so?

Hepatitis B is an insidious disease. An estimated 300,000 persons, primarily young adults, are infected each year. One-quarter become ill with jaundice; more than 10,000 patients require hospitalization; and an average of 250 die of fulminant disease each year. Between 6 and 10% of young adults with HBV infection become carriers. The United States currently contains an estimated pool of 1,000,000 hepatitis B infected carriers. Chronic active hepatitis develops in about 25% of carriers and often progresses to cirrhosis. HBV carriers also have a risk of developing primary liver cancer that is 12 to 300 times higher than that of other persons. The majority of infections are asymptomatic or more correctly subclinical in nature. This is because some of the symptoms of hepatitis B are common to the everyday life of a busy individual: headache, mild gastrointestinal upset, general fatigue and/ or a few "stiff joints." It is easy to attribute these symptoms to too much coffee, late hours and overworking, or a mild case of the flu. Rarely is that one presenting sign most believed to be pathognomonic of hepatitis present: jaundice. Most hepatitis B cases are anicteric. Depending on the route of transmission, virulence of the inoculum, and host resistance factors, only 5 to 56% of patients actually demonstrates jaundice. Approximately 80% of all hepatitis B infections are undiagnosed. Several studies indicated that only 21% of 377 patients with positive blood markers for HBV reported a positive history of hepatitis B. Thus, the patient/health care provider never knew whether the patient had hepatitis B and could not provide the dentist with a positive history of disease. Others have demonstrated that the medical history is unreliable in identifying who actually has experienced HBV infection. They showed that about half of those who reported a prior history of either hepatitis B or hepatitis A actually had serologic evidence of prior hepatitis B infection. Among those who were unsure of the type of hepatitis infection they had or even if they had experienced an HBV infection, about one-third had serologic evidence of prior hepatitis B infection. Thus, the flip of a coin is as accurate as asking a patient if they have had hepatitis (A, B, or otherwise). However, the medical history can be useful in determining what groups of patients are at a higher risk of being undiagnosed carriers. Whenever a patient from any of the groups listed in Table 2–4 sits in the dental chair, the dental staff is treating a high-risk hepatitis B patient. These high-risk, undiagnosed patients include dental staff members, the staff members of any other health care provider, and even the dentist when he sits in someone else's dental chair.

Regardless of the medical history, all patients must be regarded as potential hepatitis B carriers. With the number of undiagnosed hepatitis B cases and the unreliability of the medical history, the dentist has been misled into thinking that few of his patients have had hepatitis and thus present as potential sources of HBV infection. Additionally, hepatitis B carrier patients as well as anti-HIV positive and persons with AIDS (PWAs) are seeking places where they may have routine dental care accomplished. Some dental schools and practitioners do not routinely treat patients with hepatitis or an HIV seropositive history; therefore, these patients do not report this when seen by the next dentist. As this continues, the medical history becomes even less reliable than it is now for determining history of infectious diseases.

For the same reasons that few dentists, until recently, realized the prevalence

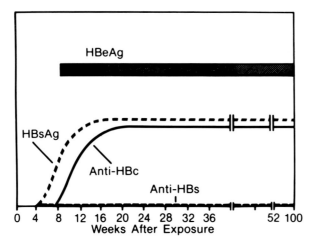

Fig. 2–7. Carrier serology.

of HBV infection in the dental profession, the medical profession believes the prevalence of HBV infection is much lower than has been documented.

The role of the HBV carrier is central in the epidemiology of HBV transmission. A carrier is defined as a person who is HBsAg-positive on at least two occasions at least 6 months apart. Carriers develop very little if any anti-HBs and therefore remain HBsAg positive. Figure 2–7 demonstrates the serology of the carrier state in chronic hepatitis. Although the degree of infectivity is best correlated with HBeAg positivity, any person positive for HBsAg is potentially infectious. The likelihood of developing the carrier state varies inversely with the age at which infection occurs. During the perinatal period, HBV transmitted from HBeAg-positive mothers results in HBV carriage in up to 90% of infected infants, whereas 6 to 10% of acutely infected adults become carriers.

Unfortunately, the hepatitis B carrier state develops more commonly via asymptomatic subclinical HBV infection versus acute infection. Additionally, carriers developing an asymptomatic subclinical infection are more likely to be HBeAg positive, indicating that they are in a more infectious contagious state, and therefore more liable to transmit the disease.

The period of jaundice usually follows the appearance of HBsAg and HBeAg in the blood. Therefore, once jaundice develops, if at all, the patient has already been potentially transmitting the disease quite effectively from one person to another including those in the dental office. Thus, the major challenge in dental practice regarding hepatitis B is to stop transmission from patient to dental staff, dental staff to practitioner, practitioner to patient, patient to patient, and dental staff to close intimate contacts (family) via appropriate infection control measures.

Prevalence of Infection in the Dental Profession

Table 2–5 lists data concerning hepatitis B infection in health care professionals in general. Table 2–6 indicates the prevalence of hepatitis B infection in US dentists from studies reported from 1975 to 1978. Unfortunately, these studies cannot be readily compared as they used different blood markers to determine their results.

The most often quoted study was performed in 1972 at the American Dental Association (ADA) annual session. At that time, 1,245 general practitioners were screened for HBsAg and anti-HBs. A positive history for hepatitis B while a dental

Table 2–5. Combined Data on Prevalence of HBV Markers in Health Care Personnel

	Prevalence of HBV Markers (%)	Annual Attack Rates (%)
General Physicians	12–19	2
Medical House Officers	8–10	—
Family Practice	15–16	—
Internal Medicine	14–18	—
Surgeons	20–28	5
Surgical Residents	10–17	4–10
Pathologists	20–27	—
Anesthesiologists	17	—
Obstetricans/Gynecologists	14–16	—
Pediatricians	13–21	—
Oral Surgeons	30	5
Dentists	14–15	2
Psychiatrists	3	—
Non-Patient Care	4–8	—

Data from Smith et al, 1976; Mosley et al, 1975; Dienstag and Ryan, 1982; Maynard, 1982.

student or in private practice was reported by 3.3% of those screened, whereas 13.6% had positive serology for previous hepatitis B infection. More recent results of health screening at the 1989 ADA annual session have indicated a decrease from 10.9% (1988) to 8.8% in natural HBV exposure *for the profession as a whole.* Although more dentists are becoming immunized against HBV via vaccine, this does not mean that the risk of infection for the *nonimmune* dental professional has decreased. Other studies looking at the dental specialties indicate that as many as 38.5% of oral surgeons had positive serology for HBV infection.

Combined studies indicate that the general dentist is at risk of hepatitis exposure at about 3 times that of the general US population, whereas nonimmunized surgical specialists are at risk about 6 times that of the general US population. HBsAg has also been detected in 76% of salivary samples of known carriers, has

Table 2–6. Prevalence of Hepatitis B Infection in US Dentists

Author	Number Surveyed History/Serology	Number Positive History/Serology	% Positive History/Serology*
Feldman and Schiff, 1975	434/236	29†/42	7†/18 5†/- (general dentists)
Mosley et al., 1975	1245/1245	90(41†)/169	7(3†)/14
Mosley and White, 1975	242/-	11†/-	5†/- (all dentists) 3†/- (general dentists) 4†/- (surgical specialists)‡
Smith et al., 1976	-/174	-/25	-/14
Weil, Lyman, Jackson, and Bernstein, 1977	511/511	63/108	12/21 (all dentists) 10/25 (surgical specialists)‡
Goldstein, Morse, and Gullen, 1978	145/145	2/13	1/9 (endodontists)
Siew, Grunenger, Chang, and Verrusio, 1989	-/1339	-/-	-/10.9 (general dentists)

*Approximately 5% of US population seropositive for prior hepatitis B infection
†Data for years of dental school and professional practice only
‡Oral surgeons, periodontists, and endodontists

Table 2–7. Prevalence of Serologic Markers of Hepatitis B Among Dental Personnel in Sera Collected From 1979–1981

Category	Number Positive	Percent Positive
Dental Hygienists	10/59	16.9
Lab Technicians	22/155	14.2
Dental Assistants	45/350	12.9
Clerical	5/56	8.9
Other	0/9	0
Total	86/629	13.0

Adapted from Schiff, E.R. et al.: Veterans Administration cooperative study on hepatitis and dentistry. J. Am. Dent. Assoc., *113*:390–396, 1986.

been transmitted by a human bite, and can be detected in nasopharyngeal secretions and gingival crevicular fluid.

The risk of HBV infection is more a factor of exposure to blood than it is to general patient contact. Intraorally the greatest concentration of the HBV is at the gingival sulcus. In most patient's mouths this area is routinely inflamed and easily allows blood to mix with saliva, thus making the saliva infectious with HBV. For this reason, the dental hygienist, who works primarily in the area of the gingival sulcus, has been demonstrated to be as highly at risk as the dentist followed closely by the lab technician and dental assistant (Table 2–7).

Prevalence of Infection in US Military Personnel

At least three studies have shown the increased prevalence of HBV infection in military personnel. Scott et al. demonstrated that during a 1-year period, the HBV markers doubled in new Army and Air Force arrivals in Thailand. James and Smith demonstrated a 20% marker positive population in an army engineer batallion in Europe, 4% of whom were HBsAg positive. Irwin demonstrated that only 10% of US soldiers were anti-HBs positive, whereas this number increased to 25% with soldiers who had at least one foreign tour of duty. Thus, military dental staff would be expected to have a higher prevalence of HBV infection than that seen in US civilian dentists especially as these dentists work primarily with a patient population demonstrated to have an increased prevalence of HBV markers. Additionally, civilian dentists and their staffs working with military dependents or personnel with a past history of active military duty should realize that these military personnel may have a higher prevalence of previous HBV infection. More recently, all the military services are reporting a decrease in their HBV infection incidence, most likely as a result of a reduction in intravenous drug use among personnel.

Prevalence of the HBV Carrier State in US Dentists

Table 2–8 demonstrates several studies concerning the prevalence of the hepatitis B carrier state in US dentists from 1975 to 1977. The range is anywhere from 3 to 10 times that of the general US population. More recent data from the ADA has shown that the carrier prevalence has decreased to 0.4% (1989 Annual Session) for the profession as a whole because of vaccine use. It has been estimated that there are 3,000 dentists and auxiliary dental workers in the United States who are

Table 2–8. Prevalence of Hepatitis B Carrier State in United States Dentists

Author	Number Surveyed	Number HBsAg +	Percentage* HBsAg +
Feldman and Schiff, 1975	236	3	1.27
Mosley et al., 1974	1245	11	0.90
Smith et al., 1976	174	3	1.70
Hollinger, Grander, Nickel, and Suarez,† 1977	94	4	3.20
Weil, Lyman, Jackson, and Bernstein, 1977	511	4	0.80
Siew, Grunenger, Chang, and Verrusio, 1989	1339	—	0.60

*Approximately 0.3% of US population HBsAg positive
†Dental students

persistent HBV carriers. Thus, susceptible dentists have a risk of developing the hepatitis B carrier state that is up to 10 times that of an average American citizen.

The potential impact of the carrier state on a dental practice is devastating. Table 2–9 summarizes the Centers for Disease Control (CDC) guidelines for a dentist who develops the HBV carrier state. To say that these guidelines are not particularly practice-building would be an understatement. On the contrary, the financial loss from one month of illness has run in the neighborhood of $40,000. And one month is the time frame for a short-term illness. It may take several months or years before complete health returns, if at all.

HBV Carrier Dentists Transmitting Disease

Table 2–10 lists studies which demonstrate that some dentists have transmitted HBV infection to their patients. Most often these cases were investigated by the CDC upon the finding of clusters of HBV infections and the determination of a common factor of dental care by a single dentist within the past 2 to 6 months before illness. To date, no health care personnel have transmitted more cases of HBV to patients than have dentists.

Table 2–9. CDC Guidelines for Hepatitis B Chronic-Carrier Dentists*

1. Determine if other factors that may facilitate hepatitis B transmission exist before resuming practice (e.g., chronic dermatitis).
2. *If* the dentist is still transmitting hepatitis, the dentist must obtain a signed informed consent from each patient stating that the patient agrees to have dental treatment with the full knowledge that the dentist carries the hepatitis B virus, but that all precautions are being taken to minimize the risk of transmission of the virus. If the dentist is not transmitting disease, signed informed consent attesting to the dentist's hepatitis B carrier state is not required.
3. Institute barrier techniques (surgical gloves and mask) for *every* dental procedure. **There is no exception to this rule.**
4. Test HBsAg serologic status of dentist periodically. Continually monitor patients to detect any possible cases of hepatitis.
5. If there is evidence of continued hepatitis B transmission despite the use of the preceding measures or, if the dentist fails to comply with the recommendations, then the state and local health departments and the state dental licensure board would likely consider more stringent actions such as suspension of the dentist's license to practice.

*Adapted from Lettau, L.A., et al. Transmission of hepatitis B with restriction of surgical practice. JAMA 255:934–937, 1986.

Table 2–10. HBV Transmission from Carrier Dentists to Patients

Author	Number of Patients	Practice
Levin, Maddrey, Wands, and Mendeloff, 1974	13	General Dentist
Williams, Pattison, and Berquist, 1975	0	General Dentist
Goodwin, Fannin, and McCracken, 1976	37	Oral Surgeon
Watkins, 1976	15	Oral Surgeon
Rimland, Parkin, Miller, and Schrank, 1977	55	Oral Surgeon
Ahtone et al., 1981	3	Oral Surgeon
Hadler et al., 1981	6	General Dentist
Reingold et al., 1982	12	Oral Surgeon
Ahtone and Goodman, 1983	4	General Dentist
Shaw et al., 1986	26	General Dentist
CDC, 1987	4	Oral Surgeon

The most outstanding case is a 46-year-old male dentist from Pennsylvania who had no history of hepatitis nor any disease with comparable symptomatology but transmitted the same subtype of hepatitis as he was found to have to 55 of his patients. He rarely wore gloves while performing dental procedures before the incident occurred. He did wear gloves during the subsequent investigation, and only two additional cases of hepatitis developed in over 4,300 patients seen. Barrier techniques (mask, gloves, protective eyewear) have been shown time and again to be effective in prevention of HBV transmission.

Additionally, in 1984, 26 cases of HBV infection were reported in the practice of a dentist in Indiana. The dentist was positive for HBsAg with the same subgroup antigen as the infected patients, but had no known history of HBV infection. Two patients developed fulminant hepatitis resulting in death. The dentist died of HBV infection sequelae in December, 1988.

Prevention of Transmission via Immunoprophylaxis

Active and Passive Immunity. Hepatitis B can be stopped in the dental office. Transmission can be prevented by neutralization of the host reservoir (irradication of all HBV sources), interruption of the modes of transmission (infection control practices), or by immunization of susceptible hosts. Immunization of susceptible hosts will be discussed first.

In order to understand immunoprophylaxis, one must understand active and passive immunization (Table 2–11). *Passive immunity* occurs by transferring pre-formed antibodies from an actively immunized host to a person in need of im-

Table 2–11. Comparison of Active and Passive Immunity

	Active	Passive
Genesis	Stimulation of immune response within a host	No host participation; transfer of performed substances from an actively immunized host
Onset of Action	Only after a latent period	Immediate
Duration	Long-lived	Transitory
Application	Acute/subclinical disease	Postexposure immunoglobulin (e.g., ISG or HBIG)

Adapted from Bellanti, J.A.: Immunology II. Philadelphia, W.B. Saunders, 1978.

munity. The protection provided is transitory, onset is immediate, and examples are injection of immune globulin (IG) or hepatitis B immune globulin (HBIG). *Active immunity* is stimulation of one's own immune response. Protection is provided only after a latent period; however, long-term immunity is provided. Examples of active immunization are actual acquisition of the disease either subclinically or acutely, and vaccination.

IG primarily provides protection against hepatitis A virus infection and is relatively inexpensive. Passive immunoprophylaxis via HBIG gives protection against HBV infection for about 2 months and is expensive. Passive immunization can occur only if the dentist or staff member knows whether they have been exposed to HBV and takes immediate action. This is seldom the case as most instances of transmission have been inapparent to the recipient. Thus, active preincident immunity is preferable. Active immunity can be conferred either through acute infection, subclinical disease, or hepatitis B vaccination.

Hepatitis B Vaccines

Plasma-Derived Vaccine. Groundwork for the success of an immunizing preparation was set by Krugman and his coworkers in a classic series of studies that found that a 1:10 dilution of hepatitis B infective serum (strain MS-2) lost infectivity, but retained its antigenicity, when boiled for 1 minute. When used as a vaccine, this preparation prevented or modified the course of hepatitis B in approximately 70% of the subjects who were later challenged with hepatitis B virus (HBV). MS-2 serum contained large quantities of hepatitis B surface antigen (HBsAg).

Subsequent vaccine work focused on the extraction and purification of this noninfectious, viral coat protein for use as the antigen preparation. This effort was fostered by the observation that HBV replication in infected individuals was not as efficient as once thought, because large amounts of excess HBsAg particles are synthesized and passed into the patient's circulation. As one recovers from infection, antibodies to this antigen (anti-HBs) are produced by the host's immune system and provide protection against recurrent viral attack.

Accumulated evidence also indicated that these HBsAg forms are present in high concentrations in the circulation of carriers of hepatitis B. Thus, carriers with high serum HBsAg titers were shown to provide a supply of viral antigen for vaccine production. This achievement was crucial to the overall effort, as HBV had yet to be cultured in vitro.

Heptavax-B, the original plasma-derived hepatitis B vaccine, had clinical tests started in 1975 and was introduced in the United States in 1982. This vaccine was developed and manufactured by Merck Sharp and Dohme, and represented a milestone in immunology, as the first clinically available vaccine derived from human sources. Over 3 million individuals worldwide have received the plasma-derived vaccine. The vaccine is given in three separate intramuscular injections: the first two doses 1 month apart and the third dose 6 months following the first dose. The immunogenicity of the vaccine is shown in Figure 2–8. Following the first dose, approximately 30% of normal, healthy, young adult vaccine recipients respond by the formation of antibodies. The response rate increases to 75% following the second dose and to 96% following the third dose. The CDC has stated that the hepatitis B vaccine has the best response rate of any vaccine ever produced in the US. Most people assume erroneously that all vaccines have a 100% response

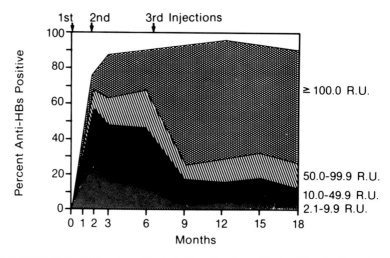

Fig. 2–8.   Hepatitis B vaccine immunogenicity. (From Szmuness, W., et al.: A controlled clinic trial of the efficacy of the hepatitis B vaccine: A final report. Hepatology, 1:377–385, 1981.)

rate; however, no vaccine produces seroconversion in one hundred percent (100%) of vaccines. Those who respond to the vaccine by the formation of protective levels of anti-HBs are 100% protected against development of active hepatitis B, asymptomatic hepatitis B infection, and development of the carrier state.

The plasma-derived hepatitis B vaccine was studied in a number of population groups both to control for modes of transmission and to study those at low and high risk to HBV infection. It was proven to be effective in protecting against HBV infection in all these studies.

The vaccine production process was designed to thoroughly ensure a safe product. The collected serum, taken from human hepatitis B carriers, was exposed to two biophysical purification steps and three chemical inactivation steps (pepsin at pH 2, 8 M urea, and 1:4000 formalin) which virtually left an entirely safe suspension of HBsAg.

Continued clinical monitoring of vaccine recipients by the CDC through 1984 and presently by the Food and Drug Administration (FDA) indicates that there is no increased incidence of any severe side effects associated with the HB vaccine.

At one time there was some concern about the possibility of the HB vaccine transmitting HIV infection. Several studies addressed this issue and supplied evidence confirming lack of HIV transmission with this vaccine. The evidence concerns four significant areas:

1. Direct testing of the inactivation steps used in the vaccine manufacturing process indicated that all three of the inactivation procedures (pepsin, pH 2; 8 molar urea; and 0.1 percent formaldehyde) inactivates HIV. Thus if HIV were in the vaccine plasma pool, it is inactivated by the vaccine production process.

2. Studies were performed looking for the HIV nucleic acid sequences in the vaccine itself, using an HIV probe. It was determined that the vaccine contained no AIDS virus-related amino acid sequences. All protein in the vaccine codes specifically for HBsAg.

3. The third approach attempted to detect seroconversion to anti-HIV in HB

vaccine recipients. No seroconversion was detected in individuals who received vaccine manufactured from plasma pools that contained plasma of donors at high risk for HIV infection.

4. Monitoring of AIDS patients reported to the CDC and FDA has continued to look for epidemiologic evidence of an association between HB vaccine and AIDS. As of June 1, 1985, 68 AIDS cases had been reported among approximately 700,000 US HB vaccine recipients; all have occurred among persons with known AIDS risk factors.

In addition, the rate of AIDS for HB vaccine recipients in CDC vaccine trials among homosexually active men in Denver and San Francisco did not differ from that for men screened for possible participation in the trials but who received no HB vaccine because they were found to be immune. Thus, the plasma-derived vaccine is not associated with HBV or HIV transmission.

Recombinant DNA Vaccines. Advances in vaccine development continued to provide clinically useful preparations and in July 1986, the first vaccine made using recombinant DNA technology was licensed. *Recombivax HB*, also from Merck Sharp & Dohme, became available for general use in the United States for the prevention of HBV infection in January 1987. This newer vaccine provided an alternative to the plasma-derived vaccine.

The recombinant vaccine is produced in cultures of *Saccharomyces cerevisiae* (common baker's yeast), into which a plasmid containing the gene for HBsAg has been inserted. HBsAg is subsequently harvested after lysis of cultured yeast cells. Purified HBsAg protein then undergoes sterile filtration and treatment with formalin prior to packaging. Administered vaccine is designed to contain 10 micrograms (μg) of HBsAg protein per milliliter (ml), absorbed with 0.5 milligrams (mg) per ml of aluminum hydroxide (alum), with thimerosal as a preservative.

The immunogenicity of *Recombivax HB* is comparable to that observed for the plasma-derived preparation. When administered in a three-dose injection regimen, *Recombivax HB* has been shown to induce protective antibody production (anti-HBs) in over 99% of healthy adults 20 to 29 years of age. Healthy adults who received either the recombinant vaccine (10 μg/dose) or the plasma-derived *Heptavax-B* (20 μg/dose) showed equal seroconversion rates. However, the geometric mean titers (GMT) of antibodies induced by the original recombinant vaccine ranged from equal to 30% lower than that developed by recipients of *Heptavax-B*.

The possibility of developing a lower antibody titer following immunization with the recombinant vaccine created some debate and also led to further investigation to improve the vaccine's immunogenicity. These changes were approved by the US Office of Biologics as amendments to the original *Recombivax HB* license. Table 2–12 summarizes the adult antibody responses to *Recombivax HB* made using original seed/original process, original seed/improved process, and new seed/improved process, respectively. It should be noted that these modifications have been associated with definite improvements in immunogenicity. The reduced immune response observed initially with early recombinant vaccine lots compared with plasma-derived vaccine has been rectified through improvements in the manufacturing process and the use of a new master seed strain of recombinant *Saccharomyces cerevisiae*. As a result, the currently licensed form of *Recombivax HB* is considered

Table 2–12. Anti-HBs Responses at 7 or 8 Months among Healthy Adults Receiving
*Recombivax HB**

Recombivax HB Seed/Process	Number of Vaccines	Anti-HBs Responders (>10 mIU/ml)	GMT of Responders
Original/original	739	95%	749
Original/improved	173	98%	1,223
New/improved	144	99%	1,823

*Anti-HBs indicates antibodies to hepatitis B surface antigen; GMT, geometric mean titers. *Recombivax HB* was administered in 10 microgram doses at 0, 1, and 6 months
Adapted from Gerety, R.J., Ellis, R.W., and Zajac, B.A.: Two superb vaccines against hepatitis B in Mexican standoff. JAMA, *259*:2403–2404, 1988.

to be superior to the early lots in ability to induce a high anti-HBs titer. The only stated contraindication for *Recombivax HB* is for those individuals who are hypersensitive to yeast or any component of the vaccine.

Another recombinant DNA hepatitis B vaccine, *Engerix-B*, has been produced by SmithKline Biologicals in Belgium. Initial observations concerning the differences between the two vaccine production processes are outlined in Table 2–13. Use of thiocyanate for conversion and folding of the antigen in *Recombivax HB* production results in a configuration that may be more immunogenic by increasing the density of antigenically active sites and overall stabilization of the structure. The use of an in situ formed alum adjuvant (Fig. 2–9) appears to promote slow release of the antigen, also related to improved immunogenicity. Another important factor concerns the formalin treatment that assists in microbial kill of any possible extraneous contaminants and antigen stabilization over time. Increased purity, achieved by decreasing the amount of remaining yeast antigen in *Recombivax HB*, also appears to increase immunogenicity. The rationale here is that the contaminating yeast protein intercalates with HBsAg aggregates and changes the configuration of antigenic sites in ways that impair immunogenicity. Thus, as the level of yeast protein is reduced, immunogenicity may be enhanced.

The amount of antigen per ml differs among the recombinant vaccines. As previously mentioned, studies have shown that the 10 μg/ml of HBsAg in *Recombivax HB* is equivalent to the 20 μg dose/ml of HBsAg found in *Heptavax-B*. *Engerix-B* is also produced with 20 μg/ml of HBsAg to compensate for the possible loss of potency during storage (Andre, FE, 1989).

In 1988, studies indicated an anti-HBs GMT following administration of *Recombivax HB* that was about twice that produced from the same regimen of *Engerix-B* despite the difference in antigen levels (see Table 2–14). Additionally, the prescribing information for *Recombivax HB* indicates that when 3 40-μg doses of the vaccine were given to dialysis patients (120 μg total), 86% seroconverted and achieved protective levels of anti-HBs ($\geq$10 mIU/ml). However, after 4 40-μg doses

Table 2–13. Production Differences Between *Recombivax HB* and *Engerix-B*

	Action	Recombivax HB	Engerix-B
Thiocyanate conversion	Antigen folding	Yes	No
Formalin treatment	Inactivation step; stabilization of antigen	Yes	No
Alum adjuvant	Increase immunogenicity	In situ	Preformed
Purity re: Yeast Protein	Increase immunogenicity	>99%	>97%

Adapted from H-B-Vax II, (hepatitis B vaccine [recombinant]) Product Monograph, 1989, Merck Sharp & Dohme.

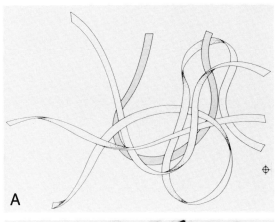

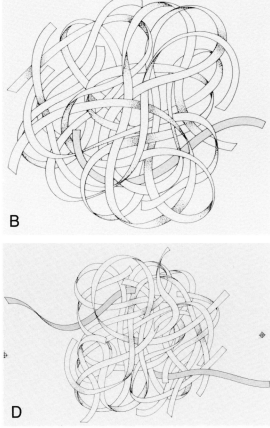

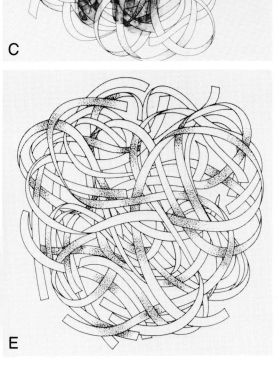

Fig. 2–9. Depiction of the thiocyanate process, which helps promote optimal immunogenicity and purity of the yeast-derived antigen in *Recombivax HB*. A, The recombinant hepatitis B surface antigen, which leaves the ribosome as a linear sequence of 226 amino acids, begins to fold. Yeast contaminant, shown shaded, is visible. B, More intricate folding occurs, creating a three-dimensional particle. Dotted areas of interchain bonding aids in antigen uniformity. C, The semistructured particle is then subjected to a thiocyanate wash. D, Through the breaking and reformation of disulfide bonds between cysteines, thiocyanate facilitates the proper three-dimensional folding of the antigen. Epitopes (antigenic active sites) are appropriately exposed. Yeast contaminants are removed as the particles expand. E, The antigen has tremendous stability because of cross-linking within the primary structure and between the individual polymers. The final vaccine product produced with this antigen is more than 99% pure with respect to residual yeast proteins. (Courtesy of Merck Sharp & Dohme.)

Table 2–14. *Recombivax HB* and *Engerix-B* in Healthy Adults

Vaccine	Time (months)	% Responding	GMT*
Recombivax HB	7	99%	1834
Engerix-B	7	99%	981

*milli International Units (mIU)/ml
Adapted from Andre, F.: Clinical experience with a recombinant DNA hepatitis B vaccine. SE Asia J Trop Med Pub Hlth, *19*:501, 1988; and Zajac, B., et al.: Improvements in the immunogenicity and purity of a genetically engineered hepatitis B vaccine. Hepatology, *8*:1322, 1988.

of *Engerix-B* (160 μg total), only 67% of dialysis patients seroconverted despite receiving an extra 40 μg of antigen.

Lastly, on June 1, 1989, the FDA approved a revised dose of *Recombivax HB* for infants and children (Table 2–15). As only half the adult dose is required in this revised dose recommendation, there is a significant cost savings for individuals immunized with *Recombivax HB* before age 20. The revised *Recombivax HB* dosing information is compared with the 1990 information concerning dosing for *Engerix-B* in Table 2–16. In some instances, the currently recommended antigen dose of *Recombivax HB* is only one fourth that of *Engerix-B* to achieve an equivalent level of protection. It appears that the quality of the antigen is most important, and only secondarily, the quantity of antigen. The biological activity (immunogenicity) of vaccines depends on the number and density of antigenic sites, which in turn depend on the tertiary and quaternary structure of the HBsAg aggregates (see Fig. 2–9). Thus, hepatitis vaccine should not be considered a generic product at this time because 1 μg of antigen significantly differs from product to product. Only clinical trials can establish the proper dosage for a given vaccine.

Table 2–15. 1989 Revised Dose Recommendation for *Recombivax HB*

Age*	Dose†
0–10	2.5 μg
11–19‡	5.0 μg
20+ above	10.0 μg

*years
†per injection
‡for infants who are immunocompetent and not born of a carrier mother

Table 2–16. Dose Recommendations for *Recombivax HB* and *Engerix-B*

Age Group*	Recombivax HB	Engerix-B
Adults over 20	10 μg	20 μg†
Adolescents, 11–19	5 μg	20 μg†
Infants and children, birth–10	2.5 μg	10 μg†
Dialysis patients	40 μg (0, 1, 6 months)	40 μg (0, 1, 2, 6 months only)
Neonates of carrier mothers	0.5 ml HBIG at birth, 5 μg vaccine within 7 days, and 1, 6 months	0.5 ml HBIG at birth, 10 μg vaccine within 7 days, and 1, 6 months†

*Age in years
†4-dose schedule (0, 1, 2 and 12 months) also available.
Adapted from Centers for Disease Control (ACIP): Protection against viral hepatitis. MMWR, *39*(RR-2):11, 1990.

Pretesting

The issue of whether to pretest an individual for anti-HBs immunity has been discussed at length since introduction of the vaccines. Pretesting can be cost effective in large groups where the proportion expected to be antibody positive is substantial, as those individuals who already are anti-HBs positive are immune to HBV infection and therefore do not need vaccine. Studies to date have shown that only 6.7% of vaccine recipients in dentistry have been already immune. Thus, pretesting is not cost effective in the average dental office although it should be offered to potential vaccinees in an immunization program in accordance with the proposed OSHA standard. Unfortunately, there can be a significant number of false-positive reports for anti-HBs, particularly in a pretesting situation.

Post-testing

Persons electing to do postvaccination testing for anti-HBs should be aware of potential difficulties in interpreting the results. Serologic testing within 6 months of completing the primary series will differentiate persons who respond to vaccine from those who fail to respond. However, the results of testing undertaken more than 6 months after completion of the primary series are more difficult to interpret. Therefore post-testing should be scheduled soon after the last inoculation.

A vaccine recipient who is negative for anti-HBs several years after vaccination can be either (1) a primary nonresponder who remains susceptible to hepatitis B, or (2) a vaccine responder whose antibody levels have decreased below detectability yet is still protected against clinical disease. Should one not have responded, three additional doses of vaccine are indicated. These extra doses will cause seroconversion in approximately 50% of the nonresponders.

Antibody Persistence and Booster Dose

Studies have shown that over 70% of those people who developed more than 100 sample ratio units (SRU) of anti-HBs are maintaining a detectable antibody titer through 7 years. Those who have lost detectable anti-HBs have demonstrated a secondary anamnestic response that was protective against clinical infection when challenged with HBV.

According to the CDC, it is not necessary to be routinely tested for anti-HBs each year after vaccination. The antibody response to properly administered vaccine is excellent for adults and children with normal immune status, and the CDC states that protection lasts for at least 7 years in these groups because of the anamnestic response.

At present, the Advisory Committee on Immunization Practices (ACIP) of the CDC is still reviewing data before a final statement will be made about a booster dose. In the absence of an ACIP statement, a 1 ml vaccine booster dose can be considered optional. There has been no documented evidence that anyone who has received either the plasma-derived or recombinant vaccines licensed in the US, and was immunocompetent, has developed clinical hepatitis (1989 statistics).

Site of Injection

There was some concern about suboptimal response to the HB vaccine when received in the buttocks. Post-testing of vaccinees early after vaccine introduction demonstrated low seroconversion rates with some response rates as low as 50%. A thorough follow-up of shipping techniques, vaccine storage techniques, retention of vaccine potency, and review of vaccine lots failed to identify any specific cause.

A breakthrough occurred when the same vaccine lot was distributed to a general hospital and a health department in a large Canadian city. The health department had 100% seroconversion whereas the general hospital had a much lower rate. The only difference was that the vaccine was given into the deltoid muscle at the health department and the hospital administered the vaccine into the buttocks. Further backtracking of the other sites reporting suboptimal responses indicated differences in site of injection to be the reason for the seroconversion discrepancies.

Any member of the dental profession who has received vaccine, particularly into the buttocks for any one or all of the injections, should be post-tested for seroconversion. Furthermore, adequate long-term studies have not been performed to demonstrate prolonged efficacy of intradermal administration or other non-FDA approved dose reductions of vaccine.

Vaccination of Pregnant Women

It is well documented that HBV infection in a pregnant woman can result in severe disease for the mother and chronic infection of the newborn. Therefore, in 1984, the ACIP recommended that pregnant women in certain groups at high risk for HBV infection be screened for HBsAg during a prenatal visit. If the mother was HBsAg positive, it was then recommended that the newborn receive hepatitis B immune globulin (HBIG) and HB vaccine at birth. Because both forms of HBV vaccine contain only noninfectious HBsAg particles, the CDC stated that the vaccination of a pregnant woman should pose no risk to either the woman or the fetus. Pregnancy should, therefore, not be considered a contraindication for vaccination of women. It must be noted that immunizations during pregnancy have not been routinely recommended, and therefore, this decision must be made in consultation with the woman's obstetrician.

The ACIP updated their earlier guidelines in June, 1988 based on further accumulated evidence and now recommends that *all* pregnant women should be routinely tested for HBsAg during an early prenatal visit in each pregnancy. This testing should be done at the same time that other routine prenatal screening tests are ordered. In special situations, such as when acute hepatitis is suspected, when there has been a history of exposure to hepatitis, or when the mother participates in a particularly high risk behavior such as intravenous drug use, an additional HBsAg test can be ordered later in the pregnancy. Enactment of these CDC recommendations will undoubtedly assist in controlling perinatal HBV transmissions in the US.

Acute Exposures

The CDC has continually published recommendations for individuals who have percutaneous or permucosal exposures to blood that contains (or might contain) HBsAg. Appendix D contains these recommendations along with those for HIV exposure. They can be summarized as stating that if you are not immunized before your next "needlestick" or other exposure, you will be after it occurs.

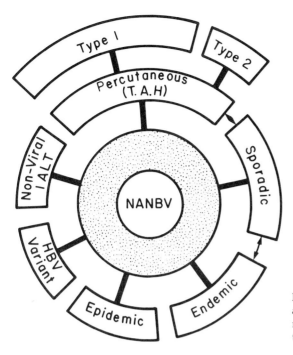

Fig. 2–10. Variants of non-A non-B hepatitis. (From Alter, H.J.: The universe of non-A non-B hepatitis. Update. Testing in the Blood Bank 2:1, 1988.)

NON-A NON-B HEPATITIS

Parenterally transmitted non-A non-B hepatitis (PT-NANB) seen in the United States has epidemiologic characteristics similar to those of hepatitis B, occurring most commonly following blood transfusions and parenteral drug use. Multiple episodes of non-A non-B hepatitis have been observed in the same individual and are most likely caused by different agents.

A major advance was reported in 1988 when Chiron Corporation reported that a portion of the genome of a 30 to 60 nm diameter enveloped RNA virus appears to be the etiologic agent for the major type of PT-NANB hepatitis. This virus appears to be responsible for the majority of hepatitis seen following a transfusion, 50% of which develops into the chronic carrier state.

Although PT-NANB hepatitis has traditionally been considered a transfusion-associated disease, most reported cases have not been associated with a blood transfusion. Although transfusion recipients, parenteral drug users, and dialysis patients are at high risk for this infection, health-care workers with frequent contact with blood, and personal contact with others who may be infected within households have also been documented as risk factors for PT-NANB. The role of sexual activity and person-to-person contact is not clear at this time.

One of the reasons this form of hepatitis is difficult to diagnose is that up to 75% of cases are anicteric. Chiron Corporation is currently developing a prototype antibody and antigen immunoassay to screen blood and has begun initial research into a vaccine. The proposed name of the PT-NANB hepatitis virus is hepatitis C virus (HCV).

It appears that as many as 150,000 may be infected with HCV per year in the United States and 700,000 infected worldwide. Approximately 1 to 3% of the US population may be HCV carriers. Figure 2–11 demonstrates how anti-HCV appears

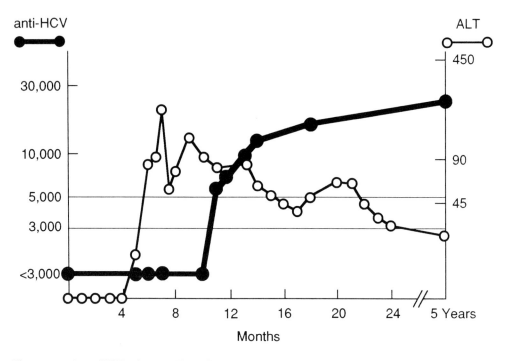

Fig. 2–11.   Acute HCV infection. (From Stevens, Update 3(2):2, 1989.)

not to become positive until several weeks or months after the first appearance of alanine aminotransferase (ALT). This delay has been reported by other investigators as well and may place a severe limit on the capability of this antibody test to detect blood infections with HCV.

Although several studies have attempted to assess the value of prophylaxis with IG against PT-NANB hepatitis, the results have been equivocal, and no specific recommendations have been made. However, for persons with percutaneous exposure to blood from a patient with non-A non-B hepatitis, it may be reasonable to administer IG (0.06 ml/kg) as soon as possible after exposure.

An outbreak of PT-NANB was reported in 1989 among parenteral drug users in Illinois. This outbreak occurred in a white, rural area rather than the usual inner city black or Hispanic population. A few household contacts were diagnosed with NANB hepatitis. The role of sexual activity in this outbreak could not be defined.

Enterically transmitted non-A non-B hepatitis (ET-NANB) was formally recognized in 1955–56 although it has been observed since ancient times. It appears to be transmitted along the fecal-oral route by a 32 to 34 nm virus-like particle. Large, well-documented outbreaks have been seen in India, the USSR, North Africa, Mexico, and Southeast Asia. There appears to be a 6 to 8 week incubation period. ET-NANB hepatitis is more common in men than in women; however, there is a high fatality rate (10 to 20%) in women who are in their third trimester of pregnancy. A low incidence of the carrier state develops following infection. There is no evidence that US-manufactured IG will prevent this infection.

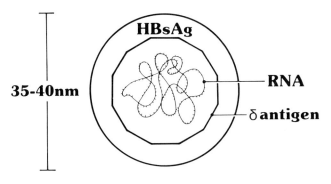

Fig. 2–12. Delta hepatitis virus.

DELTA HEPATITIS

Delta hepatitis virus (HDV) (Fig. 2–12), originally called the delta agent, was discovered in 1977 by Rizzetto and colleagues in Italy. Extensive investigations since that time have established the fact that delta hepatitis is unique and distinct from hepatitis B, although HDV depends on hepatitis B virus (HBV) for clinical expression. HDV is defective in that it requires HBV as a helper virus for an outer protein coat (HBsAg) and thus for replication.

HDV infection is worldwide in distribution and occurs in two major epidemiologic patterns. Delta is endemic in Mediterranean countries such as southern Italy, the Middle East, and parts of Africa, as it is in parts of South America. Nonpercutaneous transmission of HBV and HDV is believed to occur primarily by intimate contact and transmucosal exchange of body fluids. In areas where HDV infection is nonendemic, including North America and Western Europe, HDV infection is confined to groups with frequent percutaneous exposures such as IV drug users and hemophiliacs. Preliminary studies in the United States have found HDV to be detectable in 24% of HBsAg positive drug users in the Los Angeles area and approximately 50% of HBsAg positive hemophiliacs. Studies indicate that about 4% of US volunteer blood donors who are asymptomatic hepatitis B carriers are positive for either HDAg or anti-HD. Homosexual men, despite their high rate HBV infection, have been relatively spared HDV infection, although cases have been noted.

Hepatitis relating to delta infection occurs in two primary modes. The first mode is *simultaneous* infection with HBV and HDV. When simultaneous infection occurs, the acute clinical course of hepatitis often is limited with resolution of both hepatitis B and delta infections, although fulminant hepatitis may develop. The second mode involves acute delta *superinfection* in HBsAg carriers. In this situation, the patient already has a high titer of circulating HBsAg. These patients are more likely to have a serious and possible acute fulminant form of hepatitis that more often leads to chronic delta infection. Some of these patients will become carriers of HDV as well as HBsAg.

HDV has been associated with several US hepatitis outbreaks. The largest outbreak, in Worcester, MA, included over 700 total cases with over 200 parenteral drug users from 1983 to 1988. Over 65 of these individuals were positive for prior infection with HDV. There were 14 deaths, 11 of whom were delta positive. Four dentists and one physician were infected through this outbreak. One dentist died of fulminant hepatitis in 1986. Another dentist became a hepatitis B carrier and infected at least four patients in his practice.

Another outbreak of delta hepatitis occurred in Durham, North Carolina. Fortunately, this outbreak was limited in size with only 86 cases of hepatitis, at least 15% of which had markers for delta virus infection.

As all dental staff members are at an increased risk of HBV infection and of possibly becoming hepatitis B carriers (unless immunized), members of the dental profession are at risk of simultaneous infection with HDV and HBV. Additionally, it has been estimated there are currently 3,000 hepatitis B carriers in the dental profession in the US. These individuals are also at risk of HDV superinfection. Parenteral drug users infected with HDV are receiving routine dental treatment as many of these individuals do not report their recreational drug habits to the dentist. Immunization to hepatitis B virus also confers protection against clinical exposure of a delta hepatitis infection.

SUMMARY

All forms of hepatitis are a serious threat to members of the dental team. Hepatitis B and delta infection represent the most life threatening of these diseases; however, PT-NANB has the highest carrier rate after infection. Dental personnel who are carriers of HBV, some of whom are unaware of their status, are most at risk for delta infection.

Unfortunately, individuals who are already anti-HIV positive do not respond as well to hepatitis B vaccine and have a higher prevalence of chronic hepatitis and the carrier state. Thus, it behooves society to immunize adolescents against HBV before they start practicing high risk behaviors that could expose them to HIV infection and other infectious diseases. This is only one reason why the CDC is considering broadening recommendations for HB vaccine use to include junior high school students or a universal infant immunization program. The question is being asked, "Should hepatitis B vaccine be given to all US children?"

The problem of nonresponders and hyporesponders to immunization may be answered with new hepatitis B vaccines under development that may contain the preS2 section of the HBsAg in addition to the antigen in current vaccines. This may assist dialysis, anti-HIV positive patients, older adults, organ recipients, oncology patients, alcoholics, and possibly even chronic carriers. Only time and research will elucidate the answers.

Meanwhile, it behooves the dentist and staff to take all precautions to avoid these preventable infections by use of the hepatitis B vaccine, especially in light of the recent OSHA instruction mandating that employers provide HB vaccine free of charge to at risk employees, and by adopting appropriate infection control procedures for every patient.

SELECTED READINGS

Ahtone, J., and Goodman, R.A.: Hepatitis B and dental personnel: Transmission to patients and prevention issues. J. Am. Dent. Assoc., 106:219–222, 1983.

Ahtone, J.L., et al.: Hepatitis B association with an oral surgeon in Atlanta. In Program and Abstracts: 109th Annual Meeting of the American Public Health Association, Washington, D.C., 1981.

Andre, F.E.: Clinical experience with a recombinant DNA hepatitis B vaccine. Southeast Asian J. Trop. Med. Public Health, 19:501, 1988.

Andre, F.E.: Summary of safety and efficacy data on a yeast-derived hepatitis B vaccine. Am. J. Med., 87 (Suppl 3A): 3A–14S, 1989.

Centers for Disease Control (ACIP): Protection against viral hepatitis. MMWR, *39*(RR-2):1–26, 1990.

Centers for Disease Control (ACIP): Prevention of perinatal transmission of hepatitis B virus: Prenatal screening of all pregnant women for hepatitis B surface antigen. MMWR, *37*:341, 1988.

Centers for Disease Control (ACIP): Postexposure prophylaxis of hepatitis B. MMWR, *33*:285–290, 1984.

Centers for Disease Control (ACIP): Recommendations for protection against viral hepatitis. MMWR, *34*:313–335, 1985.

Centers for Disease Control (ACIP): Update of hepatitis B prevention. MMWR, *36*:353–366, 1987.

Centers for Disease Control: Hepatitis B vaccine: Evidence confirming lack of AIDS transmission. MMWR, *33*:685–686, 1984.

Centers for Disease Control: Outbreak of hepatitis B associated with an oral surgeon—New Hampshire. MMWR, *36*:132–133, 1987.

Choo, Q.L., et al.: Isolation of a cDNA clone derived from a blood-borne non-A, non-B viral hepatitis genome. Science, *244*:359–362, 1989.

Cottone, J.A., et al.: Manual: Clinical Management of Medically Compromised Patients at The University of Texas Dental School at San Antonio. 1989.

Cottone, J.A., and Goebel, W.N.: Hepatitis B: The clinical detection of the chronic carrier dental patient and the effects of immunization via vaccine. Oral Surg., *56*:449–454, 1983.

Cottone, J.A., and Mitchell, E.W.: Proceedings of the National Symposium on Hepatitis B and the Dental Profession: A practical guide to personal, legal and clinical issues. J. Am. Dent. Assoc., *110*:613–650, 1985.

Cottone, J.A.: Delta hepatitis: Another concern for dentistry. J. Am. Dent. Assoc., *112*:47–49, 1986.

Cottone, J.A.: Hepatitis B virus infection in the dental profession. J. Am. Dent. Assoc., *110*:617–621, 1985.

Dienstag, J.L., and Ryan, D.M.: Occupational exposure to hepatitis B virus in hospital personnel: Infection or immunization? Am. J. Epidemiol., *115*:26–39, 1982.

Feldman, R.E., and Schiff, E.R.: Hepatitis in dental professionals. JAMA., *232*:1228–1230, 1975.

Foti, S.: Death shows need for infection control. AGD Impact, *17*:12, 1989.

Francis, D.P., et al.: The safety of the hepatitis B vaccine. JAMA., *256*:869–872, 1986.

Gerety, R.J., et al.: Two superb vaccines against hepatitis B in Mexican standoff. JAMA., *259*:2403–2404, 1988.

Goebel, W.M.: Reliability of the medical history in identifying patients likely to place dentists at an increased hepatitis risk. J. Am. Dent. Assoc., *98*:907–913, 1979.

Goldstein, J., Morse, K., and Gullen, W.: Epidemiology of hepatitis B among endodontists. J. Endodont., *4*:336–339, 1978.

Goodwin, D., Fannin, S.L., and McCracken, B.B.: An oral surgeon related hepatitis B outbreak. Calif. Morbid., No. 14, April 16, 1976.

Hadler, S.C., et al.: An outbreak of hepatitis B in a dental practice. Am. Int. Med., *95*:133–138, 1981.

Hadler, S.C., et al.: Long-term immunogenicity and efficacy of hepatitis B vaccine in homosexual men. N. Engl. J. Med., *315*:209–214, 1986.

Hollinger, F.B.: Hepatitis B vaccines—to switch or not to switch. JAMA., *257*:2634–2636, 1987.

Hollinger, F.B., Grander, J.W., Nickel, F.R., and Suarez, M.: Hepatitis B prevalence within a dental student population. J. Am. Dent. Assoc., *94*:521–527, 1977.

Hoofnogle, J.H.: Type D (delta) hepatitis. JAMA., *261*:1321, 1989.

Irwin, G.R.: Passive immunization against exposure to hepatitis B virus in the military: potential and possibilities. Yale J. Biol. Med., *49*:251–257, 1976.

James, J.J., and Smith, L.: Serological markers for hepatitis type A & B among United States Army soldiers, Germany. Am. J. Public Health, *69*:1216–1219, 1979.

Kuo, G., et al.: An assay for circulating antibodies to a major etiologic virus of human non-A non-B hepatitis. Science, *244*:362, 1989.

Lettau, L.A., et al.: Transmission of hepatitis B with restriction of surgical practice. JAMA., *255*:934–937, 1986.

Levin, M.L., Maddrey, W.C., Wands, J.R., and Mendeloff, A.L.: Hepatitis B transmission by dentists. JAMA., *228*:1139–1140, 1974.

Maynard, J.E.: American Hospital Association Videoteleconference: Developing an immunization program for hepatitis B virus. Presented on Cable Health Network on October 27, 1982.

Merck Sharp and Dohme, Recombivax HB Prescribing Information, 1989.

Mosley, J.W., and White, E.: Viral hepatitis as an occupational hazard of dentists. J. Am. Dent. Assoc., *90*:992–997, 1975.

Mosley, J.W., et al.: Hepatitis B virus infection in dentists. N. Engl. J. Med., *293*:729–734, 1975.

Reingold, A.L., et al.: Transmission of hepatitis B by an oral surgeon. J. Infect. Dis., *145*:262–263, 1982.

Rimland, D., Parkin, W.E., Miller, G.B., and Schrank, W.D.: Hepatitis B outbreak traced to an oral surgeon. N. Engl. J. Med., *296*:953–958, 1977.

Schiff, E.R., et al.: Veterans Administration cooperative study on hepatitis and dentistry. JADA, *113*:390–396, 1986.

Scott, R. McN., Schneider, R.J., Snitbhan, R., and Karwachi, J.J., Jr.: Factors relating to transmission of viral hepatitis in a United States military population stationed in Thailand. Am. J. Epidemiol., *113*:520–528, 1981.

Shaw, F.E., et al.: Lethal outbreak of hepatitis B in a dental practice. JAMA., *255*:3260-4, 1986.

Siew, C., Gruniner, S.E., Mitchell, E.W., and Burrell, K.H.: Survey of hepatitis B exposure and vaccination in volunteer dentists. JADA, *114*:457, 1987.

Siew, C., Grunenger, S.E., Chang, S.B., and Verrusio, G.C.: Risk of HIV and HBV and dental professionals. J. Dent. Res., *68*:415 (abstract 1868), 1989.

Smith, J.L., et al.: Comparative risk of hepatitis B among physicians and dentists. J. Infect. Dis., *133*:705–706, 1976.

Szmuness, W., et al.: A controlled clinic trial of the efficacy of the hepatitis B vaccine: A final report. Hepatology, *1*:377–385, 1981.

Tullman, M.J., et al.: Prevalence of hepatitis B surface antigen in a dental school patient population. J. Public Health Dent., *38*:4–9, 1978.

Watkins, B.J.: Viral hepatitis B: A special problem in prevention. J. Am. Soc. Prevent. Dent., *6*:9–13, 1976.

Weil, R.B., Lyman, D.O., Jackson, R.J., and Bernstein, B.: A hepatitis serosurvey of New York dentists. NY State Dent. J., *43*:587–590, 1977.

West, D.J.: Clinical experience with hepatitis B vaccines. Am. J. Infect. Control., *17*:172–180, 1989.

Williams, S.V., Pattison, C.P., and Berquist, K.R.: Dental infections with hepatitis B. JAMA, *232*:1231–1233, 1975.

Zajac, B.A., West, D., and Meibohm, A.: Improvements in the immunogenicity and purity of a genetically engineered hepatitis B vaccine. Hepatology, *8*:1322, 1988.

Zajac, B.A., et al.: Overview of clinical studies with hepatitis B vaccine made by recombinant DNA. J. Infect., *13*(Suppl. A):39–45, 1986.

Chapter 3

HIV Infection and AIDS

In June, 1981, the Centers for Disease Control (CDC) first published reports of the unusual occurrence of five cases of *Pneumocystis carinii* pneumonia among previously healthy male homosexuals in Los Angeles. Shortly thereafter came equally surprising reports of an aggressive form of Kaposi's sarcoma occurring among young gay men in New York and California. Additional cases were identified retrospectively, as far back as 1978. Until then, pneumocystis had been observed only in severely immunocompromised patients, and Kaposi's sarcoma had been known in the United States as a rare type of skin cancer seen primarily in elderly men. Those early reports were the first glimpses of what has become known as acquired immunodeficiency syndrome (AIDS), an epidemic that has already claimed more lives in the United States than the total number of US soldiers who died during the Vietnam War. HIV infection and AIDS continues to pose a medical and social challenge unique in recent history.

AIDS has now been linked to a wide range of pernicious opportunistic infections and unusual neoplasms. No effective therapy is presently available for the underlying disease although some of the acute infections and other complications can be treated. At present, knowledge and education offer the best defense against AIDS.

The epidemic of HIV infection and AIDS has also become an epidemic of fear. Not since the polio epidemic in the 1950s has the public reacted so emotionally to a medical situation. The public's concern has intensified as each new observation has been announced. What is known about the disease process and the dental implications of HIV infection and AIDS are reviewed here.

ETIOLOGIC FACTORS

AIDS is the last stage of a complex infectious process initiated by an agent presently termed the Human Immunodeficiency Virus (HIV) (Fig. 3–1). This virus has had a variety of former names including human T-cell lymphotrophic virus type III (HTLV III), lymphadenopathy-associated virus (LAV), and AIDS-related virus (ARV).

CDC DEFINITIONS

Initially, the CDC epidemiologically defined AIDS as "the presence of a reliably diagnosed disease at least moderately predictive of an underlying cellular immunodeficiency . . . in a previously healthy patient." Thus, *Pneumocystis carinii* pneu-

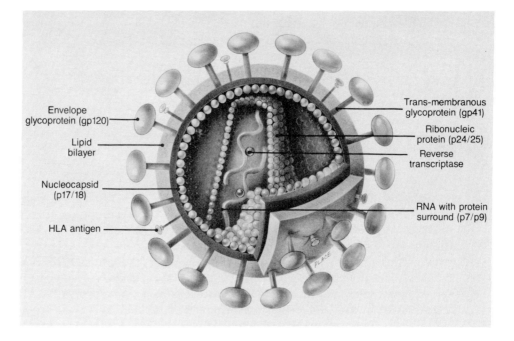

Fig. 3–1. Artist's rendition of the human immunodeficiency virus.

monia, Kaposi's sarcoma in a patient younger than 60 years old, or an opportunistic infection in the absence of any known cause of immunodeficiency met the definition.

The definition of AIDS was revised in 1985 and again in 1987 to include additional diseases in persons with laboratory evidence of HIV infection. These diseases included disseminated histoplasmosis, chronic isosporiasis, and certain non-Hodgkin's lymphomas (1985 revision), and extrapulmonary tuberculosis, HIV encephalopathy, HIV wasting syndrome, and presumptively diagnosed indicator diseases (1987 revision).

The definition of AIDS-Related-Complex (ARC) for adults applies to patients who have at least two depressed laboratory signs as well as at least two clinical signs (Table 3–1).

SEROLOGIC TESTING

Since early 1985, several serologic tests have been available to detect HIV antibody and have formed the basis of a nationwide program for screening all donated blood products for evidence of HIV infection.

The most commonly available is the enzyme-linked immunosorbent assay (ELISA) technique, which gives a spectrophotometric reading of the amount of antibody binding to HIV antigens. The different ELISA kits have been estimated to have a sensitivity of 93.4 to 99.6%, and a specificity of 99.2 to 99.8%. Sensitivity is defined as the ratio of true-positives/true-positives + false-negatives, and specificity as true-negatives/true-negatives + false-positives. Although considered highly sensitive and specific, ELISA tests underscore the imperfection of all diagnostic testing: any test that is less than 100% sensitive and specific (virtually all

Table 3–1. AIDS Related Complex (ARC)

Indicated by two signs in each of the following two areas:

Laboratory Signs
—Decreased T helper cells
—Decreased T helper/T suppressor ratio (T4/T8)
—Leukopenia
—Thrombocytopenia
—Anemia

Clinical Signs
—Lymphadenopathy Syndrome (LAS): Lymphadenopathy in two or more
    extrainguinal areas that persists for at least 3 months
—Fever
—Weight loss
—Unexplained diarrhea
—Fatigue
—Night sweats
—Hairy leukoplakia
—Unexplained oral candidiasis

tests) will necessarily generate both false-negatives and false-positives. This is an especially important consideration in the context of HIV, where extensive debate has already taken place on the issue of stigmatization and "labeling" of asymptomatic individuals with positive tests.

The Western blot test is generally considered to be more specific than the ELISA and is used as a confirmatory test. The Western blot technique uses an electrophoretic process to separate viral antigens and measure reaction of serum antibodies with specific viral protein bands.

Since March, 1985, blood banks across the country have been testing donated specimens for HIV antibody. The prevalence of positive Western blot tests among units screened by the American Red Cross in early 1985 suggested that 0.04% of all donated units may have been potentially infectious. This prevalence declined to 0.02% in early 1986 and to 0.01% in the second quarter of 1988. These rates may be artificially low because of the high self-selection of voluntary blood donors and the permanent referral system in place by the American Red Cross. Donors tested for the first time probably provide the best estimate of HIV seroprevalence in the segment of the population from which donors are drawn. The overall seroprevalence among persons donating for the first time in 1985 to 1988 was 0.042%.

Public health and medical authorities have been pleased with the results of the blood screening program and have made efforts to reassure the public that the blood supply is safe. That reassurance is justified, though with a caution: as noted, any test that is less than 100% sensitive will generate a finite number of false-negatives (an important potential consideration as more than 10 million units of blood and plasma are donated in the United States each year). In addition, several case reports have described viremic yet seronegative persons persistently infected with HIV. Screening of blood products must be accompanied by continued efforts to discourage members of risk groups from donating blood.

In early 1990, it was estimated that about 1 million persons living in the US and up to 6 million worldwide were HIV antibody positive. It is expected that as many as 480,000 persons with AIDS will have been diagnosed in the US by the end of 1993, with up to 340,000 deaths.

TRANSMISSION

HIV has been isolated from human blood, semen, breast milk, vaginal secretions, saliva, tears, urine, cerebrospinal fluid, and amniotic fluid; however, epidemiologic evidence implicates only blood, semen, vaginal secretions, and breast milk in the transmission of the virus. Preliminary studies have demonstrated that there is an unidentified factor in human saliva that appears to inactivate HIV.

Documented modes of HIV transmission include:

1. Engaging in sexual intercourse with an HIV-infected person
2. Using needles contaminated with the virus
3. Having parenteral, mucous membrane or nonintact skin contact with HIV-infected blood, blood components or blood products
4. Receiving transplants of HIV-infected organs and tissues, including bone, or transfusions of HIV-infected blood
5. Perinatal transmission from mother to child around the time of birth

HIV is *not* transmitted by casual contact. Studies evaluating nearly 500 household contacts of individuals diagnosed with AIDS reveal no cases of HIV infection of household members who had no other risk factors for the virus (including no sexual contact with or exposure to blood from the infected person). Household members were examined who lived with a person with AIDS for at least 3 months and within an 18-month period prior to the onset of symptoms in the infected person (during which time infection was presumably present). Other household members had been unaware of the infected individual's HIV status, and had not taken precautions during this time period. This study produced no evidence that HIV was transmitted by shaking hands or talking, by sharing food, eating utensils, plates, drinking glasses or towels, by sharing the same house or household facilities or by "personal interactions expected of family members" including hugging and kissing on the cheek or lips. Other studies have shown that HIV is not transmitted by mosquitoes or other animals.

Although the efficiency for most routes of HIV transmission is unknown, some routes of transmission are clearly more efficient than others. The risk of infection from receipt of transfused blood from an HIV-infected donor is approximately 90%. The risk of perinatal transmission from an HIV-infected mother is estimated to be 30 to 50%. Besides the particular route of transmission, other variables contributing to transmissibility may include susceptibility of the host, the virulence of the particular "HIV isolate" or strain, the stage of infection of the source, and the dose of virus and the size of inoculum transmitted. This last factor, the actual amount of virus, may be important in the likelihood of transmission because it appears that there is a greater probability of infection from HIV contaminated blood transfusions (890 infections per 1,000 persons transfused with contaminated blood) than there is from accidental needlesticks with needles that have been contaminated with HIV (3 to 5 infections per 1,000 persons injured with contaminated needles).

EPIDEMIOLOGY

General

The epidemiology of AIDS depends on the CDC definition and vice versa. Cases that do not meet the CDC definition are not included in the statistics. This

Table 3–2. HIV Risk Behaviors/Groups

1. Multiple sex partners: Heterosexual, homosexual, or bisexual
2. Intravenous drug use
3. Hemophiliac treatment
4. Blood transfusion before Spring, 1985
5. Steady sexual partners of persons described in 1 through 4
6. Infants born to members or sexual contacts of persons described in 1 through 5

has led to an underreporting of the disease, estimated to have been as high as 20 to 35% in some groups, particularly married bisexual males. The 1987 revision of the AIDS definition has done much to correct some of this underreporting.

Several groups were originally identified to be at high risk of acquiring AIDS. It is currently thought that risk *behaviors* versus risk *groups* are most important to emphasize. Risk behaviors/groups of concern in the US are listed in Table 3–2. Blacks and Hispanics account for an abnormally large number of persons with AIDS (PWAs). One of 8 Americans in the US is Black yet 1 of 4 PWAs is Black. Similarly, 1 of 12 Americans in the US is Hispanic and 1 of 7 PWAs is Hispanic.

Worldwide epidemiologic studies indicate three broad yet distinct geographic patterns of transmission (Fig. 3–2). Pattern I is typical of industrialized countries with large numbers of reported AIDS cases, such as North America, Western Europe, Australia, New Zealand, and parts of Latin America. In these areas, most cases occur among homosexual or bisexual males and urban intravenous drug users (IVDU). Heterosexual transmission is responsible for only a small percentage of cases, but is increasing. Transmission resulting from exposure to blood and blood products occurred between the late 1970s and 1985 in these countries but has now been largely controlled through the self-deferral of persons at increased risk for AIDS and by routine blood screening for HIV antibody. The ratio of male to female patients ranges from 10:1 to 15:1, and perinatal transmission is relatively uncommon but increasing. Overall population seroprevalence is estimated to be less than 1% but has been measured over 50% in some groups practicing high-risk behaviors, such as IV drug users and men with multiple male sex partners.

Pattern II is observed in areas of central, eastern, and southern Africa, and in some Caribbean countries. In these areas most cases occur among heterosexuals; the male to female ratio is approximately 1:1; and perinatal transmission is relatively more common than in other areas. IV drug use and homosexual transmission either do not occur or occur at a low level. In a number of these countries, overall population seroprevalence is estimated at more than 1% and in a few urban areas up to 25% of the sexually active age group is infected. Transmission through contaminated blood and blood products has been a significant problem and continues in those countries that have not yet implemented nationwide donor screening.

Pattern III is found in areas of Eastern Europe, the Middle East, Asia, and most of the Pacific. HIV appears to have been introduced into these areas in the early to mid 1980s, and only small numbers of cases have been reported. Homosexual and heterosexual transmission have only recently been documented. Generally, cases have occurred among persons who have traveled to endemic areas or who have had sexual contact with individuals from endemic areas, such as ho-

Geographic Pattern	Groups Primarily Affected	Other Groups	Blood Products	Gender Ratio (Male:Female)	Perinatal Transmission	Population Seropositivity
I. Industrial nations, North America, Western Europe, Australia, New Zealand, some Latin American countries	Homosexual and bisexual males, urban intravenous drug users	Heterosexual (small number of cases but included)	Late 1970s to 1985	10–15:1	Relative to groups	Below 1% up to 50% in some groups
II. Africa (central, eastern, south), some Caribbean countries	Mainly heterosexual	Homosexual and bisexual, a relatively small number of cases among intravenous drug users	Significant problem	1:1	Relatively common	Above 1% up to 25% in some urban areas
III. Eastern Europe, Middle East, Asia, and Pacific countries	HIV introduced in the early 1980s, a small number of cases reported. Sexual transmission only recently documented	—	Small number of cases resulting from imported blood	—	—	Cases among travelers and sexual contacts

Fig. 3–2. AIDS patterns of transmission. (From MMWR, 37:286, 1988.)

mosexual men and female prostitutes. A small number of cases caused by imported blood products have been reported.

Figures 3–3A and B give the reported global AIDS cases to the World Health Organization as of June 1, 1989. Figure 3–4 demonstrates the number of projected global AIDS cases through 1991. Figure 3–5 presents the AIDS incidence rates in the US for 1989.

Homosexual and Bisexual Men

Numerous studies have examined risk factors for exposure and the natural history of HIV infection in homosexual/bisexual men, who account for about 56% of 1989 PWAs in the United States (excluding the 6% who are also IVDUs). This is a decrease from a high of 72% in 1985 because of changes in sexual behavior patterns in this population and the increasing role of IV drug use in the transmission of HIV. Various studies have consistently identified a high number of sexual partners and a high frequency of sexual behaviors involving trauma, especially to anal mucosa, as key risk factors with the common feature of parenteral or mucous membrane exposure to infected blood or semen. Certain early reports implicated the use of nitrite-containing sexual stimulants ("poppers") as an AIDS risk factor. Subsequent analyses have indicated that their use probably only reflects high levels of sexual activity.

The risk of developing diagnosed AIDS following HIV antibody seroconversion has been studied in many groups. The largest and most comprehensive cohort study to date has involved over 6,000 subjects in San Francisco. The group was assembled initially between 1978 and 1980 as part of a study of hepatitis B among gay men attending sexually transmitted disease clinics. In 1984, the San Francisco health department and the CDC began a joint follow-up study to monitor the cohort for signs of HIV infection and disease. A representative subset of men has been followed. After 9 years of follow-ups of seropositive individuals, 33% died from HIV infection, 41% demonstrated some signs and/or symptoms, and 26% remained asymptomatic. Most current studies reveal the median time to diagnosis of AIDS is 11 years following seroconversion in individuals without therapy intervention. Improvements in therapy options already are lengthening the median time of patient survival.

Intravenous Drug Use

IVDUs represent the next largest HIV infection risk group, accounting for 23% of 1989 cases (including the 6% of gay and bisexual drug abusers). They form an important bridge for the spread of HIV infection to other segments of the population through heterosexual and vertical transmission. The extent of drug use since 1978, needle-sharing frequency, and time spent in "shooting galleries" have all been linked to seropositivity in IVDUs. Needle sharing in "shooting galleries," where addicts go to share or rent injection paraphernalia, is a relatively new phenomenon. In this setting, the same needle will be used for up to 50 injections or until it is no longer usable. Local geography also seems to play a part in HIV risk among IVDUs as the metropolitan East coast cities report a higher seroprevalence in these individuals than do West coast cities. The daily pursuit and frequent use of drugs

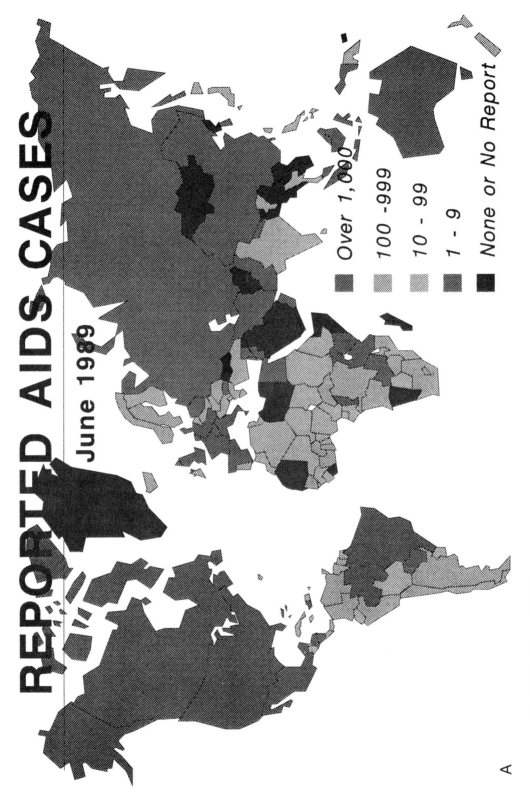

Fig. 3–3A. Reported AIDS cases: June 1, 1989. (From Mann, J.M.: Global AIDS into the 1990's. WHO, Montreal, June 4, 1989.)

Area	Cumulative number reported	Number of countries	Estimated
Africa	24,686	47	270,000
Americas	108,830	43	175,000
Asia	369	24	<1,000
Europe	21,855	28	32,000
Oceania	1,451	7	2,000
B **Total**	**157,191**	**149**	**480,000**

Fig. 3–3B. Reported and estimated global AIDS cases: June 1, 1989. (From Mann, J.M.: Global AIDS into the 1990's. WHO, Montreal, June 4, 1989.)

to avoid the symptoms of withdrawal can limit mobility of IVDUs in a way different from the lifestyle of gay and bisexual men.

It has been estimated that there are over 200,000 IVDUs in the New York metropolitan area alone and almost 1 million nationwide. The current reports of close to 60% seropositivity among IVDUs in New York, combined with even conservative estimates of projected AIDS incidence among seropositives, constitute a prediction of many thousands of new cases among this group over the coming years.

Hemophiliacs and Transfusion Recipients

The first report of AIDS in a hemophiliac (January 1982) strengthened the theory of a transmissible agent in the etiology of AIDS. Through their exposure to human plasma products, hemophiliacs had long been known to be at risk for the transmission of specific viral agents, e.g., HBV, *cytomegalovirus*, and the non-A non-B hepatitis viruses. Both heterosexual and vertical transmission in this group parallels that seen among IVDUs and their contacts. Hemophilia and coagulation disorders account for approximately 1% of the 1989 AIDS cases.

Approximately 2% of AIDS cases in the United States have been linked to the transmission of HIV through transfusion of contaminated blood and blood components (including red cells, platelets, plasma, whole blood, or tissue) in addition to the cases described among hemophiliacs. The 1983 Public Health Service recommendation that all members of AIDS risk groups refrain from donating blood

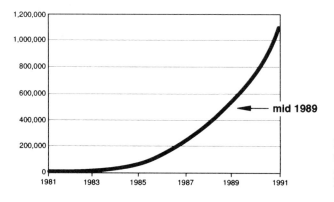

Fig. 3–4. Projected global AIDS cases. (From Mann, J.M.: Global AIDS into the 1990's. WHO, Montreal, June 4, 1989.)

Reported AIDS Patients - 1989

Per 100,000 Population (USA Mean = 14.0)

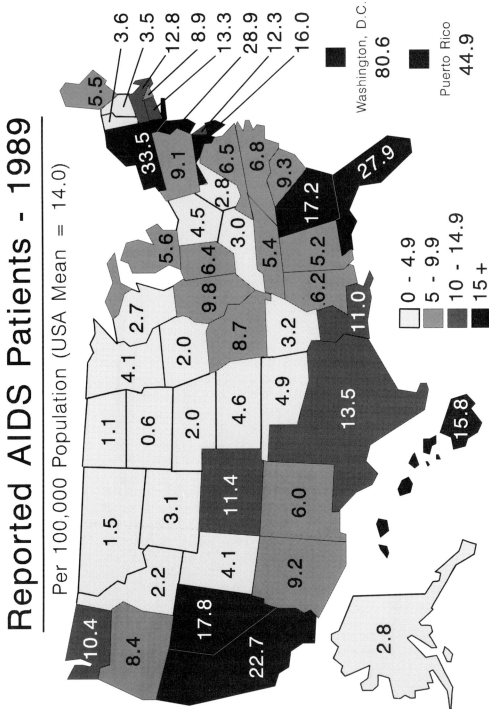

Washington, D.C.
80.6

Puerto Rico
44.9

0 - 4.9
5 - 9.9
10 - 14.9
15 +

Fig. 3–5. AIDS incidence rates per 100,000 population. (From MMWR, 39:81, 1990.)

or blood products and the testing of all donated blood in the United States for the presence of HIV antibodies since Spring, 1985 have contributed to the reduction of risk among hemophiliacs not yet exposed and transfusion recipients.

Heterosexual Cases

Heterosexual contact has been implicated in 4.5% of reported AIDS cases in the US. Cases are classified as heterosexual contacts if there are no known exposures other than heterosexual contact with someone at risk for HIV infection. The majority of these patients report sexual contacts with IV drug users. Among the adult patients born in the United States and having no known risk factors, a significant percentage of males have indicated histories of sexual contact with prostitutes.

Studies of heterosexual partners of patients with AIDS or risk-group members have suggested virus transmission rates as high as 58% as indicated by HIV seropositivity or clinical disease in their sexual partners. Limited studies among prostitutes in the United States have indicated high HIV seropositivity rates in certain regions of the country, often linked to a coexisting history of IV drug use or sexual contact with IVDUs.

Regardless of the actual efficiency of female-to-male versus male-to-female transfer, certain epidemiologic aspects of the pattern of HIV exposure in the United States may help explain the predominantly unidirectional spread. First, given the early rapid penetration of virus into the male homosexual and bisexual population, the reservoir of infected persons contains more males than females. That alone reduces the relative likelihood of female-to-male transmission on a simple probability basis. Second, the predominance of males among the estimated population of IVDUs (80% male to 20% female) enhances that effect. Adult female AIDS cases have increased from 7% before 1984 to 11% in 1989.

Pediatric Cases

The first cases suggestive of an AIDS-like illness in children were reported by the CDC in 1982. More than 82% of such cases have involved children with one or both parents at risk for AIDS; the great majority of those parents have been IV drug users. Because most pediatric cases result from perinatal transmission, the geographic, racial, and ethnic distribution parallels that seen in adult female patients with AIDS. Seventy-seven percent of pediatric patients have been black or Hispanic, and most have been reported from New York, New Jersey, Florida, and California.

Aside from major opportunistic infections, the clinical course of infants with AIDS or related conditions is marked by failure to thrive, persistent lymphadenopathy, chronic or recurrent oral candidiasis, persistent diarrhea, hepatosplenomegaly, and chronic interstitial pneumonitis on chest x-ray. Bacterial infections are common and occasionally severe and life threatening. Depressed cell-mediated immunity and T-cell function are frequently encountered. Chronic parotid swelling has also been reported. Serious central nervous system effects of HIV infection are also seen.

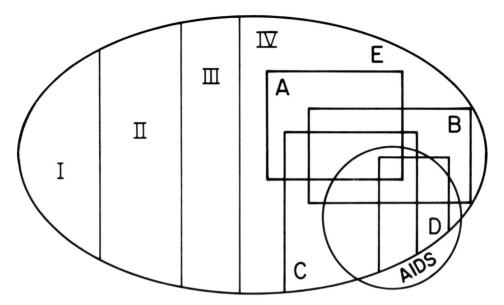

Fig. 3–6. Manifestations of HIV infection.

HIV TYPE-2

The first case of AIDS in a person from Africa, caused by another human retrovirus, human immunodeficiency virus type 2 (HIV-2), was diagnosed and reported in the United States in December, 1987. HIV-2 appears to be similar to HIV-1 in modes of transmission and natural history but has not yet been studied in as much detail. Although HIV-2 is unquestionably pathogenic, there is still much to be learned regarding its epidemiology, pathogenesis, and efficiency of transmission. Although only few cases of HIV-2 have been reported in the United States, the infection is endemic in West Africa where it was first linked with AIDS in 1986. There have also been cases of HIV-2 infection reported among West Africans living in Europe.

Serologic tests licensed for detecting HIV-1 can detect only a portion of HIV-2 infections, but HIV-2 surveillance is being conducted in the United States to monitor the frequency of occurrence using specific tests not yet available commercially.

HIV INFECTION

Until recently, all individuals with any form of HIV infection have been referred to as "having AIDS." A better understanding of the disease spectrum has allowed a fuller differentiation of the various stages of what is now termed "HIV infection" with AIDS representing only the most advanced manifestation of the disease (Figs. 3–6 and 3–7).

The full range of conditions associated with HIV infection is now appreciated to be far greater than when the first homosexual men with Kaposi's sarcoma were identified in 1981. In May 1986, the CDC issued a comprehensive classification system for categorizing patients infected with HIV according to certain clinical characteristics (Table 3–3). It includes the range of identified HIV-associated con-

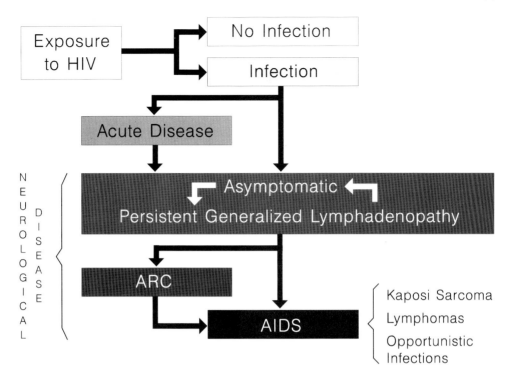

Fig. 3–7. Overview of possible outcomes after HIV exposure.

ditions, from asymptomatic infection to surveillance-definition AIDS, and it is intended to provide a unifying framework for ongoing study and clinical care of persons infected with the virus. There is also the Walter Reed System (Table 3–4) for adults and a CDC classification system for children infected with HIV (Table 3–5).

CDC Group I: Acute Infection

In an effort to describe the earliest stages of HIV exposure, investigators have identified several different syndromes associated with acute HIV infection. A mononucleosis-like illness and, less commonly, different acute neurologic syndromes have been described 3 to 6 weeks after presumed exposure. The acute syndrome is characterized by fever, lymphadenopathy, myalgias and arthralgias, diarrhea, fatigue, and transient macular erythematous rash. An inversion of the T4/T8 ratio is seen because of an increase in the number of T8 (suppressor) cells with relative preservation of T4 (helper) cells. Seroconversion occurs after the acute illness.

Clinical illness does not appear to be an inevitable consequence of acute HIV infection. Many patients who seroconvert report no associated symptoms. There have also been several case reports of patients who were consistently HIV seronegative and clinically in good health despite persistent HIV viremia documented by cultures.

Table 3-3. CDC Classification System for HIV Infection

Group I: Acute Infection
  Mononucleosis-like syndrome associated with seroconversion

Group II: Asymptomatic Infection
  Positive HIV antibody or viral culture. May be subclassified on the basis of laboratory evaluation
    (CBC, platelet count, T-cell subset studies)

Group III: Persistent Generalized Lymphadenopathy
  Palpable lymphadenopathy (>1 cm) at two or more extrainguinal sites for more than 3 months in the
    absence of a concurrent illness or infection to explain the findings. May be subclassified on the
    basis of laboratory evaluation (see above)

Group IV: Other HIV Disease
  Subgroup A: Constitutional Disease
    One or more of the following: Fever or diarrhea persisting more than 1 month or involuntary weight
      loss greater than 10% of baseline; and absence of a concurrent illness or infection to explain
      the findings

  Subgroup B: Neurologic Disease
    One or more of the following: Dementia, myelopathy, or peripheral neuropathy; and absence of a
      concurrent illness or condition

  Subgroup C: Secondary Infectious Diseases
    Infectious disease associated with HIV infection and/or at least moderately indicative of a defect in
      cell-mediated immunity

    Category C-1
      Symptomatic or invasive disease due to one of 12 specified diseases listed in the surveillance
        definition of AIDS:
      Pneumocystis carinii pneumonia
      Chronic cryptosporidiosis
      Toxoplasmosis
      Extraintestinal strongyloidiasis
      Isosporiasis
      Candidiasis (esophageal, bronchial, or pulmonary)
      Cryptococcosis
      Histoplasmosis
      Mycobacterial infection (*Mycobacterium avium* complex or *Mycobacterium kansasii*)
      Cytomegalovirus infection
      Chronic mucocutaneous or disseminated herpes simplex virus infection
      Progressive multifocal leukoencephalopathy

    Category C-2
      Symptomatic or invasive disease due to one of six other specified diseases:
      Oral hairy leukoplakia
      Multidermatomal herpes zoster
      Recurrent *Salmonella* bacteremia
      Nocardiosis
      Tuberculosis
      Oral candidiasis (thrush)

  Subgroup D: Secondary Cancers
    Diagnosis of one or more cancers known to be associated with HIV infection as listed in the sur-
      veillance definition of AIDS and at least moderately indicative of a defect in cell-mediated immu-
      nity: Kaposi's sarcoma, non-Hodgkin's lymphoma (small, noncleaved lymphoma or immunoblas-
      tic sarcoma), or primary lymphoma of the brain

  Subgroup E: Other Conditions in HIV Infection
    Clinical findings or diseases, not classifiable above, that may be attributable to HIV infection and
      are indicative of a defect in cell-mediated immunity; symptoms attributable to either HIV infec-
      tion or a coexisting disease not classified elsewhere; or clinical illnesses that may be compli-
      cated or altered by HIV infection. These include chronic lymphoid interstitial pneumonitis and
      constitutional symptoms, secondary infectious diseases, and neoplasms not listed above

From CDC: Classification system for human T-lymphotropic virus type III/lymphadenopathy-associated
virus infections. MMWR, *35*:334, 1986.

Table 3–4. Walter Reed Staging System

Stage	HIV Antibody and/or Virus Isolation	Chronic Lymphadenopathy	T Helper Cells/mm³	Hypersensitivity	Thrush	Delayed Opportunistic Infection
WR-0	−	−	>400	NL	−	−
WR-1	+	−	>400	NL	−	−
WR-2	+	+	>400	NL	−	−
WR-3	+	±	<400	NL	−	−
WR-4	+	±	<400	P	−	−
WR-5	+	±	<400	C and/or	+	−
WR-6	+	±	<400	P/C	±	+

NL = normal; P = partial cutaneous anergy (an intact response to only one of four test antigens: tetanus, Trichophyton, mumps, Candida); C = complete cutaneous anergy to the four test antigens
Adapted from Redfield, R.R., et al.: The Walter Reed staging classification for HTLV-III/LAV infection. N. Engl. J. Med., *314*:131, 1986.

CDC Group II: Asymptomatic Infection

A long period may then ensue during which the individual may have no physical manifestations of infection but will remain anti-HIV positive. Studies have shown that most, if not all, individuals will continue to be viremic and thus possible of transmitting infection to other individuals. Whether an individual progresses further than this stage may depend on the presence of infections, genetic predisposition, behavioral, or even environmental cofactors. Patients who are anti-HIV positive only have been observed to progress to a diagnosis of AIDS in a median time of 11 years without treatment in the San Francisco cohort studies. Over 20% of these individuals have remained completely asymptomatic in some studies. This is the group that will benefit most from advances in treatment research.

Table 3–5. Classification of HIV Infection in Children Under 13 Years of Age

Class P–0. Indeterminate infection

Class P–1. Asymptomatic infection
  Subclass A. Normal immune function
  Subclass B. Abnormal immune function
  Subclass C. Immune function not tested

Class P–2. Symptomatic infection
  Subclass A. Nonspecific findings
  Subclass B. Progressive neurologic disease
  Subclass C. Lymphoid interstitial pneumonitis
  Subclass D. Secondary infectious diseases
    Category D–1. Specified secondary infectious diseases listed in the CDC surveillance definition for AIDS
    Category D–2. Recurrent serious bacterial infections
    Category D–3. Other specified secondary infectious diseases
  Subclass E. Secondary cancers
    Category E–1. Specified secondary cancers listed in the CDC surveillance definition for AIDS
    Category E–2. Other cancers possibly secondary to HIV infection
  Subclass F. Other diseases possibly due to HIV infection

From CDC: Classification system for human immunodeficiency virus (HIV) infection in children under 13 years of age. MMWR, *36*:225–230, 1987.

CDC Group III: Persistent Generalized Lymphadenopathy (PGL)

PGL has been described in homosexual men since 1981. PGL is defined by the presence of lymph nodes more than 1 cm in diameter in two or more extrainguinal sites for more than 3 months in the absence of any illness or condition other than HIV infection to explain the findings.

Studies of the prognosis of patients with PGL in terms of the risk of AIDS have produced variable results. In some patients, PGL appears to have a chronic, indolent course, whereas in others it tends to accelerate rapidly along the spectrum of disease severity.

CDC Group IV: Other HIV Disease

Neurologic Manifestations. Soon after the identification and characterization of HIV in 1983 and 1984, it was discovered that the virus was not only lymphotropic but also neurotropic, with the repeated demonstration of direct viral infection of the central nervous system and other neural tissue. This complemented early observations of AIDS-related neurologic dysfunction and suggested that in some and perhaps most cases, neurologic symptoms might result from a direct effect of the virus and not to secondary opportunistic infections. Recent clinical and epidemiologic data indicates that the range of neurologic and neuropsychiatric illness related to HIV infection may be much broader than that seen in AIDS itself. It has been estimated that most patients with AIDS will manifest a characteristic dementia syndrome, which has been designated AIDS dementia complex (ADC); that many patients may present with neurologic symptoms before developing any other signs of HIV infection; and that perhaps an even larger number of infected individuals may show persistent evidence of neurologic impairment in the absence of an actual diagnosis of AIDS.

The AIDS dementia complex, which has also been characterized as subacute encephalitis or subcortical dementia, is often marked by initially subtle cognitive or behavioral changes occurring over weeks to months. Patients initially report memory loss, difficulty in concentrating, social withdrawal, and lethargy. Those early signs may often be attributed to depression and may be ignored until they eventually progress to more dramatic deficits involving severe dementia and psychomotor retardation. Motor disturbances initially include loss of coordination, tremors, and unsteady gait, and may lead to severe ataxia and paraplegia.

Opportunistic Infections. Pathogens associated with opportunistic infections commonly seen in the CDC classification system group IV C-I are listed in Table 3–6. These relatively nonvirulent organisms can cause severe and life-threatening infections in patients whose immune systems have been damaged by HIV. Commonly occurring organisms generally associated with only localized illness in immunocompetent hosts can be responsible for severe and persistent morbidity in patients with AIDS and AIDS-related conditions.

Pneumocystis Carinii Pneumonia. *P. carinii* pneumonia (PCP) is one of the most commonly diagnosed AIDS-related infections in the United States. The most common symptoms of PCP include fever, dyspnea, and dry cough, with less frequent complaints of chills, chest pain, and sputum production. Onset may be sudden or may involve gradual progression over weeks. Physical examination is often notable only for fever and tachypnea, with frequently normal auscultation

Table 3–6.   Common Opportunistic Infections in AIDS Clinical Syndromes

Organism	Syndrome
Protozoa	
Pneumocystis carinii	Pneumonia
Toxoplasma gondii	Encephalitis, brain abscess
Cryptosporidium muris	Gastroenteritis
Isospora belli	Gastroenteritis
Fungi	
Candida albicans	Oropharyngitis, esophagitis
Cryptococcus neoformans	Meningitis, pneumonia, fungemia
Viruses	
Cytomegalovirus	Chorioretinitis, pneumonia, hepatitis, colitis, adrenalitis disseminated infection
Herpes simplex	Mucocutaneous lesions, especially perianal
Varicella-zoster	Primary varicella infection, local or disseminated herpes zoster
Epstein-Barr	Oral hairy leukoplakia, lymphoid interstitial pneumonitis, B-cell lymphoma
Mycobacteria	
M. avium intracellulare	Gastroenteritis, disseminated infection (blood, liver, spleen, and marrow)

Adapted from Selwyn, P.A.: AIDS: What is now known. III. Clinical Aspects. Hosp. Pract., *21*:119–156, 1986.

of the lungs. Chest x-ray may show bilateral interstitial infiltrates but may often appear normal. Definitive diagnosis requires identification of characteristic pneumocysts with special stains of biopsy tissue obtained through fiberoptic bronchoscopy.

Fungi. *Oral candidiasis* is a common finding in HIV infection and AIDS. Its presentation is similar to that seen in other patients, with the addition of "punctate" lesions on the gingiva. Treatment with oral nystatin suspension, clotrimazole troches, or 0.12% chlorhexidine gluconate mouth rinses are generally effective. Recurrences are common and may ultimately require treatment with ketoconazole. In addition, the possible presence of other oral lesions that may resemble those of candidal infection makes diagnosis by gram stain of swabbed specimens especially important. Oral candidiasis is of additional prognostic significance; it is a frequent indicator of progressive disease among patients not yet diagnosed with AIDS.

Esophageal involvement does meet the criteria for the diagnosis of AIDS. Esophageal candidiasis may be accompanied by dysphagia, odynophagia (painful swallowing), or retrosternal pain and is usually but not always associated with oral lesions as well. Lesions may cause ulceration and bleeding, although disseminated infection is unusual. Endoscopy and biopsy are required for confirmation.

Viruses. *Herpes simplex virus* infections of the skin and mucous membranes occur commonly with HIV infection and, unlike the self-limited and well-circumscribed lesions seen in normal hosts, are often extensive and debilitating. Characteristically persistent and widespread perianal lesions have been seen in gay men, and extensive genital and oral lesions have been described in other risk groups as well. Diagnosis is made by culture of swabs from exudative lesions or tissue biopsy. Treatment for 7 days with oral or intravenous acyclovir may relieve symptoms and promote healing of lesions, although persistence of infection and relapse are common. Systemic administration of acyclovir has been associated with bone marrow suppression, elevated liver function tests, and adverse CNS effects.

Varicella-zoster virus infection may present as localized, or disseminated herpes zoster in patients with AIDS or HIV infection. Clinically, herpes zoster tends to be extremely painful, with severe ulcerations and scarring, but it is rarely widely disseminated. Treatment with acyclovir has been recommended, especially for disseminated infection. The occurrence of herpes zoster in patients at risk for AIDS may be an important marker of poor prognosis.

Epstein-Barr virus is associated with oral hairy leukoplakia, a lesion that appears as raised white areas of thickening on the lateral borders of the tongue and that increasingly has been described in patients with HIV infection. Hairy leukoplakia has been proposed as an additional marker for predicting AIDS in high-risk patients. Greenspan and co-workers reported that in a series of 143 seropositive gay men in San Francisco with hairy leukoplakia, there was a 48% predicted probability of AIDS developing by the 16th month of observation and 83% were diagnosed with AIDS in 31 months.

Nonopportunistic Organisms

There is increasing evidence that patients with AIDS and risk-group members may have an increased incidence of infection with organisms that cause disease in normal hosts. Tuberculosis, often extrapulmonary, and infection with classic pyogenic bacteria, have been consistently observed. The association between tuberculosis and AIDS appears to vary among risk groups and may represent the expression of latent infection in populations with different background exposure.

Neoplasms. Since 1981, Kaposi's sarcoma (KS) in the United States has been much more common in men with AIDS than in other risk groups. The occurrence of Kaposi's sarcoma in the absence of opportunistic infections has also been associated with a more favorable prognosis. Studies have documented a decline in the occurrence of Kaposi's sarcoma in AIDS in parallel with an increase in the occurrence of PCP.

Classically, Kaposi's sarcoma is characterized by slowly growing dark brown or purple-blue nodules and plaques found mostly on the lower legs. In AIDS, KS lesions are often multicentric, located not only on the legs but also on the trunk, arms, head, and neck, not infrequently involving the oral mucosa or the tip of the nose. The lesions may begin as pink, red, or violet macules, papules, or nodules and may often coalesce into large plaques. Involvement of internal organs is also common, particularly the lungs, gastrointestinal tract, and lymphatic system. Cases of fatal hemoptysis, intestinal bleeding, and obstruction have been reported.

ORGAN SYSTEMS IN HIV INFECTIONS

General

Clinicians must maintain a high index of suspicion of signs or symptoms affecting virtually every organ system. Many of the observed syndromes have been mentioned, although a number of other reported clinical findings will be discussed briefly.

Dermatologic

Dermatologic manifestations of AIDS are common and include not only such dramatic conditions as Kaposi's sarcoma and severe herpes zoster but also other skin lesions that may not be readily associated with HIV infection. Several of the reports describing acute HIV infection have noted that the mononucleosis-like syndrome is often accompanied by a transient maculopapular, erythematous rash, especially on the trunk. Patients with AIDS frequently complain of generalized pruritis (often with no identifiable cause); prurigo, xerosis (dry skin), and acquired ichthyosis have also been noted. Psoriasis and seborrheic dermatitis have been observed to occur with high frequency in patients with AIDS. Some investigators have postulated a possible autoimmune mechanism for the phenomenon. Of interest is the observation that patients with AIDS with severe psoriasis and seborrheic dermatitis may have spontaneous improvement in their skin lesions as their overall clinical course deteriorates and their immune systems fail.

Skin infections are also quite common in AIDS and include primary herpes simplex virus infection, varicella-zoster virus infection with herpes zoster, scabies, molluscum contageosum, miliaria, and fungal dermatoses (mucosal candidiasis, tinea pedis, and tinea faciei). The occurrence of some of these common skin conditions in a person at risk for HIV infection may be purely coincidental and of no prognostic or diagnostic importance; however, clinicians should be particularly suspicious when common skin infections present in unusual or especially severe forms.

Oral

As noted, the finding of oral candidiasis or oral hairy leukoplakia in a patient at risk for AIDS may be of great prognostic importance. The finding of intraoral Kaposi's sarcoma would establish the diagnosis of AIDS in homosexual males. Dentists are in a key position to detect many important manifestations of HIV infection merely by performing oral examinations. It has been estimated that 95% of patients with AIDS or AIDS-related conditions may have abnormal physical findings in the head and neck (including cervical lymphadenopathy and intraoral lesions), which can be easily identified through routine examination. Other oral findings include primary and recurrent herpes simplex virus infections and papillomas. Periodontal observations include HIV associated periodontitis (HIV-P) characterized by rapid loss of periodontal bone attachment and often requiring tooth extraction. HIV-P is often preceded by an HIV associated gingivitis (HIV-G). A complete list of over 30 oral lesions associated with HIV infection are listed in Table 3–7.

Gastrointestinal

Common gastrointestinal manifestations of AIDS include esophagitis, hepatitis, and gastroenteritis. Investigators have also described a chronic malabsorption syndrome in patients with AIDS characterized by weight loss, diarrhea, and steatorrhea, sometimes in the absence of specific bacterial or parasitic infection.

Table 3–7. Oral Lesions Associated with HIV Infection

Fungal infections	Neoplasms
Candidiasis	Kaposi's sarcoma
Pseudomembranous	Squamous cell carcinoma
Erythematous	Non-Hodgkin's lymphoma
Hyperplastic	Neurologic disturbances
Angular cheilitis	Trigeminal neuropathy
Histoplasmosis	Facial palsy
Cryptococcosis	Unknown etiology
Geotrichosis	Recurrent aphthous ulceration
Bacterial infections	Progressive necrotizing ulceration
HIV-necrotizing gingivitis	Toxic epidermolysis
HIV-gingivitis	Delayed wound healing
HIV-periodontitis	Idiopathic thrombocytopenia
Caused by:	Salivary gland enlargement
Mycobacterium avium intracellulare	Xerostomia
Klebsiella pneumoniae	Melanotic hyperpigmentation
Enterobacter cloacae	
Escherichia coli	
Actinomycosis	
Cat-scratch disease	
Sinusitis	
Exacerbation of apical periodontitis	
Submandibular cellulitis	
Viral infections	
Caused by:	
Herpes simplex virus	
Cytomegalovirus	
Epstein-Barr virus	
"Hairy" leukoplakia	
Varicella-zoster virus	
Herpes zoster	
Varicella	
Human papillomavirus	
Verruca vulgaris	
Condyloma acuminatum	
Focal epithelial hyperplasia	

As agreed at an EEC-sponsored meeting in Copenhagen, September 16–17, 1986, on "Oral problems related to the HIV infection"; revised edition as of October 1, 1988, by J.J. Pindborg.

Adapted from Pindborg, J.J., et al.: Classification of oral lesions associated with HIV infection. Oral Surg., 67:292, 1989.

Ophthalmologic

Complications of AIDS most often involve the effects of opportunistic infections on the retina and orbit. CMV chorioretinitis has been observed frequently in patients with AIDS, often presenting as blurred vision or loss of vision in one or both eyes. Kaposi sarcoma of the eyelid and conjunctiva is also common.

Neurologic

Neurologic assessment of PWAs is also critical, because neurologic complications may be widely distributed throughout the central and peripheral nervous system. They may include conditions ranging from isolated peripheral neuropathy to diffuse encephalitis; clinical presentations may vary from mild paresthesias and weakness to paraplegia, and mental status changes may range from subtle cognitive and behavioral deficits to severe obtundation and dementia. AIDS-related neuro-

Table 3–8. Patient Management by T-Cell Profile

| CD4# | T-Cell Profile | | Frequency of T-Cell Studies |
	CD4%	Ratio	
>400	>30%	>1.0	Annually
>400	20–30%	0.4–1.0	6 months
<400	≤20%	≤0.4	3 months
<200	≤14%	≤0.3	Expect signs and symptoms, monitor frequently

Adapted from DiGioia, R.: Physician's Notebook. AIDS/HIV Exp. Tmt. Dir., 3:31, 1989.

logic syndromes include a combination of direct HIV-associated changes and pathology resulting from opportunistic infections and neoplasms.

Hematologic

Hematologic abnormalities are central to AIDS and HIV infection, in part related to the specific effects of viral infection of the target T4 lymphocyte. Initial infection may be associated with atypical lymphocytosis or a transient increase in the number of T8 cells, with a consequent lowering of the T4/T8 ratio (an effect seen in other viral infections); the further development of immunosuppression depends on the subsequent depletion and deregulation of the T4 subset. As noted, the total number of T4 cells may be an important marker for disease progression. On routine hematologic screening, lymphopenia and neutropenia are common in patients with clinical AIDS but are generally not seen in the early stages of infection. Similarly, anemia is often seen in advanced disease but is rarely present in asymptomatic infection. A normal complete blood count may be somewhat reassuring in patients at risk for AIDS, although T-cell-subset studies and especially T4-cell enumeration may be more sensitive prognostic markers (Table 3–8).

RISK OF OCCUPATIONAL HIV TRANSMISSION TO HEALTH CARE WORKERS

Available evidence indicates a low occupational risk for HIV infection among health care workers. The cases of AIDS among health care workers in the United States have usually been classified into known transmission categories. Information on the risk of occupational infection with HIV after exposure to HIV-infected blood or body fluids has been obtained from two sources. These sources include ongoing prospective studies of health care workers after such exposures and cases reported in the medical literature.

More than 1,400 health care workers have been enrolled and most tested for antibody to HIV in CDC's ongoing study of health care workers with parenteral, mucous membrane, or nonintact skin exposures to blood and other body fluids from HIV-infected patients. Of the more than 1,000 health care workers in this study who sustained parenteral (primarily deep needlesticks) exposures to blood and for whom both acute and convalescent phase serum samples had been obtained, four showed seroconversion to HIV within 6 months of exposure.

Two other ongoing prospective surveillance studies have assessed the risk of HIV infection among health care workers in the United States. The National Institutes of Health has tested more than 100 health care workers with documented needlestick injuries and 691 health care workers with more than 2,000 cutaneous or mucous membrane exposures to blood or other body fluids of HIV-infected patients; none showed seroconversion.

A similar study at the University of California of 235 health care workers with 644 documented needlestick injuries or mucous membrane exposures identified one seroconversion after needlestick. In addition, similar prospective studies in the United Kingdom and Canada show no evidence of HIV transmission among 220 health care workers with parenteral, mucous membrane, or cutaneous exposures to HIV-infected blood or other body fluids.

The risk of transmission of the virus by saliva, as well as blood, is addressed by epidemiologic studies of dental professionals. Studies of more than 4,000 dental workers, many of whom cared for patients with AIDS or persons at increased risk for HIV infection, have shown only two dentists, without other risk factors for HIV infection, had antibodies to HIV. These studies demonstrate that in spite of infrequent use of recommended barrier techniques during most of the history of the AIDS epidemic and occupational exposure to the saliva and blood of persons at risk for HIV infection or persons who are HIV-positive, dental professionals are occupationally at very low-risk for HIV infection.

In addition to health care workers enrolled in studies, there have been about ten case reports of health care workers who despite denial of other risk factors for HIV infection, reportedly have shown seroconversion to HIV after parenteral, nonintact skin, or mucous membrane exposure to HIV-infected blood or concentrated virus in a health care or laboratory setting. Approximately six additional health care workers with no other identified risk were reported to have acquired HIV infection, but the date of seroconversion is unknown.

These data indicate that the risk of occupational transmission of HIV is very low and most often associated with percutaneous inoculation of blood from a patient with HIV infection. The prospective surveillance studies indicate that the risk of seroconversion after needlestick exposure to blood from a patient infected with HIV is less than 1.0%. The protocol to follow after an accidental needlestick is provided in Appendix D. Nonetheless, the individual case reports must be interpreted with caution because they provide no data of the frequency of occupational exposures or the proportion of exposures resulting in HIV infection. However, the level of risk associated with exposure of nonintact skin or mucous membranes is likely far less than that associated with needlestick exposures.

SUMMARY

The preceding discussion has attempted to highlight some of the varied clinical manifestations of HIV infection and AIDS. The wide range of opportunistic infections and neoplasms and the reported involvement of virtually every organ system underscore the necessity for careful clinical assessment of all patients at risk. The identification of certain prognostic markers for disease progression allows clinicians to counsel patients with HIV infection regarding their risk of developing diagnosed AIDS.

Despite the lack of available therapy for HIV infection itself, the possibility of treatment for certain related syndromes makes accurate diagnosis especially important. With the elucidation of several early intraoral manifestations, the role of

Table 3–9. Stages of AIDS Awareness

1. Avoidance
2. Demand risk-free environment
3. Recognition that AIDS "is" and that everyone is "living with AIDS"
4. Interest in self-education
5. Concern for the "person with AIDS" (PWA)

Adapted from Wofsy, C.B.: Prevention of HIV transmission. Infect. Dis. Clin. North Am., 2:308, 1988.

the dentist and the dental staff is becoming even more important in early detection of HIV infection.

The dental profession is progressing through the various stages of AIDS awareness (Table 3–9). Regrettably, some still deny the fact that anti-HIV positive patients are being treated in their dental offices unknown to them. Some are still trying to create the nonexistent "risk-free" environment or worse yet, create "separate but equal" facilities. Fortunately, most of the profession recognizes that they are living with HIV infection and AIDS in their patient population and are in the process of self-education; some of which is being forced by regulatory agencies.

Ultimately, the *emotional* challenge of the dental profession is HIV infection and AIDS; but, the *scientific* challenge is universal infection control procedures against infectious diseases using viral hepatitis as *the* target disease.

SELECTED READINGS

Abstracts of the Second International Conference on AIDS (1986). Voyages Conseil, 50 rue Sabert, Paris 75007, France.

Abstracts of the Third International Conference on AIDS (1987). Washington, DC.

Abstracts of the Fourth International Conference on AIDS (1988). Stockholm.

Abstracts of the Fifth International Conference on AIDS (1989). Montreal.

Ammann, A.J.: The acquired immunodeficiency syndrome in infants and children. Ann. Intern. Med., 103:734, 1985.

Baltimore, D., and Feinberg, M.B.: HIV revealed. Toward a natural history of the infection. N. Engl. J. Med., 321:1673–1675, 1989.

Brunet, J.B., and Ancelle, R.A.: The international occurrence of the acquired immunodeficiency syndrome. Ann. Intern Med., 103:670, 1985.

Centers for Disease Control: Estimates of HIV prevalence and projected AIDS cases: Summary of a workshop, October 31–November 1, 1989. MMWR, 39:110–119, 1990.

Centers for Disease Control: AIDS and HIV infection in the US: 1988 Update. MMWR., 38:1–38, 1989.

Centers for Disease Control: Guidelines for prevention of transmission of HIV and HBV to health-care and public-safety workers. MMWR, 38:1–37, 1989.

Centers for Disease Control: Heterosexual transmission of human T-lymphotropic virus type III/lymphadenopathy-associated virus. MMWR, 34:561, 1985.

Centers for Disease Control: Recommendations for the prevention of HIV transmission in health care settings. MMWR, 36:3S–18S, 1987.

Centers for Disease Control: Update: AIDS-Worldwide. MMWR, 37:286, 1988.

Centers for Disease Control: Update: Heterosexual transmission of AIDS and HIV infection—US. MMWR, 38:423, 1989.

Centers for Disease Control: Public Health Service statement on management of occupational exposure to human immunodeficiency virus, including considerations regarding zidovudine postexposure use. MMWR, 39(RR-1):1–14, 1990.

Cottone, J.A., and Molinari, J.A.: Hepatitis, HIV infection and AIDS: Some issues for the practitioners. Int. Dent. J., 39:103, 1989.

Friedland, G.H., et al.: Lack of transmission of HTLV-III/LAV infection to household contacts of patients with AIDS or AIDS-related complex with oral candidiasis. N. Engl. J. Med., 314:344, 1985.

Goldman, D.A., and Zuch, T.F.: AIDS: Understanding the pathogenesis of HIV infection. Infect. Control Hosp. Epidemiol., 10:248, 1989.

Greenspan, D., and Silverman, S.S., Jr.: Oral lesions of HIV infection. Can. Dent. Assoc. J., 15:28–33, 1987.

Greenspan, D., et al.: Relation of oral hairy leukoplakia to infection with the human immunodeficiency virus and the risk of developing AIDS. J. Infect. Dis., 55:475–481, 1987.

HIV Infection and AIDS: Oral manifestations. Oral Surg., 67:291– 326, 1989 and 67:396–442, 1989.

Jaffe, H.W., et al.: The acquired immunodeficiency syndrome in a cohort of homosexual men. Ann. Intern. Med., 103:210, 1985.

Levine, P.H.: The acquired immunodeficiency syndrome in persons with hemophilia. Ann. Intern. Med., 103:723, 1985.

Lewis, L.: AIDS as a chronic disease. AIDS Patient Care, 3:28, 1989.

Levy, R.M., Bredesen, D.E., and Rosenblum, M.L.: Neurological manifestations of AIDS: Experience at UCSF and review of the literature. J. Neurosurg., 62:475, 1985.

Penneys, N.S., and Hicks, B.: Unusual cutaneous lesions associated with AIDS. J. Am. Acad. Dermatol., 13:845, 1985.

Peterman, T.A., et al.: Transfusion-associated acquired immunodeficiency syndrome in the United States. JAMA, 254:2913, 1985.

Pindborg, J.J., et al.: Classification of oral lesions associated with HIV infection. Oral Surg., 67:292, 1989.

Pugliese, G., and Lampinen, T.: Prevention of HIV infection: Our responsibilities as health care professionals. Am. J. Infect. Control, 17:1, 1989.

Robertson, P.B., and Greenspan, J.S. (eds.): Perspectives on the Oral Manifestations of AIDS: Diagnosis and Management of HIV-Associated Infection. Littleton, PSG Publishing Company, Inc., 1988.

Safai, B., et al.: The natural history of Kaposi's sarcoma in AIDS. Ann. Intern. Med., 103:744, 1985.

Scott, G.B., et al: Mothers of infants with the acquired immunodeficiency syndrome: Evidence for both symptomatic and asymptomatic carriers. JAMA, 253:363, 1985.

Selwyn, P.A.: AIDS: What is now known. I. History and Immunovirology. Hosp. Pract., 21:67, 1986.

Selwyn, P.A.: AIDS: What is now known. II. Epidemiology. Hosp. Pract., 21:127–129, 1986.

Selwyn, P.A.: AIDS: What is now known. III. Clinical Aspects. Hosp. Pract., 21:119–26, 1986.

Verrusio, A.C.: Risk of transmission of HIV to health care workers exposed to HIV-infected patients: A review. J. Am. Dent. Assoc., 118:339, 1989.

Chapter 4

Rationale for Practical Infection Control in Dentistry

Dental-care professionals are routinely at an increased risk of cross-infection while providing treatment for their patients. This occupational potential for disease transmission can be initially ascertained when one realizes that most human microbial pathogens have been isolated from oral secretions (Table 4–1). As a result of repeated exposure to the microorganisms present in blood and saliva, the incidence of certain infectious diseases is significantly higher among dental professionals than observed for the general population. Hepatitis B, tuberculosis, and herpes simplex virus infections are well recognized and serve as documentation for the need for increased understanding of modes of disease transmission and infection control procedures by dental-care providers.

The general routes for transmission of microbial agents in dental medicine are:
1. Direct contact with infectious lesions or infected saliva or blood
2. Indirect transmission via transfer of microorganisms from a contaminated intermediate object
3. Spatter of blood, saliva, or nasopharyngeal secretions directly onto broken or intact skin or mucosa
4. Aerosolization, the airborne transfer of microorganisms

A portion of the problem lies in the fact that many practitioners and auxiliaries fail to comprehend or appreciate the infection potential presented by saliva and blood during treatment. Neglecting to implement effective precautions and procedures places others, including the practitioner's family and other patients, at an increased risk of disease as innocent bystanders. These dangers are often dismissed as much of the spatter coming from the patient's mouth is not readily noticed. Organic debris may be transparent or translucent, and dries as a clear film on skin, clothing, and other surfaces.

A novel demonstration was first developed by Crawford in the 1970s using the premise "if saliva were red." He had practitioners dip their fingers into red poster paint before starting their normal clinical treatment. The paint was subsequently deposited on the various surfaces of the operatory as treatment progressed. This demonstrated the cross-contamination that occurred from the practitioner's "saliva-covered" fingers.

This study was expanded in 1985 by Cottone and Glass at the University of Texas Dental School at San Antonio by coating the surface of a rubber dam placed on a mannequin with the same type of poster paint as utilized by Crawford. A Class II operative preparation was then performed on a lower second molar by a

Table 4–1.   Infectious Hazards For Both Dental Personnel and Patients in the Operatory

Infectious Organism	Habitat	Transmission	Potential Pathology	Vaccine
Bacteria				
Bordetella pertussis (B)	Nasopharynx	Nasopharyngeal secretions[1]	Whooping cough	Yes
Cardiobacterium hominis (A)	Nasopharynx	Nasopharyngeal secretions[1]	Endocarditis	No
Corynebacterium diphtheriae	Nasopharynx	Nasopharyngeal secretions[1]	Diphtheria	Yes
Enterobacteriaceae (A)				
Escherichia coli	Mouth,	Blood, lesion exudate[2]	Pneumonia, bacteremia,	No
Proteus vulgaris	gastrointestinal		abscesses, wound	
Klebsiella pneumoniae	(GI) tract		infections	
Haemophilus	Mouth,	Blood, nasopharyngeal	Pneumonia, meningitis,	Yes
influenza (C)	nasopharynx	secretions[1]	otitis	
parainfluenza (A)	"	"	Conjunctivitis, endocarditis	No
paraphrophilus (A)	"	"	Endocarditis	No
Mycobacterium tuberculosis (D)	Pharynx	Pharyngeal secretions[1]	Tuberculosis	No
Mycoplasma pneumoniae (A)	Pharynx	Pharyngeal secretions[1]	Primary atypical pneumonia	No
Neisseria	Mouth,	Blood, nasopharyngeal	Cerebrospinal meningitis	Yes
meningitidis (C)	nasopharynx	secretions[1]		
gonorrhoeae (D)	Mouth, nasopharynx	Blood, lesion exudate, nasopharyngeal secretions[2]	Oral lesions, conjunctivitis	No
Pseudomonas aeruginosa (A)	Ubiquitous, sink and drain contaminant	Lesion exudate[1]	Pneumonia, wound infections	No
Staphylococcus	Mouth, skin,	Lesion exudate[1]	Suppurative lesions,	No
aureus (A)	nasopharynx		bacteremia	
epidermidis (A)	"	"	Endocarditis	No
Streptococcus	Nasopharynx	Blood, nasopharyngeal	Rheumatic and scarlet	No
pyogenes (A)		secretions[2]	fever, otitis media, cervical adenitis, mastoiditis, peritonsillar abscesses, meningitis, pneumonia, acute glomerulonephritis	
pneumoniae (A)	"	"	Pneumonia, endocarditis	Yes
viridans group (A)	"	"	Endocarditis	No
Treponema pallidum (D)	Blood, oral mucosa	Exudate from oral lesions[2]	Syphilis	No
Actinomycosis species (sp)				
Bacteroides sp				
Eubacterium sp				
Fusobacterium sp (A)	Gingival crevice (normal oral flora)	Crevicular exudate[2]	Abscesses	No
Peptococcus sp				
Peptostreptococcus sp				
Propionibacterium sp				
Viruses				
Coxsackie virus (A)	Oropharyngeal mucosa	Ingestion	Hand/foot/mouth disease, vesicular pharyngitis	No
Cytomegalovirus (A)	Salivary gland	Saliva, blood[2]	Cellular enlargement and degeneration in immunocompromised individuals	No
Epstein-Barr (A)	Parotid gland	Saliva, blood[2]	Infectious mononucleosis	No
Hepatitis				
A (D)	Liver, GI tract	Blood (rare), ingestion	Liver inflammation, jaundice	No
B (D)	Liver	Blood, saliva, tears, semen[3]	Eventual hepatocellular carcinoma in chronic antigen carriers	Yes
non-A, non-B (C)	Liver?	Blood[3]		No
delta (A)	Liver	Blood[3]	Coinfection with hepatitis B virus (HBV) required	Yes (HBV vac)

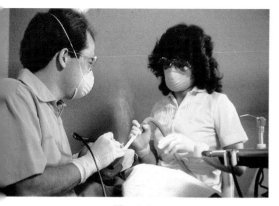

Fig. 4–1

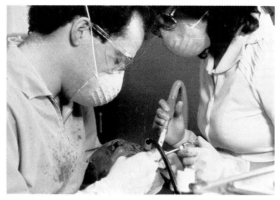

Fig. 4–2

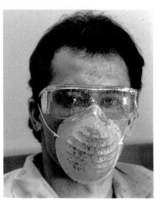

Fig. 4–3

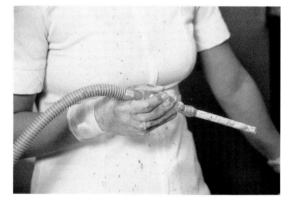

Fig. 4–4

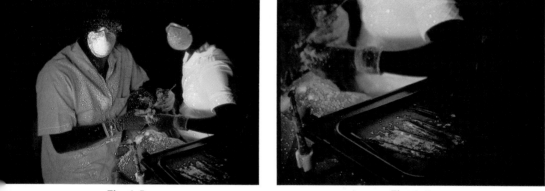

Fig. 4–5   Fig. 4–6

. 4–1.   A dentist and dental assistant using appropriate barrier techniques including mask, gloves, protective eye-
ar, clinic attire, and rubber dam on the patient.   **Fig. 4–2.**   Red dye simulating saliva splashing on the face, hair,
ves, and chest of both the dentist and the dental assistant during a single, class-II operative procedure on a mandibular
ond molar.   **Fig. 4–3.**   The dentist after completing the operative procedure.   **Fig. 4–4.**   The dental assistant after
npleting the operative procedure described in Figure 4–2.   **Figs. 4–5 and 4–6.**   The dental operatory following a
gle, class-II operative procedure on a mandibular second molar when fluorescent dye is used to trace saliva throughout
procedure.

Table 4–1. Infectious Hazards For Both Dental Personnel and Patients in the Operatory
Continued

Infectious Organism	Habitat	Transmission	Potential Pathology	Vaccine
Herpes simplex 1 and 2 (A)	Nasopharynx	Lesion exudate, saliva[2]	Oral lesions, herpetic whitlow, conjunctivitis	No
Human immunodeficiency virus (HIV) (D)	T4 lymphocyte	Blood[3]	Acquired immune deficiency syndrome (AIDS)	No
Measles				
rubeola (C)	Nasopharynx	Nasopharyngeal secretions, blood, saliva, vesicle	Generalized vesicular rash	Yes
rubella (B)		exudate[1]		Yes
Mumps virus (D)	Parotid gland	Saliva, ingestion	Parotitis, meningitis	Yes
Poliovirus (B)	Oropharyngeal mucosa, GI tract	Ingestion	CNS paralysis	Yes
Respiratory viruses (A)				
Influenza A and B			Flu,	Yes
Parainfluenza	Nasopharynx	Nasopharyngeal secretions[1]	common cold	No
Rhinovirus				No
Adenovirus				Yes
Coronavirus				No
Varicella (A)	Skin	Vesicle exudate[1]	Chicken pox	No
Fungi				
Candida albicans (A)	Mouth, skin	Nasopharyngeal secretions[1]	(Opportunistic) candidiasis, cutaneous infections	No
Protozoa				
Pneumocystis carinii (A)	Mouth	Nasopharyngeal secretions[1]	(Opportunistic) interstitial pneumonia in immuno-compromised individuals	No

[1]Infected droplet contact: inhalation, ingestion, direct inoculation.
[2]Direct inoculation to tissue surface.
[3]Inoculation into circulatory system.
Inactivation: always use heat sterilization when possible. All of the above organisms can be killed by autoclaving at 121C, 15 min, 15 psi. Dry heat sterilization: 170C, 60 min. Heat-sensitive instruments and surfaces may be disinfected using phenolic or glutar-aldehyde-based solutions.
References: Jawetz, E.; Melnick, J.L.; and Adelberg, E.A. Review of medical microbiology, ed 17. Norwalk, CT. Appleton and Lange, 1987.
Centers for Disease Control reported new US cases for 1987.
  Key
A = nonreportable.
B = less than 1,000.
C = 1,000–9,999.
D = greater than 9,999.
From: American Dental Association Research Institute, Department of Toxicology. JADA, *117*:374, 1988.

dentist using a high speed handpiece with air and water coolant. The practitioner and dental assistant were properly attired using barrier precautions during the procedure (Fig. 4–1). During the course of treatment, the dyed "saliva" was visible as spatter (Fig. 4–2) that heavily contaminated the face, hair, protective eyewear, mask, chest, arms, and clothing of the dentist by the end of the procedure (Fig. 4–3). In addition, the assistant and high-volume evacuator became laden with intraoral exudate (Fig. 4–4). The use of a fluorescent light more graphically demonstrates the spatter (Figs. 4–5 and 4–6). These figures dramatically demonstrate what occurs on an everyday basis in the dental operatory and illustrate the problem of infection control in dentistry today.

Routine examination of patients and dental prophylaxis procedures also substantially expose the dental professional and patient to potentially infectious fluids. When a red dye and water were used to simulate patient saliva at the University of Detroit by Molinari and York, cross-contamination by the simulated saliva was evident as the gloved hands of the clinician became noticeably contaminated during the intraoral examination. As a result, notations written in the patient's chart transferred secretions to the page (Fig. 4–7). Gloved hands were then washed prior to re-entering the oral cavity. They were immediately contaminated, however, when the clinician continued the examination. Commencement of other procedures, such as periodontal probing and scaling and root planing, were found to deposit salivary contamination on the instrument tray, instruments, and air/water syringe (Figs. 4–8 to 4–10). The unit light handle was also adjusted frequently throughout the session, and showed obvious contamination from the clinician's hands (Fig. 4–11). The previously sterilized sharpening stone accumulated red dye as a result of periodic instrument sharpening (Fig 4–12). When the clinician repositioned her eyewear during the polishing procedure, oral fluids were subsequently transferred to her face, glasses, and mask (Figs. 4–13 and 4–14).

As the clinician prepared to administer a topical fluoride treatment following the prophylaxis, the bottle became cross-contaminated during handling (Fig. 4–15). Finally, the "patient" showed dramatic evidence of the ease of oral fluid spread and the resultant accumulation of contamination at the conclusion of the appointment (Fig. 4–16).

The documented exposure of practitioners, auxiliaries, and patients to a variety of bacterial, viral, and other microbial pathogens led to the development of a series of infection control protocols by the ADA, CDC, and most recently by OSHA (Table 4–2).

When reviewing these guidelines, a distinction must be made between sterilization and disinfection. *Sterilization* is defined as the destruction of *all* microbial forms. The limiting factor and requirement for sterilization is the destruction of bacterial and mycotic spores. *Disinfection* properly refers only to inhibition or destruction of some but not all microbial pathogens. The term is often applied to the use of chemical agents and procedures that are unable to destroy microbial endospores and certain pathogenic microorganisms, such as *Mycobacterium tuberculosis* and hepatitis viruses. *Cleaning* refers simply to the removal of visible organic and inorganic contaminants from a surface. The use of chemical disinfectants in certain instances is warranted because it is not possible to provide sterilization for all items and surfaces contaminated during dental treatment.

When one views the red dye studies, one is tempted to institute every precaution available with no regard as to the efficacy of various modes of transmission. The CDC has stated that hepatitis B is an excellent prototype when designing infection control procedures in dentistry and has listed the principal transmission modes in order of efficiency as listed in Table 4–3.

When the efficiency of various modes of transmission is coupled with available products and techniques available today, rational decisions can be reached by the practitioner as to which products and techniques are needed to formulate an appropriate, but not excessive, infection control program. Concern about asepsis in the dental office has increased in recent years because of the danger of disease transmission, although anxiety has been almost inversely proportional to the degree of transmissibility (Table 4–4). The need for accurate objective information on infection control procedures is greater than ever.

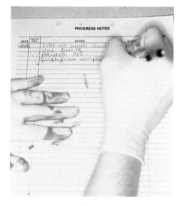

Fig. 4–7

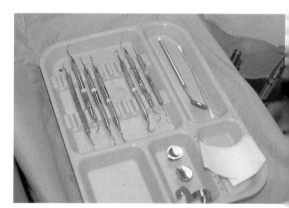

Fig. 4–8

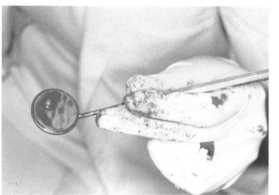

Fig. 4–9

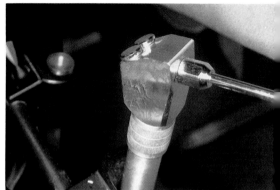

Fig. 4–10

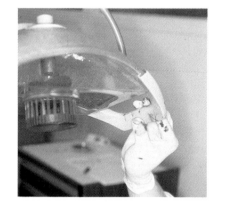

Fig. 4–11

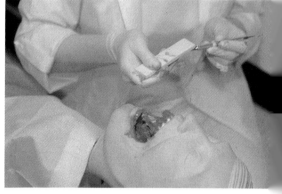

Fig. 4–12

Fig. 4–7. Recording notations in the chart may transmit oral fluids to the papers if they are handled prior to hand washing. **Figs. 4–8 to 4–10.** The instrument tray, instruments, and equipment become contaminated with accumulated "saliva" as items are handled during treatment. **Fig. 4–11.** The frequently touched light handles should properly disinfected between patient appointments. **Fig. 4–12.** The presence of oral fluids on sharpening stor requires that these materials be cleaned and autoclaved after each patient procedure.

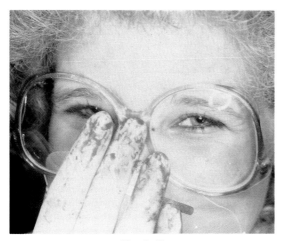

Fig. 4–13

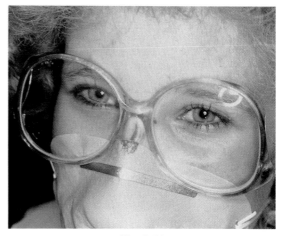

Fig. 4–14

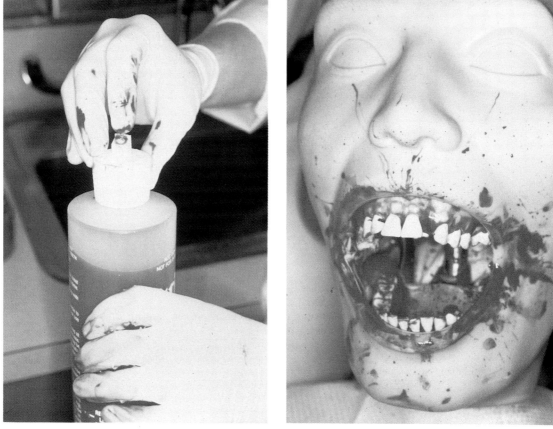

Fig. 4–15

Fig. 4–16

Figs. 4–13 and 4–14.   Saliva may be transmitted to the face, mask, and glasses of the operator by adjusting glasses and mask at chairside.   **Fig. 4–15.**   Reusable objects such as fluoride containers should not be handled until hands are washed.   **Fig. 4–16.**   Visualized saliva is also evident on the patient's face following the prophylaxis.

Table 4–2. Chronology of Infection Control Recommendations

Year	Recommendation
1972	Routine blood screening for HBsAg
1973	CDC—General infection control recommendations
1976	CDC—Rigid hemodialysis controls
1977	HBIG introduced
1978	ADA—First infection control recommendations for dentistry
1981	CDC—First reports of AIDS-related infections
1982	Plasma-derived hepatitis B vaccine (*Heptavax B*) available in US
1983	OSHA—Voluntary hepatitis B guidelines AIDS virus initially isolated
1985	ADA—Revised 1978 infection control recommendations Routine blood screening for HIV antibody
1986	HCW unions petition OSHA for hepatitis B vaccine CDC—Infection control recommendations for dentistry
1987	Recombinant hepatitis B vaccine (*Recombivax HB*) available in US CDC—Universal precautions guidelines OSHA—Joint advisory notice OSHA—Advance notice of rule-making
1988	OSHA—Draft occupational exposure to bloodborne pathogens standard ADA—Revised 1985 infection control recommendations CDC—Update: Universal precautions for prevention of HBV and HIV OSHA—Enforcement procedures for draft standard
1989	CDC—Recommendations for public safety, police, prison and emergency workers EPA—Interim final rule: Tracking and management of medical waste standard OSHA—Proposed occupational exposure to bloodborne pathogens standard
1990	OSHA—Enforcement procedures for draft standard revised
1991	OSHA—Occupational exposure to bloodborne pathogens standard becomes effective
1991–92	EPA—Tracking and management of medical waste standard becomes effective

Abbreviation Key

ADA—American Dental Association	AIDS—Acquired Immune Deficiency Syndrome
CDC—Centers for Disease Control	EPA—Environmental Protection Agency
HBIG—Hepatitis B Immune Globulin	HBsAg—Hepatitis B surface antigen
HBV—Hepatitis B Vaccine	HCW—Health Care Worker
HIV—Human Immunodeficiency Virus	OSHA—Occupational Safety and Health Administration

Table 4–3. Bloodborne Disease Transmission Efficiency

1. Direct or percutaneous inoculation by a contaminated needle or sharp object
2. Non-needle percutaneous inoculation (scratches, burns, dermatitis, i.e. nonintact skin, especially on the hands)
3. Infectious blood or serum onto mucosal surfaces (intraoral, nasal, and ocular mucosa)
4. Other infectious secretions (saliva) onto mucosal surfaces
5. Indirect transfer of infectious serum via environmental surfaces (spatter)
6. Aerosol transfer of infectious serum (theoretical)

Adapted from Bond W.: Modes of transmission of infectious diseases. From Proceedings of the National Symposium on Infection Control in Dentistry. May 13, 1986, Chicago. Atlanta, US Dept. of Health and Human Services.

Demonstration of visible patient spatter on the hands, face, and clothes of the treatment provider, as well as on numerous surfaces in the treatment area, substantiates the need for an effective infection control program in the dental office. Routine examination and prophylaxis exposes the dental professional and patient to potentially infectious fluids. Recognition of the varying degrees of infection potential by microbial-laden secretions initially led to formulation of guidelines

Table 4–4. Infectious Agents of Concern to Health Care Workers

	Transmissibility	Anxiety
Influenza		
Tuberculosis		
Respiratory syncytial virus		
Varicella-zoster virus		
Hepatitis B		
Cytomegalovirus		
Human immunodeficiency virus		
Toxoplasmosis		

Adapted from Valenti, W.M.: Infection control and the pregnant health care worker. AIDS Pt. Care, 3(3):14, 1989.

aimed at minimizing hepatitis B virus transmission. Similar protocols and procedures have been recommended regarding the routine treatment of patients with HIV infection and AIDS. Each of these guidelines mandates the use of the *SAME* appropriate infection control procedures in the management of *ALL* patients (Universal Precautions) and the treatment of every patient as if infected with an incurable infectious disease. The images of "red saliva" should come to mind during any treatment procedure, and serve as reinforcement for the routine use of appropriate and effective yet practical infection control procedures.

SELECTED READINGS

ADA Councils on Dental Materials, Instruments, and Equipment; Dental Practice; and Dental Therapeutics: Infection control recommendations for the dental office and the dental laboratory. J. Am. Dent. Assoc., 116:241–248, 1988.

ADA Councils on Dental Materials and Devices; Dental Therapeutics: Infection control in the dental office. J. Am. Dent. Assoc., 97:673–677, 1978.

ADA Councils on Dental Materials and Devices; Dental Therapeutics: Guidelines for infection control in the dental office and the commercial dental laboratory. J. Am. Dent. Assoc., 110:969–72, 1985.

Centers for Disease Control: Guidelines for prevention of transmission of HIV and HBV to health care and public safety workers. MMWR, 38(S-6):1–37, 1989.

Centers for Disease Control: Provisional PHS interagency recommendations for screening donated blood and plasma for antibody to the virus causing AIDS. MMWR, 34:1, 1985.

Centers for Disease Control: Recommendations for prevention of HIV transmission in health-care settings. MMWR, 36:1S–18S, 1987.

Centers for Disease Control: Recommended infection control practices for dentistry. MMWR, 35:237–241, 1986.

Centers for Disease Control: Recommendations for preventing transmission of infection with human T lymphotropic virus type III/lymphadenopathy associated virus in the workplace. MMWR, 34:682–6, 691–5, 1985.

Centers for Disease Control: Update: Universal precautions for prevention of transmission of HIV, HBV, and other bloodborne pathogens in health-care settings. MMWR, 37:377, 1988.

EPA: Standards for the tracking and management of medical waste: Interim final rule and request for comments. Fed. Reg., 54:12371, 1989.

Joint Advisory Notice: Department of Labor/Department of Health and Human Services; HBV/HIV; Notice. Fed. Reg., 52:41818–41824, 1987.

Occupational Exposure to Bloodborne Pathogens: Proposed rule and notice of hearing. Fed. Reg., 54:23042–23139, 1989.

Occupational Exposure to Hepatitis B Virus and Human Immunodeficiency Virus: Advance Notice of Proposed Rulemaking. Fed. Reg., 52:45438–45441, 1987.

OSHA Instruction CPL 2–2.44B. Enforcement Procedures for Occupational Exposure to HBV and HIV. February 27, 1990.

Chapter 5

Patient Evaluation: Risk Factors

The incidence of certain microbial cross-infections in the dental environment has been well established. Although the transmission of other pathogens, while highly probable, has not been definitely determined, infections do present a significant hazard to oral health care providers themselves and through them, to their families and patients. The health status of dental patients is determined primarily by using the medical history. Consequently, history taking, in the hands of experienced clinicians, should elicit information on the presence or absence of transmissible disease and identify patients at risk to harbor potentially infectious organisms and those who may have increased susceptibility to infections.

The essential elements of a medical history are those that will help clinicians to identify the patient, establish the chief complaint, determine the present health status of the patient and provide a record of major hospitalizations, a history of childhood and adult illnesses, evidence of allergies, a list of medications the patient may be taking, pertinent family and social or experiential history, and a review of major organ systems (Fig. 5–1). This process has been accepted by medical practitioners for decades, and should now be embraced by the dental profession.

The medical history should be taken by the dentist using a combined printed and oral approach. Responses should be explored to determine if the patient understands the question, is certain of the answer, and appreciates the importance of the question and the answer in the context of the care to be provided. Check marks, underlined, or circled answers are inadequate to document the medical history. The date and signature of the clinician should be filled in and there should be no blanks left on a completed history form. The circumstances of the care provided and the outcome of treatment depends on the history obtained. Failure to elicit an accurate medical history constitutes negligence.

The process of history taking usually begins the doctor-patient relationship and its primary objective is to identify those matters the patient defines as problems. Clinicians must, however, be aware of both overt and hidden concerns, and the need to assure reasonable accuracy. Patients may suppress some information either purposely or unknowingly. They may underreport other experiences or give them a context that is less disconcerting than might be appropriate. Clinicians must develop a sense for the patient's reliability as an interpreter and reporter of events. Some circumstances that should be of concern to clinicians might not be seen as unusual by patients. Practitioners have to be compulsive in compiling data, giving careful attention to the obvious and maintaining sensitivity to the less obvious, "soft" clues that may be revealed in the history. An appreciation of the patient's perspective, an attitude of friendliness, and obvious respect will go a long way in assuring the patient's cooperation in the pursuit of information.

Fig. 5–1.   SCHOOL OF DENTISTRY—CASE WESTERN RESERVE UNIVERSITY
MEDICAL HISTORY

NAME _____ Sex _____ Birth Date _____ S.S.N. _____
     last   first   middle   Phone _____
ADDRESS _____
               number and street   city   state   zip code

A. MEDICAL HISTORY
Describe your general health _____
Have you ever been hospitalized? _____
List last or present illnesses _____
Do you have any allergies or sensitivities? _____
Do you take any medications, drugs, pills? _____

B. FAMILY HISTORY
(Have any members of your family ever been treated for the conditions listed or any other medical problems?)
Diabetes _____ High blood pressure _____ Heart problem _____ Seizures _____
Other _____

C. SOCIAL HISTORY
Occupation _____ Smoking _____ Alcohol _____ Other _____

D. REVIEW OF SYSTEMS
(Have you ever had or do you now have any of the conditions listed?)

I. Skin
Itching _____
Rash _____
Ulcers _____
Pigmentations _____
Lack or loss of body hair _____

II. Extremities
Varicose veins _____
Swollen, painful joints _____
Muscle weakness, pain _____
Bone deformity, fracture _____
Prosthetic joints _____

III. Eyes
Blurring of vision _____
Double vision _____
Drooping of eyelid _____
Glaucoma _____

IV. Ear, Nose, Throat
Earache _____
Hearing loss _____
Frequent nosebleeds _____
Sinusitis _____
Frequent sore throat _____
Hoarseness _____

V. Respiratory
Cough _____
Blood in sputum _____
Wheezing, asthma _____
Tuberculosis, exposure to _____

VI. Cardiac
Shortness of breath _____
Pain, pressure in chest _____
Swelling of ankles _____
High, low blood pressure _____
Rheumatic, scarlet fever _____
Heart murmur, attack _____
Prosthetic inserts _____

VII. Gastrointestinal
Difficulty swallowing _____
Abdominal pain, ulcers _____
Hepatitis _____
Jaundice _____

VIII. Genitourinary
Difficulty, pain on urination _____
Blood in urine _____
Excessive urination _____
Kidney infections _____
STD _____

IX. Endocrine
Thyroid trouble _____
Weight change _____
Diabetes _____
Excessive thirst _____

X. Hematopoietic
Easy bruising _____
Excessive bleeding _____
G6PD deficiency _____
Anemia _____
Leukemia _____
Spleen problems _____

XI. Neurologic
Frequent headaches _____
Dizziness, fainting _____
Epilepsy, fits _____
Neuritis, neuralgia _____
Paresthesias, numbness _____
Paralysis _____

XII. Psychiatric
Nervousness _____
Irritability _____
Depression, excessive worry _____
Nervous breakdown _____

XIII. Growth or Tumor
Radiotherapy/chemotherapy _____

Student's Signature _____ No. _____ Date _____
Faculty Signature _____ Date _____

PATIENT IDENTIFICATION

The basic biographic data should include the patient's name, age, sex, ethnic extraction, marital status, occupation, and place of residence. The date of the evaluation must also be recorded. Not only are these items essential for patient identification, they may also provide invaluable background information that may place the patient in a high-risk category for infectious diseases. Health care workers, military personnel, immigrants from underdeveloped countries, and individuals who work or live in institutions should be considered potentially infectious.

HISTORY OF PRESENT ORAL CONDITION

Record, in a logical sequence, the patient's description of the signs and symptoms associated with the present oral condition. Begin with the chief complaint, stated in the patient's own words. Try to determine why the patient is consulting you today and not yesterday or tomorrow. The answer may be an important clue to the severity of the condition, underlying emotional concerns, or other matters that are important in the overall understanding of the patient and his illness. Did acute symptoms prompt the visit, or was it the desire for a "check-up"? Remember that a patient's expressed reason for seeking advice may mask underlying concerns. After an understandable statement of the chief complaint has been elicited, begin delineating the illness.

Duration and Progression

How long has the condition associated with the patient's chief complaint been present? Has the problem developed slowly or rapidly? Some conditions have a sudden onset, but others begin slowly and insidiously. Have the symptoms become worse or better? Are they better at times and worse at other times?

Domain

Does the pain or discomfort remain localized, or does it radiate to other anatomic locations? When dealing with a lesion, determine if it is found on the lips, tongue, buccal mucosa, hard or soft palate, floor of the mouth, or other areas of the head and neck.

Character

Note the character of the pain or discomfort. Is it sharp or dull? Is it pain or discomfort? Does it appear suddenly and disappear quickly, or does it gradually increase in intensity and subside slowly? Observe the lesion. Is it white, red, pigmented, ulcerative, vesiculobullous, exophytic, or is it a combination of these various characteristics?

Relation to Physiologic Function

Evaluate the effects of normal activities upon the symptoms. What is the effect of mastication? Are the symptoms worse when the patient is chewing? In some instances, mastication relieves symptoms; in others it aggravates them. The effects on eating should be noted.

Upper respiratory tract infections, pulmonary infections, sexually related conditions and diseases, and childhood diseases may all have signs and symptoms that appear typically in the dental area. A knowledge of the more common sites of involvement of a disease assists in its diagnosis. It must be remembered, however, that no diagnostic index or outline can take into consideration the capriciousness of a disease or the different reactions of an individual host to a disease. Therefore, the evaluation and integration of the clinical appearance and characteristics of a lesion with its history of development and other appropriate diagnostic findings should always determine the final diagnosis.

HISTORY OF PAST AND PRESENT ILLNESS

Inquire about the patient's perception of his/her general health status. Chronologically summarize past and present medical conditions. Note any hereditary or developmental abnormalities. Patients with hemophilia or other coagulopathies are at high risk for hepatitis and AIDS. List earlier operations, injuries, accidents, and hospitalizations, and comments about anesthesia and drug reactions. Any of the above may have been associated with blood transfusion or transfusions and predispose the patient to transmissible diseases. Investigate evidence of drugs or medications currently taken. Immunosuppressant therapy may place a patient in the high-risk category for many viral, fungal, and bacterial infections. History of repeated hospitalizations for the same condition, failure to respond normally to therapy for infection, recurrent infections with the same pathogen, and infection with unusual organisms, especially in the absence of "hard" signs of infection, should be suggestive of immune deficiency and, therefore, a high-risk patient.

FAMILY HISTORY

The family history is important in many diseases. Some conditions are always hereditary. Invariably, hemophilia has been passed on by an affected mother to her sons, diabetes shows a hereditary tendency, and allergic reactions are commonly hereditary. Similarly, acquired infectious diseases may be transmitted by one family member to another. Some of the conditions require just casual contact; others can only be transmitted through repeated, intimate encounters.

SOCIAL HISTORY

The patient's personal history should alert the clinician to the presence of environmental, cultural, or experiential factors that can significantly influence the patient's general health. It should reveal the individual as a whole, providing a basis for an assessment of personality and emotional state. Information about social, religious, and economic background, education, and feelings of achievement or frustration can be an important contribution to understanding your patient as a person. A history of frequent moves; sexual promiscuity whether homosexual, bisexual, or heterosexual; the use of recreational drugs including alcohol; frequent travels to underdeveloped countries, or recent immigration into the U.S. should alert clinicians to high-risk patients for infectious diseases.

REVIEW OF MAJOR ORGAN SYSTEMS

Record signs and symptoms related to specific organ systems. The chief complaint and medical history should guide the clinician to investigate areas of special interest. The status of organ systems may suggest the presence of concomitant systemic conditions, including infectious diseases, contribute to the diagnostic process, and influence projected treatment protocols and prognosis.

Skin

Historical evidence of alterations in the texture, color, and integrity of the skin and changes in the character of hair and nails should alert the clinician to the existence of systemic problems, including infectious processes and immunodeficiency. The most important cause of pruritus, especially in association with a bitter metallic taste and burning tongue, may be a reaction to stress and strain. Itching without a visible rash may be the only historical evidence of sensitivity to a drug, and pruritus with rash may indicate a reaction to penicillin, infectious childhood diseases, hepatitis, gonorrhea, or secondary syphilis.

A history of asymmetric loss of hair may be suggestive of developmental defects or evidence of chemical or thermal burns, but most often it is secondary to physical trauma. Symmetric loss could signify toxic alopecia or hypopituitarism but it may be scarlet fever, or syphilis. A significant percentage of patients may experience transient alopecia secondary to chemotherapy and these patients are not only susceptible to a variety of viral, bacterial, and fungal infections, but may be carriers capable of transmitting infectious disease to others.

Obvious skin lesions such as disseminated dermatitis, bullae, papules, vesicles, or ulcerations, may be indicative of endocrine, metabolic, immunologic, or infectious diseases and these patients should be referred to a dermatologist for definitive diagnosis and treatment.

Extremities

Varicose veins are dilated, tortuous vessels usually the result of incompetent valves. However, with a history of heaviness, aching, and edema of the legs, especially toward the end of the day, the condition may be secondary to thrombophlebitis, trauma, increased venous pressure, pregnancy, or heart failure. Swollen, painful joints and bone deformity may be caused by trauma, metabolic or immunologic disturbances, or neoplasia, but they may also be associated with a number of primary sexually transmissible diseases or congenital syphilis. Among the many complications after total joint replacement, infection is by far one of the most serious. Consequently, foci of odontogenic infections and transient bacteremia associated with dental procedures must be a cardinal concern both to orthopedic surgeons and dental practitioners.

Eyes

A detailed history of the patient's vision may be essential in certain situations. Make note concerning evidence of the patient wearing glasses or contact lenses. A history of hemorrhage into one or both eyes in association with evidence of trauma may be significant. A history of icteric conjunctivas in addition to hemolytic or obstructive disease may be suggestive of hepatocellular jaundice resulting from acute viral, drug-induced, or alcoholic hepatitis; subacute or chronic hepatitis; or cirrhosis. Conjunctivitis in association with burning, itching, and running eyes may be apparent with the common cold, in herpes keratitis, or with gonococcal or chlamydial infections, and should alert the clinician to the presence of a potentially transmissible disease. A shower of sparks in one quadrant of the eye followed by a curtain moving across the same eye may be suggestive of retinal detachment. Black spots moving in front of the eyes followed by nausea is the first and most common sign of migraine headache. Patients with glaucoma often omit mentioning their antiglaucoma medication in a drug history, particularly if administered as eyedrops, and this omission may lead to the inappropriate prescription of concomitants.

Ears, Nose, and Throat

Patients with a history of recurrent ear infections may at times relate their pain syndrome to the dentition or the temporomandibular joint, and pain syndromes of odontogenic myofascial origin may well mimic otitis media. Tinnitus is a common geriatric complaint associated with arteriosclerosis. Also, tinnitus, fullness, vertigo, and fluctuating hearing loss may be related to Ménière's disease.

A history of deviated septum and polyps in the nasal cavity should alert the clinician to possible mouthbreathing, leading to xerostomia and dental caries. Rhinitis, an inflammatory reaction of the nasal mucosa, is commonly initiated by an allergic response to chemical or viral irritants or may be secondary to upper respiratory tract infections. Bleeding from the interior of the nose may be caused by injuries, infectious septal perforation, tumors, blood dyscrasias, and hypertension. However, mechanical factors, such as drying of the mucosa by overheated indoor air and trauma from nose picking, account for the majority of cases and such bleeding usually originates in the anterior nasal chamber.

Sore throat is the hallmark of pharyngitis most often associated with upper respiratory tract infections but it may be the clinical manifestation of infectious mononucleosis; herpetic, gonococcal, syphilitic, chlamydial, and trichomonal infections; hepatitis; and these patients also, must be carefully evaluated for evidence of neoplasia. Hoarseness is a most commonly overlooked symptom. Always a manifestation of laryngitis if observed in a patient it must be immediately investigated to rule out the possibility of a laryngeal neoplasm.

The Respiratory System

Upper respiratory tract infections are brief illnesses most frequently of viral origin. The initial viral infection may be followed by a secondary bacterial infection which may last for weeks, especially in smokers. The prodromal manifestations of lethargy, malaise, anorexia, and rhinorrhea may be quite similar to those associated with more serious viral infections, such as hepatitis, in the early stages of the disease process.

Hemoptysis may be evidence of upper respiratory tract or pulmonary infections or pulmonary neoplasia. A productive cough in the morning characterized by hemoptysis is highly suggestive of tuberculosis especially in association with pain, dysphagia, dysphonia, and significant weight loss. Aerosols released during dental procedures may result in droplet nuclei containing highly infectious bacilli. The drug history is most useful in differentiating between patients with tuberculous infection and those with tuberculosis.

Bronchial asthma is a respiratory disease characterized by bronchial smooth muscle spasm, hypersecretion, and inflammation of alveolar epithelium resulting in cough, wheezing, and shortness of breath. An asthmatic attack may be provoked by allergens, upper respiratory tract infections, exercise, salicylates and other non-steroidal anti-inflammatory agents, and emotional stress.

Bronchitis, chronic inflammation of the alveolar epithelium, is seen most commonly in smokers. The patients are usually heavy set, blue or red-blue around the face, have distended neck veins and ankle edema, may be taking bronchodilators, and experience frequent pulmonary infections. Emphysema is usually preceded by chronic bronchitis and is characterized by irreversible obstructive disease with dilation and destruction of the walls of the acini. The patients are generally thin, pink in color, carry their shoulders high, and breathe with their intercostal muscles. Oxygen must be used with care in patients with chronic obstructive lung disease because the respiratory center readjusts so that the basic stimulus to respiration is oxygen versus carbon dioxide.

The Cardiovascular System

Historical evidence of cardiovascular disease or symptomatology (shortness of breath, pain and pressure in the chest, swelling of the ankles, high or low blood pressure, and heart murmur) suggestive of such disease should be most carefully evaluated prior to any dental procedure. The historical association of dental procedures, transient bacteremia, and subsequent infective endocarditis has prompted the American Heart Association to recommend antibiotic prophylaxis with all dental procedures that are likely to cause gingival bleeding in these patients. Patients at greatest risk for developing endocarditis (those with prosthetic heart valves) should receive antibiotics parenterally. Those without prosthetic heart valves who undergo dental treatment may be managed by oral antimicrobial prophylaxis alone.

Infective endocarditis is uncommon in children. However, children with congenital heart disease and rheumatic heart disease have a substantial lifetime risk for development of endocarditis. Recent advances in the management of these children should increase the number of patients who will survive infancy and early childhood. Any unexplained fever in a child with congenital heart disease deserves close investigation and localized bacterial infection in children at risk must be treated aggressively to prevent metastatic spread to the heart. *Staphylococcus aureus* is becoming the most common pathogen isolated in pediatric patients with endocarditis.

Infective endocarditis occurs most often in patients with structural abnormalities of heart valves and great vessels, including those with cardiac or vascular protheses (Table 5–1). In the preantibiotic era, all patients with infective endocarditis died of sepsis or the related hemodynamic consequences. Because host defense mechanisms play only a minor role in the control of infective endocarditis, in no other infectious disease does cure depend so much on prevention and the administration of adequate dosages of antibiotics.

Dental treatment of patients with well-controlled hypertension is relatively

Table 5–1. Indications for Infective Endocarditis Prophylaxis

Congenital Heart Lesions	Rheumatic Heart Disease
Ventricular septal defect	Mitral stenosis
Aortic stenosis	Mitral insufficiency
Tetralogy of Fallot	Aortic insufficiency
Aortic coarctation	Tricuspid murmurs
Patent ductus arteriosus	
Transposition of great vessels	Nonrheumatic Valvular Disease
Pulmonic stenosis	Mitral-valve prolapse
Truncus arteriosus	Idiopathic hypertrophic subaortic stenosis
Other complex lesions	Cardiac Prostheses
Other	Prosthetic heart valves
Infective endarteritis	Dacron patches
Intracardiac/extracardiac shunts	Other
Drug abuse	Dialysis

safe. However, uncontrolled hypertension may precipitate an episode of acute ventricular failure, a cerebrovascular accident, or a myocardial infarction. Dental care for these patients should consist of reduction of anxiety and control of pain, infection, and bleeding, followed by priority consultation with a physician.

Clinicians should appreciate the fact that an increase in heart rate produced by anxiety, pain, and epinephrine may provoke an anginal attack in susceptible patients. Nitroglycerine, used sublingually, should be available for the patient in the office. Repeated doses may be required, however, if the angina does not immediately resolve, the patient's physician should be contacted or the patient should be referred to a local emergency room for immediate treatment. When the medical management of angina pectoris fails, the next step is surgical correction of the blocked vessels. Bypass procedures are common and successful. Two to 6 months postsurgery, these patients are asymptomatic and can be treated in the dental milieu as normal, healthy individuals.

Congestive heart failure should preclude all but urgent dental care such as the control of anxiety, pain, infection, and bleeding followed by consultation with the patient's physician.

Stress reduction and pain control is the cardinal rule for treating postmyocardial infarction patients. For patients who are 0 to 6 months postmyocardial infarction, dental treatment should be limited to urgent care. Patients 6 to 12 months or more postmyocardial infarction will tolerate moderate sittings. In all instances, an adequate history, an appreciation for the presenting clinical signs, a complete drug review, and consultation with the patient's physician will add to timely and appropriate therapy.

The Gastrointestinal System

The gastrointestinal system is both structurally and functionally adapted for the reception, mixing, digestion, and absorption of food and the elimination of catabolic residue. Pathophysiologic disruption produces abdominal discomfort, nausea, regurgitation or vomiting, and dysphagia. Difficulty swallowing may be caused by an emotional disturbance, globus hystericus, or it may be caused by obstruction in the esophageal tract, muscular dysfunctions, or simple local irritation. Dyspepsia or indigestion is a disorder usually caused by poor dentition or a highly nervous state. Bulimia nervosa, a condition noted mostly among the young, has a psychologic basis. These patients will regurgitate food at will, causing frequent acidic reflux into the oral cavity, which in turn will cause a peculiar pattern of carious destruction. The dentist may be the one to identify this disorder first, alerting the physician to the problem.

Jaundice is caused by an increase of bilirubin in plasma as a result of (1) increased destruction of red blood cells (hemolytic anemia); (2) hepatitis, cirrhosis, infectious mononucleosis, or other liver disease, and (3) cholelithiasis, or carcinoma of the head of the pancreas. Most patients may not be aware of the fact that they had hepatitis, as many of the cases of hepatitis are subclinical. Consequently, past medical or social histories may not help identify high-risk patients and dictate office protocol.

The Genitourinary System

Dental care is seldom complicated by diseases of the genitourinary tract; however, there are a few instances that the clinician should keep in mind. One of the most common types of infection is the urinary tract infection. Patients with such infections are on highly specific drugs (e.g., sulfonamides, nitrofurantoin, methamine, mandelic acid, and phenozopyridine) that have to be carefully identified. Many sexually transmissible diseases have also reached epidemic proportions. When we discuss venereal diseases, we must therefore, take into account the increase in orogenital activity that can be accompanied by corresponding increases in oral manifestations of sexually related diseases. The extent to which the recognition of these conditions requires modification of dental therapy, and the clinical implications for office personnel, are obvious.

The Endocrine System

An obese patient who relates symptoms of fatigue, drowsiness, intolerance to cold, poor memory, and presents with physical signs to include dry, coarse skin and hair, decreased heart rate, and slow reflexes may have hypothyroidism. Conversely, a patient who relates symptoms of headache, increased appetite, weight loss, heat tolerance and presents with physical signs to include exophthalmia, increased heart rate, and agitation may have hyperthyroidism.

In an adult, increase in body weight may reflect an increase in adipose tissue or an accumulation of fluid. The increased fluid retention may be the result of increased salt and fluid intake or decreased sodium and water excretion (e.g., cardiovascular, renal, hepatic, or adrenal problems).

Diabetes mellitus is the most prevalent of all endocrine dysfunctions. Concerns from the dental standpoint include insulin shock, diabetic coma, and the patient's inability to limit infection. Polyuria and concurrent polydipsia should alert the clinician to the possibility of diabetes mellitus or insipidus, and excessive thirst may also be secondary to severe primary aldosteronism, Cushing's disease, or diuretic therapy.

Hematopoietic System

The oral manifestations of blood dyscrasia are varied, and they are not pathognomonic. Any disease that causes immunosuppression, bone marrow suppression, or other abnormalities of the blood-forming organs may present with similar oral findings. Historical evidence of easy bruising, excessive bleeding, anemia, or leukemia should, however, prime the clinician for a greater appreciation of such clinical findings as lymphadenopathy; erythema or pallor of the oral mucosa, gingivitis, necrotic ulcerations, petechiae, ecchymoses, hemorrhage; fungal, viral, and bacterial infections; tooth mobility, toothache in apparently healthy teeth; and neurologic abnormalities in the head and neck area. The presence of these signs and symptoms is a clear indication for hematology screening and evaluation of hemostasis as part of urgent care. G6PD deficiency should preclude prescribing salicylates or other NSAIDs for the management of pain. The asplenic patient, who is at high risk of massive infections through the hematogenous route, should receive antimicrobial prophylaxis prior to dental treatment.

The Nervous System

Headaches, along with fatigue, hunger, and thirst represent man's most frequent discomfort. From a medical standpoint, the significance of headaches is often obscure; however, it may be symptomatic expression of tension and fatigue. Dizziness and lightheadedness may be related to a hypoglycemic state, anemia, or a disturbance in the vestibular component of the eighth cranial nerve. Fainting is associated with the sensation of impending loss of consciousness. Epileptic seizures may occur at any time of night and day and the patient will be characteristically confused and exhausted following convulsion. Neuralgias of interest to the dental practitioner include trigeminal neuralgia, glossopharyngeal neuralgia, sphenopalatine neuralgia, and Bell's palsy, which represents the most common cause of paralysis in the head and neck area, and may be associated with viral infections.

Psychiatric Evaluation

The majority of patients who enter a dentist's office will admit to being nervous or anxious. If this is in direct relationship to a stressful event or circumstance, it is accepted as a normal response. When nervousness or anxiety is uncontrollable and accompanied by physical effects, they become the basis for a medical consultation.

SUMMARY

Sir William Osler once said one should "never treat a stranger." His statement is especially applicable to the practice of dentistry in which the physical and emotional stability of the patient is determined primarily by using the medical history. However, patients do not always appreciate the significance of medically related questions asked by a dentist. The accomplished clinician must, therefore, not only master the science of inquiry and the art of observation but must also establish the rapport that precedes the unguarded flow of pertinent information from the patient. This information is germinal to successful treatment and to minimize the potential for cross-infections in the dental environment.

SELECTED READINGS

Bottomely, W.K.: The importance of a detailed drug history for the dentist. U.S. Navy Med., 62:18–20, 1973.

Brady, W.F., and Martinoff, J.T.: Diagnosed past and present systemic disease in dental patients. Gen. Dent., 30:494–499, 1982.

Brady, W.F., and Martinoff, J.T.: Validity of health history data collected from dental patients and patient perception of health status. J. Am. Dent. Assoc., 101:642–645, 1980.

Collen, M.F., et al.: Reliability of a self-administered medical questionnaire. Arch. Intern. Med., 123:664–681, 1969.

Cottone, J.A., and Kafrawy, A.H.: Medications and health histories: A survey of 4365 dental patients. J. Am. Dent. Assoc., 98:713–718, 1979.

Council on Dental Education: Guidelines for Teaching Physical Evaluation in Dental Education. Chicago, American Dental Association, 1976.

Falace, D.A.: Physical evaluation of the dental patient: Current practices and opinions. J. Dent. Educ., 42:537–540, 1978.

Langlais, R.P., et al.: Oral Diagnosis, Oral Medicine, and Treatment Planning. Philadelphia, W.B. Saunders Co., 1984.

Lewis, D.M., Krakow, A.M., and Payne, T.F.: An evaluation of the dental-medical history. Milit. Med., 143:785–787, 1978.

Little, J.W., and King, D.R.: The significance of physical diagnosis, patient history data, and medical screening in the dental office. Ann. Dent., 3:42–55, 1971.

McCarthy, F.M., and Malamed, S.F.: Physical evaluation system to determine medical risk and indicated dental therapy modifications. J. Am. Dent. Assoc., 99:181–243, 1978.

Owens, W.D., Fets, J.A., and Spitznagel, E.L., Jr.: ASA physical status classifications: A study of consistency of ratings. Anesthesiology, 49:239–243, 1978.

Rothwell, P.S., and Wragg, K.A.: Assessment of the medical status of patients in general dental practice: A comparative survey of a questionnaire and verbal inquiry. Br. Dent. J., 133:252–255, 1972.

Sonis, S.T., Fazio, R., Setkowicz, A., et al.: Comparison of the nature and frequency of medical problems among patients in general, specialty, and hospital dental practices. Ann. Dent., 41:42–45, 1982.

Taybos, G.M., Terezhalmy, G.T., and Pelleu, G.B., Jr.: Assessing patient's health status with the Navy Dental Health Questionnaire, U.S. Navy Med., 74:24–32, 1983.

Terezhalmy, G.T., and Sazima, H.J.: Medical evaluation of the dental patient; A science and an art. Milit. Med., 146:423–426, 1981.

Thorn, G.W., et al.: Harrison's Principles of Internal Medicine, 8th Ed. New York, McGraw-Hill Book Co., 1977.

Trieger, N., and Goldblatt, L.: The art of history taking. J. Oral Surg., 36:118–124, 1978.

Truelove, E.L.: Preventive health screening in dentistry: Is it feasible? J. Prevent. Dent., 5:24–28, 1978.

section two

Personal Protection

Chapter 6

Recommendations for Immunization of Oral Health Care Providers

Childhood immunization programs have significantly reduced the incidence of vaccine preventable diseases. Today, a substantial portion of the morbidity and mortality from these conditions are manifested in older adolescents and adults. Individuals who have escaped natural infection or proper immunization against childhood diseases may be at increased risk for such diseases and their complications as adults. Special attention should be given to immunizing health care personnel because of their documented increased risk of exposure to certain preventable diseases and to minimize the likelihood of transmitting infectious diseases to other susceptible health care personnel, patient, family, and other contacts.

Dental educators have an obligation to educate, to continuously make aware, and to provide balanced assessments of benefits, costs, and risks on the antigens that are routinely recommended for the immunization of health care personnel. Infection control programs in dentistry are to be designed to assess and minimize communicable disease risk in the dental environment through these programs. Immunizations and other prophylaxis against preventable diseases should be made available to all oral health care providers. At the time of employment, each person should be asked to provide documentation of previous immunizations. A review of this documentation will indicate which immunizations are needed, saving valuable time and emotional stress in the event that exposure occurs on the job. The following recommendations, developed to assist in the prevention of illness among oral health care providers and patients, cover immunizations in three areas of concern:

1. Immunizations recommended at the time of employment for susceptible oral health care providers
2. Immunization regimens which require booster doses
3. Immunizations and chemotherapeutic agents administered only in the event of inadvertent exposure to a communicable disease

The recommendations are based on the characteristics of immunobiologics, scientific knowledge about the principles of active and passive immunization, and judgments by public health officials and specialists in clinical and preventive medicine.

RUBELLA (GERMAN MEASLES)

Universal immunization against the rubella virus is generally recommended for all health care providers, but particularly for previously unimmunized women of childbearing age who do not have laboratory evidence of immunity. Not only are susceptible health care providers themselves at risk of acquiring rubella, but they may transmit the disease to associates and patients, some of whom might be pregnant. Fetal infection can occur in up to 80% of fetuses during the first trimester of pregnancy, to some extent in the second trimester, and may produce serious birth defects.

The rubella vaccine contains live attenuated rubella virus that is prepared in human cell cultures. Women should receive the vaccine only if they are not pregnant and must be counseled not to become pregnant for 3 months after immunization because of the potential risk of infecting the fetus in vitro with the vaccine virus. Adverse reactions to the vaccine are infrequent in healthy persons. The most common complication is joint pain, usually of the small distal joints, reported by up to 40% of adult vaccinees. Rarely, arthralgias may occur 3 to 25 days after vaccination and persist for up to 10 days. As with all live virus vaccines, the rubella vaccine should not be given to immunocompromised patients.

RUBEOLA (MEASLES)

Universal immunization against rubeola is recommended for all young adults, particularly health care providers born after 1956, unless there is a physician-documented history of infection or vaccination after the age of one, or laboratory evidence of immunity. Those vaccinated between 1963 and 1967 with inactivated rubeola vaccine should be revaccinated to prevent severe atypical measles. Giving rubeola vaccine to an individual who is already immune, either from natural infection or previous vaccination, is safe. Nonpregnant, susceptible persons exposed to the rubeola virus may receive protection if immunized within 72 hours following exposure.

The rubeola vaccine contains live attenuated measles virus that is prepared in cell cultures made from chicken embryos. However, the chance of allergic reactions occurring in persons allergic to eggs, chickens, or feathers is low. Because the rubeola vaccine contains live attenuated virus, it should not be given to immunocompromised or pregnant individuals. Rubeola may be prevented or modified in susceptible pregnant personnel by administering immune globulin within 6 days following exposure. About 5 to 15% of the vaccine recipients develop symptoms of attenuated measles, characterized by fever, beginning 5 to 12 days after vaccination. A transient rash may occur in about 5% of vaccines.

MUMPS

Health care workers are likely to be exposed to mumps and suffer the consequences of infection characterized by the involvement of major salivary glands, possibly meningitis, and in males, painful swelling of the testicles or orchitis.

The vaccine contains live attenuated mumps virus grown in chicken embryo cell cultures. Reactions to the vaccine are rare; however, individuals with a history of anaphylactic reaction after eating eggs should not be vaccinated. Boosters are not required.

POLIOMYELITIS

Occasional cases of poliomyelitis caused by wild virus still occur in the US and, therefore, all health care providers should have completed a primary series of trivalent oral polio vaccine (OPV) which contains live attenuated polioviruses, types 1, 2, and 3. Inactivated poliovirus vaccine (IPV) is indicated in persons over 18 years of age because of the slightly increased risk of vaccine-associated paralysis in adults following the administration of OPV. In addition, the virus may be shed following the receipt of the OPV vaccine, inadvertently exposing immunocompromised contacts to live vaccine virus.

After ingestion of the OPV, the attenuated polioviruses infect the mucosa of the small intestine and stimulate the production of both circulating and surface antibodies. A recipient of the OPV, if exposed later to virulent polioviruses, is protected against intestinal infection and against poliomyelitis. Persons who receive the IPV which induces only the production of circulating antibodies, if exposed later to virulent poliomyelitis, are protected against poliomyelitis, but not against the intestinal infection.

OPV or IPV boosters are recommended for fully immunized health care providers only if there has been direct contact with oral secretions or feces of a person with poliomyelitis. OPV is recommended for unimmunized health care providers, regardless of age, who have direct contact with a case of polio.

HEPATITIS B (HB)

The risk of HB infection among health care workers is well established and correlates directly with the degree of exposure to blood or blood products. Consequently, HB vaccine is recommended for all health care providers.

Primary immunization with HB vaccine consists of three intramuscular (IM) doses of 1.0 ml of vaccine each. The second and third doses should be given 1 and 6 months, respectively, after the first. The deltoid muscle is the preferred site because injections given into the buttocks have yielded a lower seroconversion rate than expected. Because the vaccine contains only noninfectious HBsAg particles, there should be no risk to the fetus. In contrast, HBV infections in a pregnant woman may result in severe disease for the mother and chronic infection for the newborn. Pregnancy should not be considered a contraindication to the use of this vaccine for persons who are otherwise eligible. Soreness at the site of the infection is the most common adverse effect that has been associated with the HB vaccine.

A combination of hepatitis B immune globulin (HBIG) and HB vaccine therapies is the HB postexposure prophylaxis of choice for persons who have not been immunized with HB vaccine.

Susceptible personnel who have had a single parenteral, oral, or mucosal exposure to blood, secretions, or excretions *known* to be positive for hepatitis B surface antigen (HBsAg) should be administered a single dose of HBIG (0.06 ml/ kg IM) within 24 hours (see Appendix D). This is followed by a complete course of the HB vaccine, with the first dose of vaccine administered within 7 days of exposure and the remaining two doses given according to the recommended schedule for the vaccine. The first dose of vaccine may be given at the same time as the single dose of HBIG if administered at a different site. However, the HB vaccine should be given into the deltoid rather than the buttocks. Use of the HB vaccine eliminates the need for a second dose of HBIG.

If the person chooses not to take the HB vaccine, the regular, two-dose schedule for HBIG should be followed, with the first dose (0.06 ml/kg IM) administered ideally within 24 hours of exposure and the second identical dose given 25 to 30 days after the first dose. If HBIG is not available, IG can be given in the same dosage and schedule. Persons known to have antibodies to hepatitis B virus antigens or whose blood contains HBsAg do not need immunoprophylaxis. More information about hepatitis and hepatitis B vaccine is contained in Chapter 2.

INFLUENZA

Immunization of health care providers with the influenza vaccine is strongly recommended. Not only will vaccination reduce time lost from work, but it will also minimize the transmission of influenza from health care providers to patients. Annual immunization is recommended, particularly for health care providers with diabetes and other metabolic diseases, severe anemia, chronic pulmonary, cardiovascular, or renal disease, immunocompromised individuals, those over 65 years of age, and all other health providers who may have contact with high-risk patients.

Adult immunization with the influenza virus vaccine consists of 1 IM (intramuscular) dose of 0.5 ml of vaccine. Local tenderness for 1 to 2 days at the site of injection is the most common associated side effect of the vaccine observed in fewer than one-third of the recipients. Malaise and low-grade fever for up to 48 hours are infrequent, and hypersensitivity reactions are rare.

The viruses contained in the influenza vaccine are grown in chicken embryo and are inactivated with formalin to minimize the amount of residual egg protein in the vaccine. Although allergic reactions are rare, persons who have had signs and symptoms of an anaphylactic reaction to eggs should not be given the vaccine. However, the vaccine will not cause influenza because the viruses that it contains are not infectious.

The virus content of the vaccine is revised each year to incorporate the new strains that are expected to be prevalent. When the vaccine contains the prevalent strains of viral organisms in a given year, the incidence of influenza is reduced by up to 90% in immunized persons. However, the immunity produced by the vaccine is temporary and annual reimmunization with the appropriate strains is necessary.

TETANUS-DIPHTHERIA (Td)

Health care providers not previously immunized should receive a series of two doses of tetanus-diphtheria (adult) vaccine 4 to 8 weeks apart, followed by a booster 6 to 12 months later. Subsequent to the primary series of immunizations, a Td booster should be administered every 10 years.

Previously vaccinated health care providers with puncture wounds or lacerations should receive a Td booster if more than 10 years have elapsed since their last booster. Those with severe or heavily contaminated wounds may require adsorbed tetanus toxoid *and* human tetanus immune globulin if their history of previous primary tetanus immunizations is uncertain or inadequate. If boosters are given too often, tetanus toxoid can cause severe local pain and swelling.

SUMMARY

The high degree of success of routine childhood immunization programs, recognition of the fact that most vaccines routinely recommended for use in adults are poorly utilized, the introduction and subsequent underutilization of the hepatitis B vaccine targeted primarily for adult use, and the weight of evidence to date distinctly in favor of the cost-effectiveness of disease prevention by immunization rather than by disease treatment should bring about an acute interest in the immunization status of oral health care providers.

As no vaccine is completely safe or completely effective, benefits and risks are associated with the use of all immunobiologics. Benefits may range from partial to complete protection against the consequences of disease, while the risks range from common, trivial, and inconvenient side effects to rare, severe, and life-threatening conditions. Consequently, the recommendations for immunization practices must balance scientific evidence of benefits, costs, and risks to achieve optimal levels of protection against infectious diseases.

SELECTED READINGS

Centers for Disease Control (ACIP): Recommendations for protection against viral hepatitis. MMWR, 34:313–324, 329–335, 1985.

Centers for Disease Control (ACIP): Suboptimal response to hepatitis B vaccine given by injection into the buttock. MMWR, 34:105–108, 113, 1985.

Centers for Disease Control (ACIP): Recommendations for protection against viral hepatitis. MMWR, 34:313–324, 329–335, 1985.

Centers for Disease Control (ACIP): Immune globulins for protection against viral hepatitis. MMWR, 30:423–428, 433–435, 1981.

Centers for Disease Control (ACIP): Postexposure prophylaxis of hepatitis B. MMWR, 33:285–290, 1984.

Centers for Disease Control (ACIP): Prevention and control of influenza. MMWR, 34:261–268, 273–275, 1985.

Centers for Disease Control (ACIP): Measles prevention. MMWR, 31:217–224, 229–231, 1982.

Centers for Disease Control (ACIP): Rubella prevention. MMWR, 33:301–310, 315–318, 1984.

Centers for Disease Control (ACIP): Rubella vaccination during pregnancy— United States, 1971–1983. MMWR, 33:365–368, 373, 1984.

Centers for Disease Control (ACIP): Adult immunization: Recommendations of the Immunization Practices Advisory Committee (ACIP). MMWR, 33:1S–68S, 1984.

Committee on Immunization. Council of Medical Societies. Guide for adult immunizations. Philadelphia: American College of Physicians, 1985.

Hayden GF: Measles vaccine failure. A survey of causes and means of prevention. Clin. Pediatr., 18:155–167, 1979.

Chapter 7

Practical Barrier Techniques

All infectious diseases begin with an initial exposure of the body to potentially pathogenic microorganisms. This exposure may result from inhalation, ingestion, percutaneous inoculation, or direct contact with mucous membranes. Not all exposures result in disease because the dose of the microorganism may be too low or the resistance of the body may be great enough to ward off the infection. Thus, it follows that one effective approach to the prevention of disease is to reduce the dose of potentially dangerous microorganisms that may contaminate the body. The techniques used to interfere with this initial step in the infectious disease process are called barrier techniques. They provide a physical barrier between the body and a source of contamination. The barrier techniques discussed here include those that protect the body (gloves, masks, eyeglasses, clinic attire, dental dam) and those that protect environmental surfaces (surface covers).

GLOVES

The skin harbors resident and transient bacterial flora. The resident flora of *Staphylococcus epidermidis*, micrococci, and diphtheroids can be cultured repeatedly from the hands. The transient flora, acquired from the environment, is only present on the hands for short periods of time. More than 100 years ago, Semmelweis and Lister implied that the hands of medical personnel were sources of pathogenic bacteria. Few practitioners, however, consider their hands as threats to the health of their patients. Even fewer practitioners consider that their patients may be infecting them.

Pathogenic microorganisms that are present in blood, saliva, and dental plaque can contaminate the hands of dental health care personnel. These microorganisms can infect the host by passing through dermal defects, and they can contaminate sterile instruments, dental equipment, and other environmental surfaces. The fingernails are common areas for blood impaction and evidence strongly suggests that this blood is not easily removed by dentists' hand-washing techniques. Blood from patients can remain impacted under a practitioner's fingernails for 5 days or longer.

Even the most carefully washed hands (Table 7–1) will not be totally free of resident or transient bacterial florae. Fingernails should be kept short. Orange wood or rounded plastic sticks can be used to clean under the fingernails. When tests were conducted among nurses to simulate hand washing using a skin-coloring dye, results showed that parts of the thumb and areas of the finger tips were missed by a large number of test subjects. The benefits of careful hand washing

Table 7–1.   Suggested Hand Washing Procedures

At the Beginning of the Work Day

1. Remove ALL jewelry and check the surfaces of the hands for hangnails, small cuts/abrasions and sores
2. Clean fingernails with a plastic or wood stick
3. Scrub hands, nails and forearms with a liquid germicidal agent and sterile brush or sponge for 2 minutes and rinse well with cool-lukewarm tap water for 10 seconds
4. Lather hands and forearms with the cleaning agent by rubbing for 10 seconds
5. Repeat lathering and rinsing procedures
6. Dry hands first, then forearms with clean paper towels and use the paper towels to turn off hand-controlled sink faucets

Between Nonsurgical Patients

1. Vigorously lather hands and forearms with a liquid soap and water by rubbing for 10 seconds and rinse with cool lukewarm tap water for 10 seconds
2. Repeat lathering and rinsing procedures 2 times
3. Dry hands first, then forearms with clean paper towels and use the paper towels to turn off hand-controlled faucets

Before Surgery

1. Remove ALL jewelry and clean fingernails with a clean plastic wood stick
2. Scrub nails, hands and forearms with a germicidal agent and a sterile brush or sponge for a total of 7 minutes, using multiple scrub and rinse cycles
3. Rinse hands and forearms with cool, lukewarm tap water, starting with the fingers and keeping your hands above the level of the elbows. Let the water drip from your elbows not your hands
4. Dry with sterile towels
5. Put on sterile gloves by inserting hands into the gloves held around the wrist by an assistant wearing sterile gloves
6. Check gloves for defects

can be negated by practitioners and assistants who turn off contaminated taps or touch trash bin lids to discard used paper towels. Although hand washing helps protect patients from cross-contamination, it can make oral health care providers more susceptible to infection by causing dry, chapped hands. Soaps containing chlorhexidine gluconate, parachlorometaxylenol (PCMX), or iodophors are effective and usually do not irritate the skin. Substituted phenol preparations, such as chlorhexidine gluconate (a bis-phenol) and PCMX are used routinely by many health-care professionals. Although with a single application they significantly lower the concentration of microorganisms on the skin, both require repeated washings throughout the day to attain maximal effectiveness. Active forms of the antimicrobial chemicals accumulate and remain in the epithelial tissues for prolonged periods, thus leaving a residual effect after each wash procedure. This property is called *substantivity* and fosters the build-up of an antimicrobial "barrier" against many common skin contaminants.

When minor trauma occurs to the hands, visual inspection cannot disclose all of the breaks in the epidermis. Any abrasion, cut, or minor trauma can compromise the integrity of the skin, and minor traumata can be portals for a variety of viral and bacterial organisms. To prevent cross-contamination to patients and to protect the hands of oral health care providers, the ADA recommends that gloves be *routinely* worn for the treatment of all patients.

Several types of gloves are available today. The least expensive type is non-sterile, fits both hands, and comes in small, medium, and large sizes. The disadvantage of these gloves is that the fit can be too tight or too loose. The most expensive types of gloves are sterile surgeon's gloves, but their cost is minor when compared to the protection provided.

Table 7–2.   Skin Irritation

Cause	Possible Solution
Excessive multiplication of skin bacteria	Wash hands before gloving and after removing gloves
Irritation to hand washing agent	Change hand washing agent
Irritation to component in the latex compound	1. Change glove manufacturer 2. Use vinyl glove 3. Use underlying cotton glove

The type of gloves to be worn is dictated by the task to be performed. Inexpensive, nonsterile vinyl gloves can be used for examination and charting. Nonsterile but properly fitting latex gloves can be used for operative procedures or for tasks that require a greater tactile sense. The more expensive, sterile surgeon's gloves should be used in surgical procedures.

Utility gloves, such as neoprene or polynitrile gloves, are too thick and bulky for intraoral use, but their puncture-resistant nature makes them excellent for handling contaminated instruments and for operatory clean-up.

Gloving does not replace hand washing. Hands must be washed before gloving and after the gloves are removed. This keeps the level of skin bacteria to a minimum and reduces the irritating build-up of skin bacteria that multiply under the gloves. It also removes most transient bacteria that may contaminate the hands through pinholes and tears. Double gloving reduces the chances of contamination through inherent pinholes.

Examination and surgeon's gloves are manufactured as single-use disposable items—to be used on one patient and then discarded. Reuse of gloves increases infection risks to dental personnel and to the patient. Microorganisms from the first patient may enter inherent pinholes or tears. They may begin to multiply under the glove or enter small cuts or abrasions on the skin. They may also exit through the same defect into the next patient's mouth. Washing latex gloves also begins to weaken them and makes most gloves tacky. Gloves should be stored in a cool dark place.

Some people develop skin irritations or hypersensitivity after wearing gloves. These skin reactions may be caused by one of several factors that must be identified by trial and error, using different types of gloves (Table 7–2).

MASKS

When a tooth is cut with a high-speed turbine handpiece or cleaned with an ultrasonic scaler, blood, saliva, and other debris are atomized and expelled from the mouth. Dental aerosols, therefore, can be defined as solid and/or liquid airborne particles that are a source of microorganisms capable of inducing illness. Particles larger than 50 μm in diameter have inertial forces greater than the frictional force of air, and are ballistic in nature. The highest concentration of microorganisms is found 2 feet in front of the patient, where practitioners and dental hygienists are usually positioned. When the droplets that contain organisms evaporate, residual droplet nuclei form and remain in the operatory. These aerosol particles are usually smaller than 50 μm in diameter and cannot be seen.

Infectious aerosols are composed of dust or droplet nuclei. The dust-borne aerosols can be removed from the air by sedimentation, but droplet nuclei remain suspended in the air for a long time. Droplet nuclei settle slowly and are spread through the operatory by air currents, contaminating the atmosphere. Ninety-five percent of dental aerosols are 5 μm or less in diameter. It has been shown that when an isolated tooth was contaminated with a tracer organism, *Serratia marcescens*, 60% of the generated aerosols contained viable particles capable of direct penetration into the alveoli. Larger droplets and debris, 50 μm to 100 μm in diameter, will fall to the floor and mix with dust within a 2-foot range. Activity in the operatory disturbs settled, contaminated dust, and airborne particles settle on skin and clothing, releasing as many as 1000 particles per minute.

Bacterial counts of one viable particle (VP) per cubic foot of air are considered acceptable in surgical operating rooms. During the use of high-speed turbines, bacterial counts may reach 109 to 300 VPs per cubic foot of air, and a 250% increase over background counts can be measured 35 minutes after a 1.5-minute to 50.0-minute operative procedure. Thirty minutes after instrumentation with an ultrasonic scaler, 5000 VPs per cubic foot of air were noted, representing a 3000% increase in the bacterial count. Ninety percent of the bacterial shower released by ultrasonic scalers has been associated with alpha hemolytic streptococci, which can remain airborne and viable for as long as 24 hours. To date, these have not been associated with airborne infections.

Microorganisms discovered in dental aerosols include staphylococci, streptococci, diphtheroids, pneumococci, tubercle bacilli, influenza virus, hepatitis virus, *Herpesvirus hominis*, and neisseria. These organisms, with the exception of staphylococci, are not usually found in the air.

Masks that cover the mouth and nose reduce inhalation of potentially infectious aerosol particles. They also protect the mucous membranes of the mouth and nose from direct contamination. Masks should be worn whenever aerosols or spatter may be generated.

It has been demonstrated that the filtering efficiencies of commercially available surgical masks varied from 14 to 99% and the glass fiber mat and the synthetic fiber mat were the most effective filters. However, if a mask is worn longer than 20 minutes in an aerosol environment, the outside surface of the mask becomes a nidus of pathogenic bacteria rather than a barrier. It is recommended that a new mask be worn for each patient, and that masks be routinely changed at least once every hour and more often in the presence of heavy aerosol contamination. Masks selected for use should have at least a 95% bacterial filtering efficiency for small particle aerosols (3–5 μ) and must be comfortable and fit well over the nose.

PROTECTIVE EYEGLASSES

During dental procedures, large particles of debris and saliva can be ejected toward the practitioner's face. These particles can contain large concentrations of bacteria and can physically damage the eyes. Protective eyewear is indicated, not only to prevent physical injury, but also to prevent infection. Of particular concern are the herpes simplex viruses and *Staphylococcus aureus*; however, most members of the normal oral flora must be considered as opportunistic pathogens. Recent evidence has shown that hepatitis B can be transmitted to a chimpanzee by gentle placement of contaminated fluid under the eyelid. Infection through the eye may also occur in humans, but this has not yet been documented.

Eyeglasses that give the best protection have both top and side shields, and some models are made to fit over the regular corrective glasses. Clear plastic face shields are also available.

Contaminated protective eyewear should be thoroughly washed with soap and water, rinsed well and sterilized, if possible, or disinfected in an agent that does not damage eyeglasses.

Disposable eyeglasses for the patient also should be considered for protection from accidentally dropped instruments, chemical splashes, and other foreign object injury.

RUBBER DAMS

It has also been demonstrated that the use of a rubber dam consistently reduced bacterial counts with or without an air-water spray combination. The rubber dam was most effective in reducing bacterial counts when water spray and high-volume evacuation were used. Water further reduced the number of microorganisms in aerosols when a spray was used.

CLOTHING

Dental aerosols and spatter can contaminate clothing worn by dentists and by the clinical staff. Gowns or clinic jackets should be worn to avoid contamination of street clothing. To prevent cross-contamination to family members, operatory clothing should be removed in the office and laundered separately from street clothes.

SURFACE COVERS

Many operatory surfaces become contaminated during patient care by dental aerosols, salivary spatter, or contaminated fingers. If these surfaces are not protected during treatment or disinfected after treatment, they may serve as sources for cross contamination of the next patient.

Examples of operatory surfaces that lend themselves to barrier protection with disposable covers are:

light handles	unit controls
chair switches	bracket/instrument tables
head rests	handpiece shafts
handpiece hoses	air-water syringe controls

An effective cover must be impermeable to water. A material manufactured and advertised as a surface barrier should be accompanied with evidence of the impermeable nature of the product. In general terms, paper items are not effective covers, whereas disposable knobs and handles, plastic wrap, vinyl latex, and aluminum foil materials are probably effective if corroborated by permeability test results. If moisture is absorbed through the cover to the underlying surface, then the purpose of the barrier is defeated and the surface must be disinfected. The protective covers must be replaced after each patient and must be disposed of properly as contaminated items.

OTHER MEASURES

The use of high-volume aspiration during operative procedures reduces further the production of both spatter and aerosols. The ejection of particulate matter during polishing procedures can be further minimized by avoiding the use of bristle brushes. Rubber caps should be used instead.

It has been shown that having the patient rinse with water before operative procedures can reduce the bacterial count in the aerosols generated by 75%. Brushing the teeth can reduce the bacterial count in aerosols by 90%, and the use of a mouthwash can reduce the bacterial count by 98%. A study tested four commercially available mouthwashes of different formulations (quaternary ammonium compound base, phenol base, essential oil base, and zinc chloride base). The results showed that water and the four chemical types of mouthwash, when used with toothbrushing, were equally effective in reducing aerosols. A recently developed formulation contains 0.12% chlorhexidine gluconate. This type of rinse effects a prolonged suppression of oral microorganisms over a 5-hour period when compared with other alcohol-containing mouthwashes or water.

Microorganisms that are retracted up into the handpiece or water spray hose can be transmitted in the aerosol when the handpiece or water spray is used. The American National Standard—American Dental Association Specification No. 47 (April 21, 1984) states that the handpiece should not retract more than 2.032 centimeters back into the handpiece to minimize cross-contamination between patients. Antiretraction valves that are inserted into the water hose are now available that meet or exceed this standard.

Flushing water through the handpiece can also lessen the chance of cross-contamination. Flushing does not eliminate the possibility that the handpiece will be a source of contamination, so additional measures are necessary. The handpiece should be autoclavable or chemically disinfected.

SUMMARY

The barrier techniques of using gloves, masks, protective eyeglasses, clinic attire, rubber dams, and surface covers are among the most efficient approaches to disease prevention. They interfere with the initial step (exposure) in the development of an infectious disease.

SELECTED READINGS

Abel, L.C., et al.: Studies on dental aerobiology: IV. Bacterial contamination of water delivered by dental units. J. Dent. Res., 50:1567–1579, 1971.

Belting, C.M., Haberfelde, G.C., and Juhl, L.K.: Spread of organisms from dental air rotor. J. Am. Dent. Assoc., 68:648–651, 1964.

Brown, R.V.: Bacterial aerosols generated by ultra-high speed cutting instruments. J. Dent. Child., 32:112–117, 1965.

Davies, P.A.: Please wash your hands. Arch. Dis. Child., 57:647–648, 1982.

Grenby, T.H., and Saldanha, M.G.: The antimicrobial activity of modern mouthwashes. Br. Dent. J., 157:239–244, 1984.

Hausler, W.J., and Madden, R.M.: Microbiological comparison of dental handpieces: 2. Aerosol decay and dispersion. J. Dent. Res., 45:52–58, 1966.

Langmuir, A.D.: Contact and airborne infections. In: Preventive Medicine and Public Health, 10th Ed. Edited by K.E. Maxcy and M.J. Rosenau. New York, Appleton-Century-Crofts, 1973, p. 248.

Larato, D.C., et al.: Effect of a dental air turbine on the bacterial counts in air. J. Prosthet. Dent., 16:758–765, 1966.

Lu, D.P., and Zambito, R.F.: Aerosols and cross-infection in the dental practice: A historic view. Gen. Dent., 29:136–143, 1981.

Madden, R.M., Hausler, W.J., and Leaverton, P.E.: Study of some factors contributing to aerosol production by the air turbine handpiece. J. Dent. Res., 48:341–345, 1969.

Micik, R.E., et al.: Studies on dental aerobiology: I. Bacterial aerosols generated during dental procedures. J. Dent. Res., 48:49–56, 1969.

Mills, S.E., et al.: Disinfection of dental unit water lines with 10 percent providone iodine. J. Dent. Res., 64:195, 1985.

Palenki, M.S., and Miller, C.H.: Approaches to preventing disease transmission in the dental office. Dent. Asepsis Rev., 5(9), 1984.

Pistocco, L.R., and Bowers, G.M.: Demonstration of an aerosol produced by air-water spray and air-turbine pieces. US Navy Med., 40:24, 1962.

Pokowitiz, W.M., and Hoffman, H.: Dental aerobiology. NY J. Dent., 37:337–351, 1971.

Register-General of Great Britain: Death from Respiratory Tuberculosis. London: H.M. Printing Office, 1931.

Scheid, R.C., et al.: Reduction of microbes in handpieces by flushing before use. J. Am. Dent. Assoc., 105:658–660, 1982.

Shreve, W.B., Wachtel, L.W., and Pelleu, G.B.: Air cleaning devices for reduction in number of airborne bacteria. J. Dent. Res., 49:1078–1082, 1970.

Spendlove, J.C., and Fannin, K.F.: Source, significance, and control of indoor microbial aerosols: Human health aspects. Public Health Rep., 98:229–244, 1983.

Stevens, R.E.: Preliminary study—Air contamination with microorganisms during use of air turbine handpieces. J. Am. Dent. Assoc., 66:237–239, 1963.

The American Dental Association: Dentist's Desk Reference: Materials, Instruments, and Equipment. Chicago, American Dental Association, 1981, pp. 16–17.

Underhill, T.E., and Terezhalmy, G.T.: Epidemiologic aspects of infectious diseases important to dentists. Comp. Cont. Educ. Dent., 7:48–57, 1986.

Underhill, T.E., Terezhalmy, G.T., and Cottone, J.A.: Prevention of cross-infections in the dental environment. Comp. Cont. Educ. Dent., 7:260–269, 1986.

Wyler, D., Miller, R.L., and Micik, R.E.: Efficacy of self-administered preoperative oral hygiene procedures in reducing the concentration of bacteria in aerosols generated during dental procedures. J. Dent. Res., 50:509, 1971.

Sterilization and Chemical Disinfection

Chapter 8

Instrument Sterilization and Monitoring

A basic guideline for infection control is: **Do not disinfect when you can sterilize.** In fact, sterilization is the most important component of an infection control program. In this regard, a distinction between important outcomes such as sterilization and disinfection is essential. *Sterilization* is defined as the destruction or removal of all forms of life, with particular reference to microorganisms. The limiting requirement and basic criterion for sterilization is the destruction of bacterial and mycotic spores, because these are the most heat-resistant microbial forms. In contrast, *disinfection* refers only to the inhibition or destruction of pathogens. Spores are not killed during disinfection procedures and, in fact, the use of disinfectants constitutes a compromise from the above guide. By custom, the term disinfectant is reserved for those chemicals applied to inanimate surfaces.

The following chapter will consider the application of sterilization procedures and equipment in dental medicine. These include such physical modes as steam under pressure, dry heat, and unsaturated chemical vapor sterilization. Gas sterilization with ethylene oxide and chemical sterilization using glutaraldehyde or chlorine dioxide chemical solutions will also be discussed, although the latter chemicals will be considered in a later chapter. Because the preparation of items for sterilization can affect the actual sterilizing process, instrument recirculation will comprise a segment of the discussion. In the last portion of the chapter, the importance of and the mechanisms for sterilization monitoring will also be included.

PHYSICAL METHODS OF STERILIZATION

The utilization of heat has long been recognized as the most efficient, reliable method of achieving instrument sterilization. The CDC and the ADA Council on Dental Therapeutics have repeatedly stressed this in their recommendations. Accordingly, heat sterilization is required for all instruments and items that can withstand repeated exposure to high temperatures.

The following section will primarily consider the most appropriate physical methods of sterilization. A summary of the standard conditions for each of these, as well as the requirements for ethylene oxide are presented in Tables 8–1 through 8–4.

Steam Sterilization

Efficient sterilization can be accomplished by the use of moist heat at higher temperatures in the form of saturated steam under pressure. This method is the

Table 8–1.   Characteristics of Autoclave Sterilization

Temperature: 121°C (250°F)	Temperature: 134°C (273°F)
Pressure: 15 psi	Pressure: 30 psi
Cycle Time: 15 to 20 minutes	Cycle Time: 3 to 5 minutes
Packaging material requirements Must allow steam to penetrate	
Acceptable materials Paper, plastic, or surgical muslin	
Unacceptable materials Closed metal and glass containers	

Advantages
  1. Short cycle time
  2. Good penetration
  3. Wide range of materials can be processed without destruction	

Disadvantages
  1. Corrosion of unprotected carbon steel instruments
  2. Dulling of unprotected cutting edges
  3. Packages may remain wet at end of cycle
  4. May destroy heat-sensitive materials	

oldest of the acceptable physical modes for instrument sterilization. In its usual application, an autoclave is used for this purpose. A temperature of 121°C (250°F) is applied for 15 to 20 minutes. These conditions yield 15 pounds pressure of steam at sea level (Table 8–1). Direct exposure to saturated steam at 121°C for 10 minutes normally destroys all forms of microbial life. In practice, an additional "safety factor" interval must be allowed for the temperature to reach this point in the center of thick packages of instruments. Sterilization intervals may vary with load size, the use of different instrument wraps, and the nature of the materials to be sterilized. Most surgical wrap materials and commercial bags will allow the steam to penetrate sufficiently to kill all microbial forms. Even when thick wrapping materials are used, a maximal sterilization period of 30 minutes usually suffices. Advances in sterilizer technology have allowed for the application of higher temperatures and pressures for shorter intervals in newer equipment used in many dental facilities.

As efficient as autoclaving can be, this procedure is effective only when suitable conditions are present in the pressured chamber. Areas of preparation and operation that pose problems for steam sterilization include: faulty preparation of materials for sterilization (packaging that does not allow for penetration of steam), improper loading of the instrument chamber, improper functioning of the sterilizer (failure to reach temperature and/or pressure), the presence of air in the chamber (may delay microbial destruction up to 10 times longer), and excess water in the steam (can serve as passageway for microorganisms to get through wet instrument packages).

Corrosion or accumulation of rust on metallic instruments also comprises a major problem when an autoclave is used for sterilization. Even the best autoclaves contain sufficient oxygen to cause carbon steel corrosion. A preventive solution using chemicals that vaporize in the autoclave and protect metal from oxidation by hydrolysis can be used. A common agent for this purpose contains 1% sodium nitrite.

Table 8–2. Characteristics of Dry Heat Sterilization

Temperature: 160°C (320°F)	Temperature: 170°C (340°F)
Cycle Time: 2 hours	Cycle Time: 1 hour

Packaging material requirements
  Must not insulate items from heat. Must not be destroyed by
    temperature used

Acceptable materials
  Paper bags, muslin, aluminum foil, aluminum trays, and pans

Unacceptable materials
  Plastic bags

Advantages
  1. Effective and safe for sterilization of metal instruments and mirrors
  2. Does not dull cutting edges
  3. Does not rust or corrode

Disadvantages
  1. Long cycle required for sterilization
  2. Poor penetration
  3. May discolor and char fabric
  4. Destroys heat-labile items

Dry Heat

The destruction of all forms of microbial life in the absence of moisture requires different conditions than those discussed previously. As proteins dry, their resistance to denaturation increases. Thus, at a given temperature, dry heat sterilizes much less efficiently than moist heat, and, as shown in Table 8–2, higher temperatures are required for a properly functioning hot air oven. Sterilization of instruments with dry heat is the least expensive form of heat sterilization. A complete cycle involves heating the oven to the appropriate temperature and maintaining that temperature for the proper interval.

Practical destruction of microorganisms by dry heat in a dental facility is accomplished by using a unit that has been tested and approved by the FDA as a commercial sterilizer. Because dry air is not as efficient a heat conductor as moist heat at the same temperature, a much higher temperature is required for sterilization. The usual recommended practice is to hold the temperature at 160°C for 2 hours. A 1-hour exposure at 170°C will also be effective. These conditions are suitable for sterilizing metal instruments that rust or dull in the presence of water vapor. Many dental practitioners prefer the use of dry heat sterilizers in their offices because of the preservation of sharp cutting edges on their surgical instruments. However, these high temperatures will destroy many rubber and plastic-based materials, melt the solder of most impression trays, and weaken some fabrics, as well as discolor other fabrics and paper materials. As with the design of newer generations of autoclaves, advances in the technology for dry heat sterilization are continuing. Dry heat convection units are currently available that use higher temperatures and require substantially shorter sterilization intervals.

One of the most common problems with the employment of a dry heat sterilizer is the failure of clinical personnel to properly time the sterilization interval. Because the penetration of dry heat into the center of an instrument pack is slow and depends both on the size of packages and the type of wrapping material, one must be certain that appropriate preheating of the chamber is accomplished before beginning the sterilization cycle. A common misuse of this apparatus can occur when the oven is opened and an instrument is quickly removed during the timed cycle.

Table 8–3.   Characteristics of Unsaturated Chemical Vapor Sterilization

Temperature: 131°C (270°F)
Pressure: 20 psi
Cycle Time: 30 minutes

Packaging material requirements
    Vapors must be allowed to precipitate on contents
    Vapors must not react with packaging material
    Plastics should not contact sides of sterilizer

Acceptable Materials   Perforated metal trays or paper
Unacceptable materials   Solid metal trays and sealed glass jars

Advantages
    1. Short cycle time
    2. Does not rust or corrode metal instruments, including carbon steel
    3. Does not dull cutting edges
    4. Suitable for orthodontic stainless wires

Disadvantages
    1. Instruments must be completely dried before processing
    2. Will destroy heat-sensitive plastics
    3. Chemical odor in poorly ventilated areas

This interrupts the cycle, and thus, timing must begin all over again. In addition, it is important to keep a space between instrument packs during dry heat sterilization. Because the air does not circulate well, failure to ensure uniform hot air distribution during the cycle may cause some packages to become sterilized, while others in the same load are not. Thick wraps and larger than normal packages can also significantly increase the interval required for assured sterility. Some individuals also view the prolonged exposure times for dry heat as a disadvantage. The argument is made that if only one sterilizer is available, the 1- to 2-hour period plus cooling time disrupts a smooth flow of instrument recirculation.

Unsaturated Chemical Vapor

This system depends on heat, water, and chemical synergism for its efficacy; a mixture of alcohols, formaldehyde, ketone, acetone, and water is employed. As shown in Table 8–3, the temperature and pressure required with chemical vapor sterilizers are greater than those for the autoclave. The principle of operation has similarities with steam sterilizers, but also some important distinctions. The solution of premixed chemicals added to the unit reservoir must be purchased from the manufacturer, because the ratio of each in the preparation is critical. After the apparatus is preheated, the clean, dry, loosely wrapped instruments are placed in the chamber. The package wraps must be loose to allow the chemical vapors to condense on the instrument surfaces during the cycle. Thick, tightly wrapped items will require longer exposure because of the inability of the unsaturated chemical vapors to penetrate as well as saturated steam under pressure. Metal instruments must be dry prior to sterilization, or chemicals will accumulate on the wetted surfaces and corrosion will occur.

The major advantages of chemical vapor sterilization are: a short cycle time similar to that for the autoclave, no rusting of instruments and burs in contrast to steam sterilization, the removal of dry instruments at the end of the cycle, and

Table 8–4. Characteristics of Ethylene Oxide Sterilization

Temperature: Room temperature (25°C/75°F)

Cycle Time: 10 to 16 hours (depending on material)

Packaging material requirements
  Gas must be allowed to penetrate

Acceptable materials
  Paper, plastic bags

Unacceptable materials
  Sealed metal or glass containers

Advantages
  1. High capacity for penetration
  2. Does not damage heat-labile materials (including rubber and handpieces)
  3. Evaporates without leaving a residue
  4. Suitable for materials that cannot be exposed to moisture

Disadvantages
  1. Slow—requires long cycle times
  2. Retained in liquids and rubber materials for prolonged intervals
  3. Causes tissue irritation if not well aerated
  4. Requires special "sparkshield"—explosive in presence of flame or sparks

automatic, preset cycle timing. The presence of only about 8 to 9% water vapor in the chemical solution is significantly below the 15% minimum for rusting and dulling, and this property prevents destruction of dental items such as endodontic files, orthodontic pliers, wires and bands, burs and carbon steel instruments. Thus, a wide range of items can be routinely sterilized. However, the requirement of adequate ventilation can constitute a problem for practitioners who use this type of apparatus. Chemical vapors, particularly formaldehyde, can be released when the chamber door is opened at the end of the cycle, and these leave a temporary unpleasant odor in the area. Although numerous toxicity studies by the manufacturer indicate little chance of eye irritation from these residual vapors, dental personnel may occasionally report some discomfort if the sterilizer is in an area with poor air circulation. To counteract this detrimental aspect, later models were equipped with a special filtration device that further reduces the amount of vapor left in the chamber at the end of the cycle.

Ethylene Oxide

Ethylene oxide is actually a chemical sterilant. The use of this gaseous agent is recognized by the ADA and CDC as an acceptable method of sterilization, especially for those items that can be damaged by heat and/or moisture. Ethylene oxide is a highly penetrative colorless gas at room temperature. This chemical is effective as sporicidal agent, is virucidal, does not damage materials, and evaporates without a residue. Table 8–4 summarizes some of the features that characterize its clinical use. Materials such as suction tubing, all handpieces, radiographic film holders, and prosthetic appliances may be sterilized without adverse effect.

Pure ethylene oxide is rather toxic, allergenic, slow in its action, and forms explosive mixtures with air. Commercial preparations therefore contain carbon dioxide or an inert gas to form a more stable active combination. Ethylene oxide functions as an alkylating agent by irreversibly inactivating cellular nucleic acids and proteins. Multiple chemical sites on these molecules are most susceptible to this binding, including exposed $-NH_2$, $-COOH$, $-SH$, and $-OH$ groups. Be-

Table 8–5.   Recommendations For Operation of an Ultrasonic Cleaner

1. Whenever possible, clean instruments ultrasonically before hand scrubbing
2. Always wear heavy duty gloves and protective eyewear
3. Prerinse all instruments
4. Clean only 8 to 10 loose instruments at a time
5. Use a cleaning solution sold by a cleaner manufacturer
6. Use separate breakers for special cleaning solutions
7. Keep the solution level at least 1½ inches from the top of the tank
8. Clean loose instruments in basket for 5 to 8 minutes
9. Clean instruments for 10 to 15 minutes unless the manufacturer recommends another time
10. Rinse the instruments well
11. Inspect and dry instruments before wrapping or packaging
12. Change cleaning water at least once a day
13. Disinfect unit tank and dry well at the end of the work day
14. Test ultrasonic unit for cleaning efficiency at least once a month

Adapted from Dent. Asepsis Rev., 9:9, 1988 Rouse, M. Health Sonics Corp. (Personal Communication)

cause the toxic effects are not selective for microorganisms and a potential for explosion remains during the sterilization cycle, materials must be processed in a special container (i.e., spark shield), which is placed in a well-ventilated area.

The slow penetration of gas throughout the holding container signals a prolonged sterilization interval, subsequently followed by an aeration interval. In most cases, 10 to 16 hours are sufficient for sterilization of nonrubber-based items. For those containing rubber or porous plastic, an additional 24 to 48 hours may be required to allow for complete dissipation of ethylene oxide from the porous material. Residual gas can cause painful burns when improperly aerated items come into contact with epithelial tissues. For those liquids that can be sterilized by ethylene oxide, aeration may have to occur over even longer intervals.

INSTRUMENT PROCESSING AND RECIRCULATION

Routine processing of reusable instruments and other items includes cleaning, packaging, sterilizing, monitoring, and storage of sterilized packages. Any method of sterilization can be overchallenged by accumulated debris such as blood or saliva. At the very least, the interval required for sterilization may be extended, or the bioburden may actually prevent sterilization in some instances. The initial requirement for processing thus involves thorough cleaning by removing any collected organic matter. Hand scrubbing can accomplish this step, although caution must always be exercised to prevent puncture accidents. Heavy duty, puncture-resistant utility gloves should be worn when cleaning, scrubbing, or otherwise handling instruments during processing. Latex examination or surgical gloves are not to be substitutes as they may tear and not provide adequate protection. An alternative or additional method for instrument cleaning utilizes an ultrasonic cleaner (Table 8–5). The removal of saliva and/or blood is significantly enhanced by this method when compared to the results following hand scrubbing. Ultrasonic cleaners should be operated with a cover to prevent aerosolization of contaminants. One should also use only cleaning solutions that are designed for use in an ultrasonic apparatus. Finally, the metal container within the unit should be wiped and cleaned with a suitable cleaner/disinfectant at frequent intervals. This can be accomplished periodically during the day or after each use, depending on the size of the instrument load.

The packaging of items prior to heat or gas sterilization will depend on the type of sterilizer used and the nature of the items to be sterilized. Cleaned instruments should be placed in heat-stable wraps or bags, then sealed and dated. Sterilized instruments should also remain wrapped until used. A general guideline would be to consider many commercial wraps and sealed pouches as capable of maintaining sterility for 1 month. Removal of sterilized instruments from a package and placement in cabinet drawers for later use is not recommended. A list published by the ADA concerning the application of various forms of sterilization for instruments and other intraoral items is presented in Table 8–6 and Appendix A.

STERILIZATION OF DENTAL HANDPIECES

Advances in technology have impacted on the area of handpiece sterilization. Heat sterilization of this important piece of equipment was not possible for many years, because many of the unit's components could not withstand the elevated temperatures required. Ethylene oxide sterilization will accomplish the task, but is not currently practical for routine use. As a result of this dilemma, dental professionals usually only disinfected the outer surfaces of their handpieces. Neither cleaning, disinfection, nor sterilization of the internal components was accomplished, even though these areas were also exposed to saliva and blood. The manufacture and sale of heat sterilizable handpieces resolved many of these problems. As a result, current infection control guidelines include a statement for the sterilization of handpieces after use with each patient.

The current recommended methods for heat sterilization prescribe the use of an autoclave or an unsaturated chemical vapor sterilizer. Newer generation, shorter cycle time, dry-heat ovens may also be feasible, and are being tested for their applicability with dental handpieces. For those handpieces that cannot withstand heat, the CDC has outlined a compromise protocol involving appropriate precleaning and subsequent disinfection. It must be noted that handpieces should never be immersed in a disinfectant solution or treated with chemical sterilants such as 2.0 to 3.2% glutaraldehyde solutions. This misuse of chemical preparations substantially shortens handpiece life and increases the chances for glutaraldehyde toxicity reactions during operator handling.

Manufacturers also provide extensive, step-by-step instructions for maintenance of their handpieces. For example, proper lubrication is required prior to wrapping the handpiece for sterilization. Failure to maintain the unit in this manner can diminish its efficiency. The same basic principles and precautions apply for other similar items, such as air/water syringes and tips and ultrasonic scalers.

MONITORING OF STERILIZATION

An integral component of office sterilization procedures is monitoring the efficiency of the system. In 1986, the CDC published their recommended infection control guidelines for dentistry, which stated that "heat and steam-sensitive indicators may be used on the outside of each pack to assure it has been exposed to a sterilizing cycle." A more stringent requirement was included later where the

Table 8–6. Sterilization and Disinfection of Dental Instruments, Materials, and Some Commonly Used Items*

	Steam Autoclave	Dry Heat Oven	Chemical Vapor	Ethylene Oxide	Chemical Disinfection/ Sterilization	Other Methods/Comments
Angle attachments·	+	+	+	+ +	+	
Burs						
Carbon steel	−	+ +	+ +	+ +	−	
Steel	+	+ +	+ +	+ +	+	
Tungsten-carbide	+	+ +	+	+ +	+	
Condensers	+ +	+ +	+ +	+ +	+	
Dapen dishes	+ +	+	+	+ +	+	
Endodontic instruments (broaches, files, reamers)						Hot salt glass bead sterilizer 10 to 15 seconds, 218 C (425 F)
Stainless steel handles	+	+ +	+ +	+ +	+	
Stainless with plastic handles	+ +	+ +	−	+ +	−	
Fluoride gel trays						
Heat-resistant plastic	+ +	− −	−	+ +	−	
Nonheat-resistant plastic	− −	− −	−	+ +	−	Discard (+ +)
Glass slabs	+ +	+ +	+ +	+ +	+	
Hand instruments						
Carbon steel						
Stainless steel	+ +	+ +	+ +	+ +	+	
Handpieces·						Sterilizable preferably
Sterilizable·	(+ +)·	−	(+)·	+ +	− −	
Contra-angles·	−	−	−	+ +	+	Combination synthetic phenolics
Nonsterilizable·	−	−	−	+ +	+	or iodophores (−)
Prophylaxis angles·	+	+	+	+	+	
Impression materials						Table 2
Impression trays						
Aluminum metal	+ +	+	+ +	+ +	−	
Chrome plated	+ +	+ +	+ +	+ +	+	
Custom acrylic resin	− −	− −	− −	+ +	+	
Plastic	− −	− −	− −	+ +	+	Discard (+ +): preferred
Instruments in packs	+ +	+ Small packs	+ +	+ + Small packs	− −	
Instrument tray setups	+	+	+	+ +	− −	
Restorative or surgical	Size limit		Size limit	Size limit		
Mirrors	−	+ +	+ +	+ +	+	
Needles						
Disposable	− −	− −	− −	− −	− −	Discard (+ +) Do not reuse
Nitrous oxide						
Nose piece	(+ +)·	− −	(+ +)·	+ +	(+)·	
Hoses	(+ +)·	− −	(+ +)·	+ +	(+)·	
Orthodontic pliers						
High quality stainless	+ +	+ +	+ +	+ + −	+	
Low quality stainless	−	+ +	+ +	+ +	−	
With plastic parts	− −	− −	− −	+ +	+	
Pluggers	+ +	+ +	+ +	+ +	+	
Polishing wheels and disks						
Garnet and cuttle	− −	−	−	+ +	− −	
Rag	+ +	−	+	+ +	− −	
Rubber	+	−	−	+ +	+	
Prostheses, removable	−	−	−	+	+	

Hand instruments, Carbon steel: [Steam autoclave with chemical protection (1% sodium nitrite)]

Table 8–6. Sterilization and Disinfection of Dental Instruments, Materials, and Some Commonly Used Items* *Continued*

	Steam Autoclave	Dry Heat Oven	Chemical Vapor	Ethylene Oxide	Chemical Disinfection/ Sterilization	Other Methods/Comments
Rubber dam equipment						
Carbon steel clamps	−	+ +	+ +	+ +	−	
Metal frames	+ +	+ +	+ +	+ +	+	
Plastic frames	−	−	−	+ +	+	
Punches	−	+ +	+ +	+ +	+	
Stainless steel clamps	+ +	+ +	+ +	+ +	+	
Rubber items						
Prophylaxis cups	−	−	−	+ +	−	Discard (+ +)
Saliva evacuators, ejectors						
Low melting plastic	−	−	−	+ +	+	Discard (+ +)
High melting plastic	+ +	+	+	+ +	+	
Stones						
Diamond	+	+ +	+ +	+ +	+	
Polishing	+ +	+	+ +	+ +	−	
Sharpening	+ +	+ +	+ +	−		
Surgical instruments						
Stainless steel	+ +	+ +	+ +	+ +	+	
Ultrasonic sealing tips	+	− −	− −	+ +	+	
Water-air syringe tips	+ +	+ +	+ +	+ +	+	
X-ray equipment						
Plastic film holders	(+ +)·	− −	(+)·	+ +	+	
Collimating devices	−	− −	− −	+ +	+	

*Reprinted with permission from Council on Dental Therapeutics: Infection control recommendations for the dental office and the dental laboratory. J. Am. Dent. Assoc., *116*:241–248, 1988.

The table is adapted from *Accepted Dental Therapeutics* and *Dentists' Desk Reference Materials, Instruments, and Equipment.*

·As manufacturers use a variety of alloys and materials in these products, confirmation with the equipment manufacturers is recommended, especially for handpieces and the attachments.

+ + Effective and preferred method.

+ Effective and acceptable method.

− Effective method, but risk of damage to materials.

− − Ineffective method with risk of damage to materials.

periodic use of spore testing devices was designated as the definitive verification of sterilization. Thus, routine monitoring of sterilization includes the use of heat-sensitive indicators with each sterilization cycle, as well as use of a biological monitoring system. The CDC has suggested weekly monitoring of dental sterilizers, modeling their recommendations after long-standing protocols used in hospitals.

A multitude of factors may diminish the effectiveness of an autoclave, dry heat sterilizer, or unsaturated chemical vapor apparatus. Frequent problems include: improper wrapping of instruments, which can prevent adequate penetration onto the instrument surface; human error in timing the cycle; defective control gauges that do not reflect actual conditions inside the sterilizer; worn door gaskets and seals; internal chamber temperature variations; and sterilizer malfunction.

One may employ chemically treated tapes that change color or biological controls to check for the proper functioning of an office sterilizer. Materials that change color generally inform the practitioner that sterilizing conditions have been reached, but do not necessarily indicate that sterilization of the chamber contents has been achieved. In addition, certain indicators change color long before sterilization occurs and before appropriate conditions are met. Autoclave tape is probably the worst offender in this regard, as it will change to show the striped markings following brief exposure to steam.

Heat-sensitive indicators consist of paper strips impregnated with chemicals designed to change color when exposed to heat or chemical vapor. The chemical formulation of the indicator ink on a strip used to monitor autoclaves, for example, makes it sensitive to the correct combination of the three factors necessary for sterilization: time, temperature, and saturated steam. It appears that specific chemical indicators to monitor sterilization are used mainly as a routine check for each load of items processed through the sterilizer. Gross malfunctions can be usually detected quickly by utilization of indicator labels, strips, and steam-pattern cards.

Even though the sterilizer gauges may display correct values for internal conditions, and indicator tapes are used, the employment of calibrated biological controls remains the main guarantee of sterilization. These preparations contain bacterial spores that are more resistant to heat than are viruses and vegetative bacteria. Because a spore vehicle designed for one sterilization method is not necessarily the proper mode to use for other procedures, manufacturers produce both glass vials containing spores and biological test strips in glassine envelopes. The organisms most used are calibrated concentrations of either *Bacillus stearothermophilus* or *Bacillus subtilis* spores. *B. stearothermophilus* spores are the appropriate biologicals for monitoring autoclaves and chemiclaves, while *B. subtilis* preparations are more resistant to the conditions in dry heat ovens and ethylene oxide units.

Bacterial test preparations are either suspended in a nutrient medium (ampule form) or are impregnated onto a test strip with the broth in an adjacent capsule. A pH indicator in the medium is also present; this changes color when spores germinate and produce acids, thereby visually demonstrating a failure to sterilize. Because the spore preparations are relatively heat-resistant, the proof of their destruction after exposure to the sterilization cycle is used to infer that all microorganisms exposed to the same conditions have been destroyed. The demonstration of sporicidal activity by an office sterilizer thus represents the most sensitive check for efficiency.

SELECTED READINGS

ADA Council on Dental Materials and Devices, Council on Dental Therapeutics: Infection control in the dental office. J. Am. Dent. Assoc., 97:673–677, 1978.

ADA Council on Dental Therapeutics: Current status of sterilization instrument devices and methods for the dental office. J. Am. Dent. Assoc., 102:683–689, 1986.

ADA Council on Dental Therapeutics: Infection control recommendations for the dental office and the dental laboratory. J. Am. Dent. Assoc., 116:241–248, 1988.

Block, S.S. (ed.): Disinfection, Sterilization and Preservation. 4th Ed. Philadelphia, Lea and Febiger, 1983.

Centers for Disease Control: Recommended infection control practices for dentistry. MMWR, 35:237–242, 1986.

Crawford, J.J.: Clinical Asepsis in Dentistry. Dallas, R.A. Kolstad, 1978.

Crawford, J.J.: State-of-the-art: Practical infection control in dentistry. JADA, 110:629–633, 1985.

Ernst, R.R., and Shull, J.J.: Ethylene oxide gaseous sterilization. I. Concentration and temperature effects. Appl. Microbiol., 10:337–341, 1962.

Favero, M.S.: Sterilization, disinfection and antisepsis in the hospital. *In* Manual of Clinical Microbiology. 4th Ed. Washington, D.C., American Society for Microbiology, 1985, pp. 129–137.

Joslyn, L.: Sterilization by heat. *In* Disinfection, Sterilization and Preservation. 4th Ed. Edited by S.S. Block. Philadelphia, Lea & Febiger, 1983, pp. 3–46.

Molinari, J.A., Campbell, M.D., and York, J.: Minimizing potential infections in dental practice. J. Mich. Dent. Assoc., *64*:411–416, 1982.

Molinari, J.A., Gleason, M.J., and Merchant, V.A.: Infection control. An overview for dentistry. Calif. Dent. Assoc. J., *16*:14–21, 1988.

Runnells, R.R.: Heat and heat/pressure sterilization. Calif. Dent. Assoc. J., *13*:46–49, 1985.

Runnells, R.R.: Dental Infection Control. Update '88. North Salt Lake, I.C. Publications, 1988.

Whitacre, R.J., Robins, S.K., Williams, B.L., and Crawford, J.J.: Dental Asepsis. Seattle, Stoma Press, 1979.

Chapter 9

Chemical Disinfectants: Use, Reuse, and Misuse

Published guidelines for infection control include the use of chemical sterilants and disinfectants when it is not possible to sterilize or dispose of items that become contaminated during treatment. In addition, numerous operatory surfaces routinely become coated with saliva, blood, and exudate (i.e., bioburden), and require cleaning and disinfection when it is not feasible to use disposable covers.

A variety of commercial products are available as disinfectants, and many may be used in certain instances. It is important to recognize at the outset that the effectiveness of both immersion and surface disinfectants depends on a number of factors. These include (1) concentration and nature of contaminant microorganisms, (2) concentration of chemical, (3) length of exposure time, and (4) amount of accumulated bioburden. Disinfection is defined as the destruction of pathogenic microorganisms on inanimate surfaces. When used as disinfectants, chemicals are not effective against highly resistant forms such as bacterial and mycotic spores. This use of these chemicals thus represents a compromise from the guideline: *Do Not Disinfect When You Can Sterilize.* Available product formulations include immersion or surface solutions, sprays, foams, and wipes, each with a specific rationale for use. Chemical germicides manufactured for disinfection are regulated and registered by the Environmental Protection Agency (EPA), in contrast to those products marketed as antiseptics, which are formulated for use on living tissues and regulated by the Food and Drug Administration (FDA). It is important to note that the procedures and criteria for product approval are different between these two agencies. Thus, one should not attempt to interchange the use of disinfectants and antiseptics. Unfortunately, this misuse of products is common and has led to numerous tissue toxicity reactions and equipment failures.

DISINFECTANT CRITERIA AND ACTIVITY

Choosing appropriate immersion and surface disinfectants has become confusing for many dental professionals because of exaggerated manufacturer claims and misleading assays reported in the literature. The actual performance capabilities of individual agents may therefore be obscured. Confusion also arises when dentists and other treatment providers are not aware of guidelines that assist in the selection of appropriate chemicals. This can be initially alleviated by comparing the efficacy of available agents with published criteria for an *ideal* disinfectant (Table 9–1). As shown in this table, properties to be considered include penetration and

Table 9–1.   Properties Of An Ideal Disinfectant

Broad spectrum
  Should always have the widest possible antimicrobial spectrum

Fast acting
  Should always have a rapidly lethal action on all vegetative forms and spores of bacteria and fungi, protozoa, and viruses

Not affected by physical factors
  Active in the presence of organic matter such as blood, sputum, and feces
  Should be compatible with soaps, detergents, and other chemicals encountered in use

Nontoxic

Surface compatibility
  Should not corrode instruments and other metallic surfaces
  Should not cause the disintegration of cloth, rubber, plastics, or other materials

Residual effect on treated surfaces

Easy to use

Odorless
  An inoffensive odor would facilitate its routine use

Economical
  Cost should not be prohibitively high

Adapted from Molinari, J.A., Campbell, M.D., and York, J.: J. Michigan Dent. Assoc., *64*:411–416, 1982.

activity in the presence of bioburden, a broad antimicrobial spectrum, residual activity that becomes reactivated when surfaces are moistened, minimal toxicity, and compatibility with disinfected surfaces. The most desirable disinfectant would also be tuberculocidal and virucidal. None of the available products fulfills all of these criteria. This will be demonstrated when the properties of available classes of disinfectants are compared with the features of an ideal agent in a later section.

A standard system of classification for chemical sterilants and disinfectants was proposed by Spaulding in 1972. This system was originally developed for classifying hospital instruments according to their use and degree of contamination, but can be adapted to dental instruments and equipment. Patient care items and equipment are placed into one of three categories: critical, semicritical, and non-critical (Table 9–2). In addition, three levels of disinfection are defined: high, intermediate, and low (Table 9–3). Different classes of disinfectants are defined based upon their efficacy against vegetative bacteria, tubercle bacilli, fungal spores, lipid- and nonlipid-containing viruses, and bacterial endospores (Table 9–4). High-level disinfectants are analogous to EPA-registered sporicides, because they are capable of inactivating resistant bacterial spores as well as all other microbial forms. These chemical sterilants are exemplified by ethylene oxide gas (discussed in an earlier chapter) and immersion glutaraldehyde solutions. Both are useful for sterilization

Table 9–2.   Spaulding Classification of Inanimate Objects

Critical: Sterilization Required
  Items that penetrate or touch broken skin or mucous membranes
  Needles, scalpels, surgical instruments, mirrors, and dental explorers

Semicritical: Sterilization or High-Level Disinfection Required
  Items that touch mucous membranes but do not enter sterile body areas
  Amalgam condensers, handpieces, and ultrasonic scalers

Noncritical Items: Tuberculocidal Intermediate-Level Disinfection
  Surfaces that do not touch mucous membranes
  Countertops, light handles, and chair surfaces

Table 9–3. Levels of Germicidal Action

	Efficacy Against					
	Bacteria				Viruses	
Level	Vegetative Bacteria	Tubercle Bacillus	Spores	Fungi[a]	Lipid and Medium-Sized	Nonlipid and Small
High	+[b]	+	+[c]	+	+	+
Intermediate	+	+	±[d]	+	+	±[e]
Low	+	−	−	±	+	−

[a]Includes asexual spores but not necessarily chlamydospores or sexual spores

[b]+, Killing effect can be expected when the normal-use concentrations of chemical disinfectants or pasteurization are properly employed; −, little or no killing effect

[c]Only with extended exposure times are high-level disinfectants capable of actual sterilization

[d]Some intermediate-level disinfectants, e.g., iodophors, formaldehyde, tincture of iodine, and chlorine compounds, can be expected to exhibit some sporicidal action

[e]Some intermediate-level disinfectants, e.g., alcohols and phenolic compounds, may have limited virucidal activity

of those materials that are unable to withstand heat sterilization procedures. Prolonged immersion times of 6 to 10 hours are often required to achieve sterilization with 2.0 to 3.2% glutaraldehyde preparations, however, and the interval can be even longer under conditions of heavy contamination. The ability to kill bacterial spores is an essential criterion for inclusion of a chemical into the high-level disinfectant class.

Even though high-level disinfectants are capable of sterilizing immersed items, these chemicals are often misused. Instead of immersing items in the solution for the required interval (i.e., 6 to 10 hours at room temperature), personnel may use only a 20 to 30 minute exposure and rinse the "sterilized" materials in nonsterile, sanitized water. These items are at best disinfected, and use of such "cold sterilization" represents one of the most abused aspects of infection control. Because the solutions routinely employed in this procedure may not be able to guarantee destruction of all microbial forms present, cold sterilization is actually a misnomer. This term should not be confused with accepted methods of sterilization.

Intermediate-level disinfectants may not inactivate bacterial endospores, but do kill other microbial forms, especially tubercle bacilli. *Mycobacterium tuberculosis* presents a severe challenge to chemical disinfectants, and is considered to be the most resistant microorganism after bacterial endospores. Formaldehyde, chlorine compounds, iodophors, alcohols, and phenolic disinfectants are included in this class. It should be noted that there can be differences between intermediate-level disinfectants with regard to their ability to inactivate small, nonlipid viruses (hydrophilic), which are much more resistant than medium-sized, lipid-coated viruses (Table 9–5). Thus, the ability to destroy *M. tuberculosis* does not necessarily signify that a chemical solution is able to inactivate all viruses. When an intermediate-level disinfectant is selected for use in dentistry, it should be EPA registered as a

Table 9–4. Spaulding Classification of Chemical Disinfectants

Bacterial endospores *Mycobacterium tuberculosis* Small non-lipid viruses Fungi Medium-sized lipid viruses Vegetative bacteria	Resistance

Table 9–5. Major Virus Categories

Hydrophilic Viruses	Lipophilic Viruses
Rotavirus WA	Herpes simplex - 1
Rotavirus SA 11	Herpes simplex - 2
Poliovirus type 2	Influenza A_2
	Human immunodeficiency virus

tuberculocidal, hospital disinfectant, with appropriate virucidal activity. The designation "hospital disinfectant" is given by the EPA to those products which are documented to kill the three species of basic test bacteria: *Staphylococcus aureus*, *Salmonella typhimurium*, and *Pseudomonas aeruginosa*.

Chemical agents with the narrowest antimicrobial range are classified as low-level disinfectants. Examples of common disinfectants in this group include quaternary ammonium compounds, simple phenolics, and detergents. They are suitable for cleaning environmental surfaces in a treatment area but are unacceptable for disinfection of routine items and equipment that are classified as critical or semicritical. Although low-level disinfectants may inactivate certain viruses and vegetative bacteria, they will not kill tubercle bacilli, nonlipid viruses, or fungi.

MECHANISMS OF ANTIMICROBIAL ACTION

Most chemical disinfectants disrupt target cells by acting as cytoplasmic poisons. This general lack of specificity limits the usefulness of these agents to inanimate objects. Any part or all of three major portions of microbial cells can be affected: cell wall, cytoplasmic contents (particularly enzymes), and nuclear material. Resultant microbial destruction is accomplished by one of a number of possible reactions, or a combination of multiple reactions. These will be further discussed for each class of chemical disinfectant.

DETERGENTS (SURFACE-ACTIVE SUBSTANCES)

Detergents are those preparations that alter the nature of interfaces to lower surface tension and increase cleaning. The antimicrobial effect occurs primarily on the cell membrane by alteration of the osmotic barrier. This results in increased cell permeability. Target cells are subsequently unable to maintain their integrity. Common surface-active agents are classified as nonionic, anionic, or cationic. Nonionic chemicals do not possess any antimicrobial properties. Anionic preparations are represented by soaps and synthetic anionic detergents. Soaps are salts of long-chain aliphatic carboxylic acids of animal and plant fats. Most synthetic anionic detergents contain alkyl and/or aryl sulfates or sulfonates. The alkali content and sodium salt are responsible for the cidal effects of soaps on streptococci, treponemes, pneumococci, gonococci, and influenza viruses. Despite these effects, the primary value of anionic detergents appears to be caused by their mechanical cleansing action.

Cationic surface-active disinfectants are exemplified by the quaternary ammonium preparations. These agents are germicidal in a much lower concentration than anionic detergents, and can remain bacteriostatic in relatively high dilutions. The most probable site of antimicrobial action for quaternary ammoniums is the cell membrane. Alteration of the membrane triggers release of enzymes and cellular

Table 9–6. Disinfectant Characteristics of Quaternary Ammonium Compounds

Advantages	Disadvantages
1. EPA registered	1. Not tuberculocidal, sporicidal, or virucidal against hydrophilic viruses
2. Bactericidal against gram-positive bacteria	2. Inactivated by anionic detergents, i.e., soaps and hard water
3. Pleasant odor	3. Inactivated by organic matter, i.e., blood, plaque, saliva, and exudate
4. Nonirritating	4. Solutions sometimes support the growth of gram-negative bacteria
5. Economical	5. NOT APPROVED FOR INSTRUMENT OR SURFACE DISINFECTION BY THE ADA

metabolites, with gram-positive bacteria being most susceptible to destruction. Little or no cidal effects occur on many gram-negative bacteria, bacterial spores, most viruses, and fungi. Severe limitations in the use of cationic detergents have been noted because of their inability to penetrate organic debris on inanimate surfaces, and their incompatibility with anionic agents, calcium, magnesium, and iron of hard water, and organic matter (i.e., bioburden). Quaternary ammonium solutions also easily become contaminated by gram-negative bacteria such as *Pseudomonas* species (Table 9–6).

A substantial amount of scientific data has demonstrated the ineffectiveness of these chemicals against many pathogens that may be transmitted during the practice of dentistry. These include the etiologic agents for tuberculosis and hepatitis B. In what amounted to removing any doubt concerning the feasibility of quaternary ammonium preparations, the ADA Council on Dental Therapeutics in 1978 eliminated these agents from the ADA Acceptance Program as disinfectants. Thus, benzalkonium chloride, dibenzalkonium chloride, cetyldimethylethylammonium bromide, and other similar chemicals are not recommended for routine use as disinfectants in dentistry. They are, however, good cleaning agents and are marketed in the health professions as "disinfectant cleansers" on the basis of this cleaning ability. The word disinfectant here refers to their action against only gram-positive bacteria.

ALCOHOLS

Ethyl alcohol and isopropyl alcohol have been extensively used over many years as surface disinfectants and skin antiseptics. Both of these agents are effective protein denaturants and lipid solvents. The latter property probably enhances their antimicrobial range because of the destructive effect on enveloped viruses, such as Herpes simplex viruses, and tubercle bacilli. In general, alcohols exhibit a fairly broad antimicrobial spectrum of activity under certain conditions (Table 9–7). They are not recommended for use as surface disinfectants, however, because of a number of serious problems inherent with their chemical actions. They are not effective in the presence of tissue proteins, such as those found in saliva and blood. Thus, alcohols are poor cleaning agents in the presence of bioburden. Exposure to alcohol denatures proteins thereby making them insoluble and adherent onto most surfaces. A coating of denatured bioburden can then protect contaminant microorganisms from the cidal effects of alcohols for prolonged intervals. Rapid evaporation from treated environmental surfaces also limits alcohol activity on protein-coated

Table 9–7.   Characteristics of Alcohols* As Surface Disinfectants

Advantages	Disadvantages
1. Rapidly bactericidal	1. Not sporicidal
2. Tuberculocidal and virucidal (lipophilic viruses only)	2. Diminished activity with bioburden
	3. Cidal activity reduced below 60%
3. Economical	4. Damages certain materials including rubber and plastics
4. Only slightly irritating	5. Rapid evaporation rate with diminished activity against viruses in dried blood, saliva, etc. on surfaces
	6. NOT ACCEPTED BY THE ADA FOR SURFACE OR INSTRUMENT DISINFECTION

*Applies to 70% isopropyl and 70% ethyl alcohol

bacteria and viruses, which are commonly found in the spatter generated during dental procedures. Other problems include the corrosiveness of alcohols on metal surfaces, lack of sporicidal activity, and destruction of certain materials (i.e., plastics and vinyl coverings).

Vegetative bacteria are killed by exposure to high concentrations of alcohol (70% optimum), the most notable pathogen being *Mycobacterium tuberculosis*. The concentration of an alcohol preparation is critical to its antimicrobial effectiveness. When the 70% concentration is exceeded, the initial dehydration of microbial proteins allows these cell components to resist the subsequent detrimental denaturation effects. Thus, the exposed microorganisms are able to remain viable for longer periods of time. Ethyl alcohol is relatively nontoxic, colorless, nearly odorless and tasteless, and readily evaporates without residue. Isopropanol is less corrosive than ethanol, because it is not oxidized as rapidly to acetic acid and acetaldehyde.

In summary, neither is regarded as an effective cleansing agent, an important first step in the preparation for disinfection and sterilization procedures. For these reasons, neither the ADA nor the CDC currently recommends alcohol as a surface disinfectant for dental practice.

IODINE AND IODOPHORS

Iodine is one of the oldest antiseptics for application onto skin, mucous membranes, abrasions, and other wounds. The high reactivity of this halogen with its substrate provides iodine with potent germicidal effects. It acts by iodination of proteins, and subsequent formation of protein salts. Because iodine is insoluble in water, it has been routinely prepared as a tincture by dissolving an iodide salt in alcohol. Iodine in this form continues to be an effective antiseptic, as shown by the fact that at different concentrations, tinctures of iodine are toxic for both gram-positive and gram-negative bacteria, *Mycobacterium tuberculosis*, spores, fungi, and most viruses. However, this chemical suffers from some serious drawbacks. It is irritating, allergenic, corrodes metals and stains skin and clothing. Hypersensitivity reactions to iodine are also not uncommon, and range from mild to severe.

Attempts to utilize the powerful germicidal action of iodine, while reducing its caustic and staining effects, have led to the synthesis of later generation iodine compounds. The basis for these formulations is the preparation of an agent in which iodine is held in dissociable complexes. These compounds, called iodophors, retain a similar broad antimicrobial spectrum as iodine tinctures, but have the following added features: less irritation to tissues, significantly less allergic, do not

Table 9–8. Disinfectant Characteristics of Iodophors

Advantages	Disadvantages
1. EPA registered and ADA accepted as a surface disinfectant	1. Not a sterilant
2. Broad spectrum: Bactericidal, tuberculocidal, and virucidal against hydrophilic and lipophilic viruses	2. Unstable at high temperatures
	3. Dilution and contact time are critical
3. Biocidal activity within 5–10 minutes	4. Must prepare fresh daily
4. Economical	5. May discolor some surfaces
5. Effective in dilute solution	6. Rust inhibitor necessary
6. Few side reactions	7. Inactivated by hard water (1:200)
7. Surfactant carrier maintains surface moistness	8. Inactivated by alcohol
8. Residual biocidal action	

stain skin or clothing, and have a prolonged activity after application (Table 9–8). Iodophors are prepared by combining iodine with a solubilizing agent or carrier. One of the most common carriers for iodophors is polyvinylpyrrolidone (PVP). This agent stabilizes the iodine, minimizes its toxicity, and slowly releases the halogen to the tissues. The carriers themselves are surfactants (usually nonionic) that are water soluble and react with epithelial areas to increase tissue permeability. Thus, the active iodine that is released is better absorbed.

Iodophor *antiseptics* are useful in preparation of the oral mucosa for local anesthesia and surgical procedures. Iodophors have also been found to be effective handwashing antiseptics. In addition to removing microbial populations from the skin in large numbers, these cleansers are not rinsed off completely; therefore, a residual antimicrobial effect may remain in the scrubbed areas.

Other iodophor preparations serve as *disinfectants* in hospitals, clinics, and similar health care facilities. Their surfactant properties make them excellent cleaning agents prior to disinfection, and newer iodophor commercial formulations have received EPA-approved tuberculocidal activity within 5 to 10 minutes of exposure. (See Appendix E.) Fresh solutions must be prepared daily to ensure this tuberculocidal activity. It must be noted here that diluting iodophor disinfectants in hard water may cause rapid loss of antimicrobial activity. The general recommendation is, therefore, to use distilled, or at least softened water, to dilute the iodophors prior to use.

CHLORINE-CONTAINING AGENTS

Chlorine acts primarily by oxidation, as hypochlorous acid, into which it is quickly converted by water. As a result, chlorine is more active in acid solutions. Elemental chlorine is a potent germicide, killing most bacteria in 15 to 30 seconds at concentrations of 0.10 to 0.25 p.p.m. Accepted chlorine-containing compounds in common use are hypochlorite solutions (Table 9–9) and chlorine dioxide preparations (Table 9–10). Diluted bleach (1:10 to 1:100) in water was shown in the 1970s to be useful as a disinfectant, especially in areas considered to have been contaminated with hepatitis viruses. The Centers for Disease Control has recommended the use of 500 to 5,000 p.p.m. (0.05 to 0.5%) sodium hypochlorite as an effective agent in destroying hepatitis B viruses. Because this chemical is unstable, fresh solutions must be prepared daily. Despite its effectiveness as a disinfectant,

Table 9–9.   Disinfectant Properties of Chlorines

Advantages	Disadvantages
1. Some products are EPA registered and ADA accepted	1. Sporicidal only at high concentrations
2. Rapid antimicrobial action	2. Cannot be reused
3. Broad spectrum: Bactericidal, tuberculocidal, and virucidal	3. Must be prepared fresh daily
4. Economical	4. Activity diminished by organic matter
5. Effective in dilute solution	5. Unpleasant, persistent odor
	6. Irritating to skin and eyes
	7. Corrodes metals and damages clothing
	8. Degrades plastics and rubber

this chlorine-releasing preparation has some obvious disadvantages. It is corrosive to metals and irritating to skin and other tissues, and destroys many fabrics. See Appendix E for product names in this category.

PHENOLS AND DERIVATIVES

The classical antiseptic for surgical procedures was carbolic acid. It was first thought that postoperative infections would be virtually eradicated with widespread use of this phenol. However, because of the severe toxicity reported in individuals exposed to carbolic acid, its application was curtailed. Subsequent generations of phenolic compounds have filled roles as effective disinfectants or antiseptics. These agents act as cytoplasmic poisons by penetrating and disrupting microbial cell walls, leading to denaturation of intracellular proteins. The intense penetration capability of phenols is probably the major factor associated with their antimicrobial activity. Unfortunately, they can also penetrate intact skin causing local tissue damage and possible systemic complications. Thus, with the exception of the bisphenols, most phenolic derivatives are used primarily as disinfectants.

Complex (Synthetic) Phenols

In the mid-1980s a new class of phenolic compounds was approved by the EPA as surface disinfectants (Table 9–11). These contain more than one phenolic agent. Currently, most products contain two, but newer formulations have three phenols as the active compounds. After appropriate dilution in water, these phenolics act in a synergistic manner to offer a broad antimicrobial spectrum, including tuberculocidal activity. They also serve as good surface cleaners and are effective in the presence of detergents. Unfortunately, the penetration properties of phenols tend to cause epithelial toxicity in exposed tissues. Appropriate utility gloves should

Table 9–10.   Characteristics of Chlorine Dioxide

Advantages	Disadvantages
1. Instrument or environmental surface disinfectant/sterilant	1. Discard daily
2. Rapid acting: 3 minutes for disinfection 6 hours for sterilization	2. 24 hours sterilant use-life
	3. Does not readily penetrate organic debris
	4. Protective eyewear/gloves required
	5. Closed containers
	6. Adequate ventilation for surface disinfection
	7. Corrodes aluminum containers

Table 9–11.   Disinfectant Characteristics of Synthetic Phenols

Advantages	Disadvantages
1. EPA registered and ADA accepted as both an immersion and a surface disinfectant	1. Not sporicidal
2. Synergistic	2. Must prepare fresh daily
3. Broad antimicrobial spectrum	3. Can degrade certain plastics and etch glass with prolonged exposure
4. Tuberculocidal	4. Film accumulation
5. Useful on metal, glass, rubber, and plastic	5. Skin and eye irritation
6. Less toxic and corrosive than glutaraldehyde	
7. Economical	

be worn when these or any other disinfectant is to be handled in order to prevent this. See Appendix E for product names in this category.

GLUTARALDEHYDES

Glutaraldehyde ($C_5H_8O_2$) has two aldehyde units, one at each end of the carbon chain. Different commercial preparations are formulated to exhibit maximal activity at either alkaline, acidic, or neutral pH. Those products that are active at alkaline or neutral pH utilize an activator that brings the final 2.0 to 3.2% glutaraldehyde to the desired pH. At these concentrations, glutaraldehydes are effective against all vegetative bacteria, including *M. tuberculosis,* fungi and viruses, and are able to destroy microbial spores in 6 to 10 hours (Table 9–12). They therefore offer an alternative as immersion sterilants, for those few items that cannot withstand repeated heat sterilization and are not disposable.

In addition to their wide antimicrobial range, glutaraldehydes also offer other important advantages as disinfectants. Their low surface tension permits them to penetrate blood and exudate to reach instrument surfaces and facilitates rinsing. Rubber and plastic items are not degraded during prolonged immersion, and, in fact, these chemicals may be useful in removing blood from suction hoses. Unfortunately, glutaraldehydes can damage many metallic items if misused. For example, nickel-coated impression trays and carbon steel burs will often discolor and corrode when immersed in a 2.0 to 3.2% glutaraldehyde for prolonged periods.

Sterilization of instruments by immersion in glutaraldehyde solutions can be useful in certain specified conditions, but can also represent the most abused aspect

Table 9–12.   Characteristics of Glutaraldehydes As Immersion Chemical Sterilants/ Disinfectants

Advantages	Disadvantages
1. EPA registered and ADA accepted	1. Not an antiseptic
2. High biocidal activity	2. Not a surface disinfectant
3. Broad antimicrobial spectrum	3. Severe tissue irritation
4. Sporicidal at room temperature after 6 to 10 hours	4. Allergenic
5. Generally noncorrosive	5. Discolors some metals
6. Penetrates blood, pus, and organic debris	6. Biologically nonverifiable
7. Prolonged activated life	7. Reuse life varies with bioburden
8. Useful for rubber and plastic items	8. Cannot package items
9. Instrument sterilant or disinfectant	9. Corrosive activity can increase with dilution

of office asepsis. The potentially misleading term "cold sterilization" was derived from such practices. Chemical sterilization techniques and the use of chemical holding solutions are not acceptable substitutes for heat sterilization. Important considerations that directly relate to glutaraldehyde biocidal activity include their shelf life, use life, and reuse life. *Shelf life* is the time that a product may be safely stored. *Use life* is the life expectancy for the solution once it is activated, but not actually put into use with contaminated items. *Reuse life* is the amount of time a solution can be used and reused as it is challenged with instruments that are wet or coated with bioburden. Reuse life takes into account a dilution factor because of added water from wet instruments, the effects of soap and other detergents, and evaporation. The EPA started accepting reuse claims from glutaraldehyde manufacturers in 1985. Acceptance allows the manufacturer to include a reuse statement on the product label. See Appendix E for glutaradehyde product names and reuse information.

Although glutaradehyde formulations are effective as sterilants/disinfectants, they are not functional as antiseptics. Irritation of hands is common and thus, direct physical contact between glutaraldehyde solutions and tissues should not occur. Utility gloves should always be worn when handling any glutaraldehyde solution. Contact with this potent chemical can induce hypersensitivity and other dermatologic reactions with repeated exposures. For these reasons, immersed items should be thoroughly rinsed with sterile water prior to use.

A class of glutaraldehyde surface disinfectants was developed in the mid-1980s. Currently available products contain 0.25 to 0.50% glutaraldehyde and have received EPA approval as intermediate hospital-surface disinfectants. Other chemicals in these preparations may add to the disinfectant activity of the product (i.e., addition of low concentrations of phenols) or lower the potential toxicity of the active ingredient.

SUMMARY

The ADA Council on Dental Therapeutics recognizes many commercial products as being effective for use in dentistry as disinfectants or sterilants. Some of these only disinfect and do not sterilize, some have an odor that is unpleasant, others stain or bleach surfaces, and some of the formulations are corrosive to metallic surfaces. The EPA and ADA currently list iodophors, synthetic phenolics, and chlorine-containing compounds as acceptable intermediate hospital-surface disinfectants. With regard to liquid sterilants, most dental offices currently use a 2 to 3.2% glutaraldehyde solution or a chlorine dioxide preparation for chemical sterilization. It is therefore essential that before purchasing a chemical sterilant/ disinfectant and a surface disinfectant for routine use, the practitioner, dental hygienist, assistant, and laboratory technician obtain as much information as possible. This will then allow for subsequent decisions to be based on appropriate efficacy criteria, and reduce the potential for product misuse.

SELECTED READINGS

ADA Council on Dental Therapeutics: Quaternary ammonium compounds not acceptable for disinfection of instruments and environmental surfaces in dentistry. J. Am. Dent. Assoc., 97:855–856, 1978.
ADA: Infection control recommendations for the dental office and the dental laboratory. J. Am. Dent. Assoc., 116:241–248, 1988.

Block, S.S.: Disinfection, Sterilization and Preservation. 4th ed. Philadelphia, Lea & Febiger, 1983.

Bond, W.W., Petersen, N.J., and Favero, M.S.: Viral hepatitis B: Aspects of environmental control. Health Lab. Sci., 14:235–252, 1977.

Bond, W.W., Favero, M.S., Petersen, N.J., and Ebert, J.W.: Inactivation of hepatitis B virus by inter-mediate-to-high level disinfectant chemicals. J. Clin. Microbiol., 18:535–538, 1983.

Centers for Disease Control: Recommended infection control practices for dentistry. MMWR, 35:237–242, 1986.

Centers for Disease Control: Recommendations for prevention of HIV transmission in health-care settings. MMWR, 36:1–18, 1987.

Cottone, J.A.: Infection control in dentistry. In Proceedings: National Conference on Infection Control in Dentistry. Edited by E.W. Mitchell and S.B. Corbin. Chicago, United States Public Health Service, 1986, pp. 34–46.

Crawford, J.J.: State-of-the-art: Practical infection control in dentistry. J. Am. Dent. Assoc., 110:629–633, 1985.

Environmental Protection Agency: Advocacy of pesticide uses which do not appear on registered pesticide labels; amendment to the statement. Fed. Reg., 51:19174–19175, 1986.

Favero, M.S.: Sterilization, disinfection and antisepsis in the hospital. In Manual of Clinical Microbiology. 4th ed. Washington, D.C., American Society for Microbiology, 1985, pp. 129–137.

Garner, J.S., and Favero, M.S.: Guideline for handwashing and hospital environmental control. Am. J. Infect. Control, 14:110–126, 1985.

Kobayashi, H., et al.: Susceptibility of hepatitis B virus to disinfectants or heat. J. Clin. Microbiol., 20:214–216, 1984.

Lister, J.: On the antiseptic principle of the practice of surgery. Br. Med. J., (Sept. 21, 1867).

Mitchell, E.W.: Chemical disinfecting-sterilizing agents. Calif. Dent. Assoc. J., 13:64–67, 1985.

Molinari, J.A., Campbell, M.D., and York, J.: Minimizing potential infections in dental practice. J. Mich. Dent. Assoc., 64:411–416, 1982.

Molinari, J.A.: Surface disinfection and disinfectants. Calif. Dent. Assoc. J., 13:73–78, 1985.

Runnells, R.R.: Infection Control in the Former Wet Finger Environment. North Salt Lake, I.C. Publications, 1987.

Rutala, W.A.: Draft guideline for selection and use of disinfectants. Am. J. Infect. Control, 17:24A–38A, 1989.

Rutala, W.A., and Cole, E.C.: Ineffectiveness of hospital disinfectants against bacteria: a collaborative study. Infect. Control, 8:501–506, 1987.

Spaulding, E.H.: Chemical disinfection and antisepsis in the hospital. J. Hosp. Res., 9:5–31, 1972.

Spaulding, E.H.: Chemical disinfection of medical and surgical materials. In Disinfection, Preservation and Sterilization. Edited by C.A. Lawrence and S.S. Block. Philadelphia, Lea & Febiger, 1968, pp. 517–531.

section four

Environmental Surface and Equipment Disinfection

Chapter 10

Environmental Surface Disinfection

In addition to recommending an increased use of disposable covers, infection control guidelines routinely address cleaning and disinfection of operatory surfaces that become contaminated with bioburden as a result of treatment procedures. The use of chemical disinfectants is warranted in certain instances because it is not possible to sterilize all contaminated items and surfaces. When one then considers the large number of operatory surfaces that may become coated with saliva, blood, or exudate (see Chapter 4), it becomes readily apparent that environmental surface disinfection comprises a major portion of an effective asepsis program. The present discussion will consider the rationale and procedures for surface disinfection by utilizing information presented for chemical disinfectants in the previous chapter.

BASIC CRITERIA AND CONSIDERATIONS

The simplest way to approach the subject of environmental surface disinfection is to adhere to a basic premise of aseptic technique, that is, <u>Clean It First!</u> As straightforward and logical as this statement appears, operatory disinfection has become a source of confusion for some dental professionals. Available chemical products include concentrates, premixed solutions, sprays, wipes, foams, and impregnated disposable wipes. Unfortunately, choosing an appropriate general purpose surface cleaner and disinfectant may be difficult because of exaggerated claims by manufacturers and misleading assays reported in the literature. These analyses can obscure the actual performance capabilities of individual agents and may also yield information that is neither clinically applicable nor readily reproducible. The importance of initial cleaning cannot be overemphasized, and is routinely included in all infection control recommendations. For example, the CDC regularly reinforces this concept in their published infection control guidelines for all healthcare professionals. The ADA has also repeatedly stressed this, as exemplified by the following section from the recently published "Infection Control In The Dental Environment" instructional program:

> Cleaning is the physical removal of debris. It has two major effects. First, it results in a reduction in the number of microorganisms present. Second, it removes organic matter, such as blood and tissue, and other debris which may interfere with sterilization and disinfection. In some instances, cleaning is all that is necessary. Most often, however, it is the preliminary step before sterilization or disinfection. In these instances it is referred to as pre-cleaning. Pre-cleaning is an essential step because sterilization and disinfection procedures may not be effective if items have not been cleaned first.

Initial cleaning and disinfection are important not only for aesthetic reasons,

Table 10–1. Guidelines for Selection of Liquid Disinfectants and Sterilants

All chemicals used for disinfection or sterilization in dental practice MUST meet the first three of the following guidelines to prove product efficacy and user compliance:

1. **The product must display an Environmental Protection Agency number on the label of the product.**

   Display of this number is proof that the product is registered with the EPA in compliance with federal law and that the product performs as claimed by the manufacturer. The EPA number also affords reasonable legal protection for the user in that only products in compliance with federal law are to be used in patient treatment.

2. **The product must be used in strict compliance with the printed instructions on the label.**

   Chemical and microbiological considerations require use of the product in a *disciplined* manner to assure that the representations of the manufacturer will be accomplished. Ignoring instructions nearly always reduces microbial control.

3. **The product should state on the label that it kills** *Mycobacterium tuberculosis*.

   The tubercle bacillus is a "benchmark" organism and is comparatively difficult to destroy. Tuberculocidal action assures that the product is an intermediate or higher level disinfectant and that it will destroy all pathogens potentially threatening to dentistry.

4. **The product should display the American Dental Association Seal of Acceptance.**

   While not mandatory, compliance with the ADA Acceptance Program is very desirable and provides additional assurance that products are efficacious for use in dentistry.

From R.R. Runnells: Dental Infection Control—Update '88. Fruit Heights, I.C. Publications, Inc.

but primarily because effective disinfection minimizes the potential for cross-infection from environmental surfaces. It must also be noted here that manufacturers are required to state on the product label that the disinfectant be used on precleaned surfaces. Although separate cleaners and disinfectants may be applied, chemical agents that accomplish both functions offer a more efficient approach. Thus, a fundamental consideration for chemical selection should be the agent's ability to penetrate and preclean surfaces contaminated with saliva, blood, and/or exudate. EPA and ADA approved surface disinfectants, such as iodophors, synthetic phenolics, and chlorine compounds, can both clean and disinfect (see Appendix E for product names).

It is also advisable to compare the products under consideration with the properties of an "ideal" disinfectant discussed in Chapter 9 and adhere to a series of other important guidelines outlined in Table 10–1. Criteria for effective disinfection call for preparation and use of products according to their label directions, which have been approved by the EPA. Manufacturers' directions that call for dilution of disinfectants in water rather than alcohol must be followed, as the cleaning ability of the active agent will be impaired and the alcohol may actually increase the deleterious effects of some disinfectants, such as the iodophors. Hands should also be protected with puncture-resistant utility gloves when cleaning and disinfecting items, and protective eyewear worn if splashing of the chemical may occur.

DISINFECTION PROCEDURES

Disinfection of environmental surfaces involves a two-step procedure, termed a "spray-wipe-spray" technique. As mentioned above, all surfaces to be disinfected must be precleaned before disinfection can occur. Water-based disinfectants, particularly those that contain a detergent, are effective in the initial precleaning step. For the most part, pump spray bottles are appropriate for cleaner/disinfectants,

Table 10–2.   Tips on Surface Disinfection

1. Surfaces that are difficult to disinfect (such as chair buttons, control buttons on the air/water syringe, switches on the unit, light handles, hoses, and handpiece and air/water syringe holders) should be covered with plastic wrap, aluminum foil, or other material impervious to water. Replace with fresh covers between each patient. It takes less time to replace a cover than to disinfect the uncovered surface between patients.

2. Disinfecting electrical switches on the chair or unit may damage or cause a short in the switch. Cover them!

3. Choose an EPA-registered, ADA-accepted surface disinfectant, and use this agent for both the cleaning step and the disinfecting step for uncovered surfaces. Using a water-based agent (e.g., iodophors or combinations synthetic phenolics) with both cleaning and disinfecting properties provides some protection during the cleaning step, helps sanitize any debris splattered by the cleaning procedure, and helps keep the number of different products that need to be ordered at a minimum.

4. The primary difference between surface cleaners and disinfectants used in hospitals and surgery suites versus those used in dentistry is the capability of achieving a hydrophilic virus kill (**Rotavirus, Poliovirus**). Surface disinfectants used in dentistry **must** achieve this broader virus bill in order to meet ADA acceptance standards.

5. Follow the manufacturer's directions on the disinfectant product label.

6. Water, rather than alcohol, must be used to dilute those agents requiring dilution before use.

7. Use heavy, puncture-resistant nitrile rubber utility goves during surface cleaning and disinfection to reduce chances of direct contamination of the hands.

8. Use protective eyeglasses to protect eyes from splashes or splatter created when mixing solutions or cleaning surfaces with a brush.

9. Use a mask when cleaning an item with a bristle brush to prevent inhalation or direct mucous membrane contamination from splatter.

10. Paper towels, rather than more expensive gauze sponges, are appropriate for surface cleaning.

11. The time required for operatory clean-up between patients can be shortened if extra handpieces are cleaned and disinfected or heat sterilized in advance for a quick interchange with the contaminated handpiece. Heat sterilization of handpieces between patients is preferred.

Adapted from Miller, C.H.: Disinfection of surfaces and equipment. Dent. Assist., 8:21–22, 1988, and Dent. Asepsis Rev., 9:9, 1988.

with a major exception being the application of hypochlorite solutions. When spray bottles are used, they provide the following advantages: (1) allow active chemicals to better penetrate equipment crevices, (2) protect the germicide from being inactivated or absorbed by gauzes, paper towels, or sponges, and (3) minimize the cost of gauze and other applicator materials. The prepared disinfectants should not be stored in containers with gauze, as this may shorten the effective life of the disinfectant. A summary of the some of the above suggestions, as well as other "tips" for surface disinfection, are presented in Table 10–2. Once a routine is established, a unit can be cleaned and disinfectant applied in 3 minutes. The time specified by most disinfectant manufacturers for keeping surfaces wet after precleaning is usually 10 minutes. Chemicals that require a 20-minute or longer tuberculocidal kill time are of limited value. Most disinfectants currently approved by the EPA were required to supply kill data of 5 minutes, in order to be able to recommend 10-minute exposure interval. This provides a 5-minute safety factor. Wetted, clean surfaces are usually ready to use by the time the patient is seated and prepared for treatment. Any excess disinfectant can be wiped away with a clean paper towel.

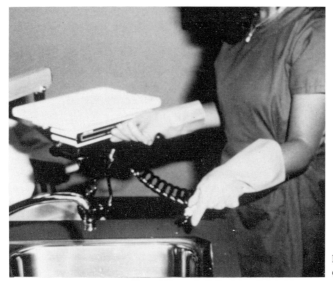

Fig. 10–1. Flushing water lines of the unit.

Infection Control of the Dental Unit

Each Morning Before the First Patient of the Day. Flush the water lines of the unit for 3 to 5 minutes (Fig. 10–1). Use the spray-wipe-spray technique on all nonsterilizable surfaces and equipment. First, clean (with an approved cleaner/disinfectant) items such as the operatory cabinets, counters, sinks, bracket table, dental chair, chair control unit, air/water syringe, and light controls. After cleaning, disinfect these areas with an EPA-approved, hospital-level, tuberculocidal disinfectant, which will kill hydrophilic and lipophilic viruses (Fig. 10–2). Alternatively, surface covers are applied after cleaning.

Between Patients. Flush water lines for at least 15 seconds. Sterilize, or disinfect if not sterilizable, the handpiece and air-water syringe tip. If the handpiece cannot be heat sterilized, it can be disinfected as follows: clean to remove organic debris,

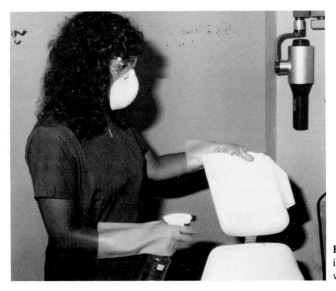

Fig. 10–2. Disinfecting nonsterilizable surface areas with spray-wipe-spray techique.

spray and wrap in a paper towel or gauze impregnated with an approved compatible disinfectant, and keep in contact with the disinfectant for the approved exposure time. Clean and disinfect all "high touch" areas with an approved surface cleaner/disinfectant. Alternatively, covers are removed and discarded, and clean surface covers are applied.

End of Day. Flush the water lines for 3 minutes. Evacuate a generous amount of cleansing solution through the evacuation lines and clean or replace the unit's solid waste filter trap. Clean and disinfect the floor around the dental chair, and all counter and "high touch" areas.

Weekly. Clean and disinfect the main evacuation system trap. Clean and disinfect the inside and outside of drawers and cabinets. In addition, as part of the routine asepsis protocol, the operatory and laboratory floors should be thoroughly cleaned and disinfected.

SUMMARY

Because it is not currently possible to provide absolute asepsis for all surfaces and objects during dental treatment, cleanup procedures should attempt to decontaminate those that are potential sources of cross-infection. It is not necessary to sterilize surfaces such as counter tops, light handles, chair buttons, and unit controls, as these are not considered "critical items," requiring sterilization between each appointment. A thorough cleaning followed by appropriate intermediate-level disinfection according to chemical use instructions provides effective environmental surface disinfection. The most desirable disinfectants are virucidal for both hydrophilic and lipophilic viruses, and tuberculocidal. Properties of available classes of disinfectants and the "how to's" for their use, have been considered in this and the previous chapters.

SELECTED READINGS

ADA: Infection control recommendations for the dental office and the dental laboratory. JADA, *116*:241–248, 1988.

Crawford, J.J.: Sterilization, Disinfection, and Asepsis in Dentistry. *In* Disinfection, Sterilization and Preservation. 3rd Ed. Edited by S.S. Block. Philadelphia, Lea & Febiger, 1983

Department of Veterans Affairs, American Dental Association, Department of Health and Human Services: Infection Control in the Dental Environment. Instructional Program, VA Medical Center, Washington, D.C., 1989.

Favero, M.S.: Sterilization, disinfection and antisepsis in the hospital. *In* Manual of Clinical Microbiology. 4th Ed. Washington, D.C., American Society for Microbiology, 1985, pp. 129–137.

Molinari, J.A., et al.: Comparison of dental surface disinfectants. Gen. Dent., *35*:171–175, 1987.

Molinari, J.A., et al.: Cleaning and disinfectant properties of dental surface disinfectants. JADA, *117*:179–182, 1988.

Runnells, R.R.: Practical How To's of Dental Infection Control. North Salt Lake, I.C. Publications, 1987.

Runnells, R.R.: Dental Infection Control—Update '88. Fruit Heights, I.C. Publications, 1988.

Chapter 11

Aseptic Considerations In Dental Equipment Selection

Dental equipment has been traditionally designed with operator efficiency and esthetics as the primary considerations. Little attention was paid to the potential for cross-contamination. More recently, however, the profession has become increasingly aware of the real potential for transfer of pathogenic microorganisms via treatment equipment.

Transfer of organisms may occur primarily through direct contact, or indirectly, by exposure to blood or saliva on contaminated equipment. Aerosolization and wide dispersal of blood and saliva also appear to be factors. As a component of this, air dispersal and/or subsequent settling out of other environmental contaminants (e.g., water and oil mists, tooth and material particles) are possible. It is thus necessary to assume that adjacent surfaces and equipment may become contaminated, and should be made to withstand routine cleaning and disinfection.

Manufacturers are upgrading major equipment items, with a trend toward maintenance of a clean working environment, by realizing that absolute sterility in the dental workplace is neither practical nor necessary. It is essential, however, to maintain a disinfected environment within the working area of treatment providers. There are no "critical" items associated with general treatment equipment, i.e., no items come into contact with sterile body areas and thus do not need to be sterilized. The exception to this is the handpiece, which should be heat sterilized between patients. The majority of treatment equipment are semi- or noncritical items (Table 11–1).

MAJOR EQUIPMENT AND DELIVERY SYSTEMS

At present, most major equipment items are not designed for use without contaminating the surfaces, switches, and handles during routine patient treatment. Efficient cleaning and disinfection is often difficult because of the large numbers of crevices, uneven surfaces, knurled knobs, porous finishes, and surfaces that may be damaged by disinfecting chemicals (Fig. 11–1).

The delivery system itself is often subject to the greatest amount of direct microbial transfer. There are countless configurations of systems, however, the same principles apply to all. Maximum use of barrier materials and meticulous cleansing and disinfection of nonbarrier areas is recommended. Nonpermeable, single layer covers and barriers may be used for each patient. These are to be discarded and replaced between patient appointments. Such covers as plastic bags,

Table 11–1. Dental Equipment Disinfection

| | Contamination Risk | | | Disinfection Procedure | | |
| | Semicritical | Noncritical | | | | |
	High	Medium	Low	Cover (each patient)	Wipe (each patient)	Wipe (daily)
Unit						
handles	x			x	x	
switches	x			x		
hangers		x			x	
surfaces	x				x	
arms			x		x	x
hoses		x			x	
syringes	x			+x	x	
handpieces	critical			+	x	
Light						
reflector			x			x
shield		x			x	
handles	x			x	x	
switches	x			x	x	
arms			x			x
Chair						
upholstery			x			x
arms	x	x		x	x	
headrest	x	x		x	x	
switches	x			x		
Stool						
upholstery			x			x
arms	x	x		x	x	
controls	x			x	x	
X-Ray (PA)						
head	x			x	x	
arm			x			x
control	x			x		
switch	x			x		
X-Ray (PANO)						
head			x			x
cassette		x			x	
positioners		x			x	
bite blocks	x			+x		
controls		x		x	x	
switch		x		x		
X-Ray Processor						
loader	x				x	
surfaces			x			x
Cabinetry						
counter	x	x		x	x	
drawer (inside)			x			#
handles	x			x	x	
sink	x				x	
faucet (man)	x				x	
faucet (auto)			x			x
soap dispenser (man)	x				x	
soap dispenser (auto)			x			x

Legend
+ sterilize for each patient
# periodic sanitizing

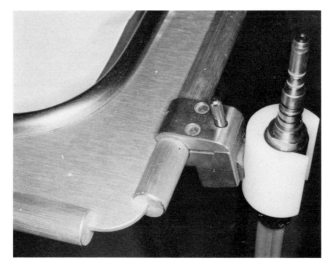

Fig. 11–1. Seams and crevices common to older treatment equipment, making it difficult to disinfect.

aluminum foil, or plastic wraps may be used. Special attention must be given to control knobs and switches that are touched during treatment. Knobs should be covered with wraps and switches protected with disposable covers to ensure cleanliness (Fig. 11–2).

Controls for handpieces and coolant sprays are generally arranged for the convenience of the operator. However, in practice, most dentists seldom adjust these controls once they are set. Units are available that protect these controls from the environment and make disinfection between patients unnecessary (Fig. 11–3). Handpiece hangers are subject to direct contamination, but do not readily lend themselves to barrier protection. Therefore, they must be carefully cleaned and disinfected between patients. Each system should be analyzed by the staff to determine the most efficient approach for minimizing contamination.

The underside edges of cart tops and unit heads are especially prone to contamination during movement. Basically, equipment should be moved with attached handles, which are generally easily disinfected and/or protected with barrier materials. Older equipment that is not fitted with handles should be modified by placing handles in convenient locations.

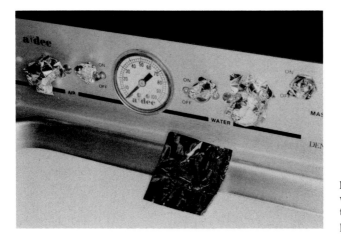

Fig. 11–2. Use of aluminum foil, which is changed between patients, as a barrier material for protection of operating controls.

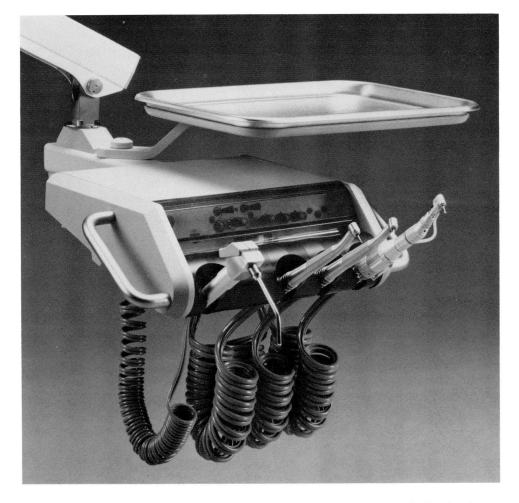

Fig. 11–3. *A,* Use of a transparent shield to protect controls from contamination. *B,* Seamless "membrane" control switches that are easy to disinfect between patients. (Photos courtesy of A-dec, Newberg, OR, and Siemens, Charlotte, NC.)

Exposed surfaces that are not practical to cover should be constructed of materials that will withstand repeated cleaning and disinfection procedures. Natural metal finishes will normally tolerate most cleaners and disinfectants, although sodium hypochlorite solutions may corrode some metal surfaces. Modern powder paints and epoxy finishes generally hold up well, but should be smooth and free from irregularities. Adhesive trims and decorations should be avoided. Attached tubs and trays are also not recommended. Work areas should be seamless and smooth, with trays and other articles brought in as needed. Bulk storage of patient treatment materials in tubs attached to delivery equipment, or in reach of the staff during treatment, should be discouraged. The potential exists for contamination of the entire supply of items if the cover is opened in the treatment area, or if items are selected using contaminated hands or instruments. Unit dose dispensing of disposable items during tray preparation is recommended to prevent this.

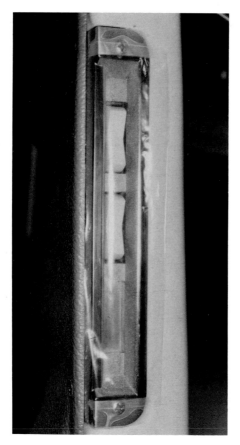

Fig. 11–4. Use of plastic barrier material taped over chair controls and changed between patients.

Operatory Chair

The greatest potential for dental chair cross-contamination occurs from chair-mounted control switches. Common finger-operated switches or latches normally contain a multitude of crevices that are impossible to clean, let alone disinfect. One cannot use copious amounts of liquid cleaner and/or disinfectant on the switches because of the possibility of an electrical short. A practical method for solution of this problem is through diligent use of barrier materials. Small pieces of plastic wrap taped onto the switch area usually provide the best protection (Fig. 11–4). It is also strongly recommended that all dental chairs be fitted with foot-operated controls. These are available through local supply distributors for retrofitting to most chairs.

Headrest controls and chair arms are other areas of concern. These are sites that are often overlooked during chair cleaning and disinfection. The use of disposable headrest covers will often eliminate this problem, but it is not feasible to cover the underside of chair arms where patients and health professionals are likely to grip. Arm slings tend to trap debris and provide crevices for accumulation of dirt. These are being eliminated in future equipment designs, with arm support being built into the main frame of the chair (Fig. 11–5).

A modern dental chair should be constructed of durable, nonorganic materials. Upholstry should be easily removable, impervious to moisture, and essentially seamless for maximum asepsis. There is no question that the arm/hand rests should

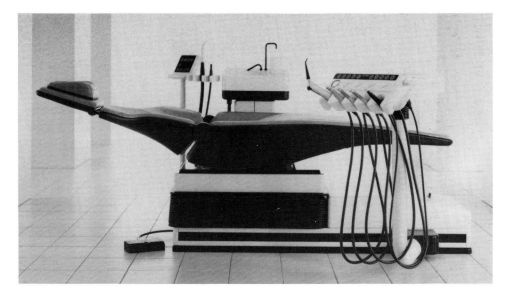

Fig. 11–5.   Patient chair with no separate armrests and completely seamless upholstery. (Photo courtesy of Siemens, Charlotte, NC.)

be able to withstand repeated cleaning and disinfection. The seat upholstery should also meet the same criteria if the chair is used routinely with medically compromised patients or with patients where incontinence may be a problem. There is some question, however, about the necessity of a moisture-proof material for the entire seating surface for the majority of patients. As dental procedures become more exacting and the patient sits in the chair for longer periods, comfort becomes a concern. Molded or carved foam cushions provide outstanding ergonomic support for the patient, and breathable fabric covers tend to allow air circulation for comfort (Fig. 11–6). If a fabric centered cushion with vinyl bolsters is used, there is little potential for either direct transfer or aerosol fallout of pathogenic material onto fabric surfaces during treatment.

X-Ray Equipment

Periapical x-ray units are subject to gross contamination as a result of individuals operating units with contaminated hands after placing and removing films from the patient's mouth. Barrier materials should be placed around the x-ray cone and/or tube head, depending on which surfaces are touched when positioning the head. The timing controls should be protected with a transparent cover and the exposure switch protected with a disposable plastic sleeve. These items should also be replaced between patient appointments. In contrast, panoramic x-ray units are relatively clean. The patient does not contact the film in any manner, and often only guiding planes touch facial surfaces. Some units, however, have "bite" blocks, used by the patient to aid in alignment. These blocks are usually protected with a disposable sleeve and/or are sterilized between patients. Operator controls on the equipment itself are usually simple and may be easily covered with barrier materials. These units normally need little more than cleaning and disinfection of the handles and contact surfaces. The control console may have knobs and switches

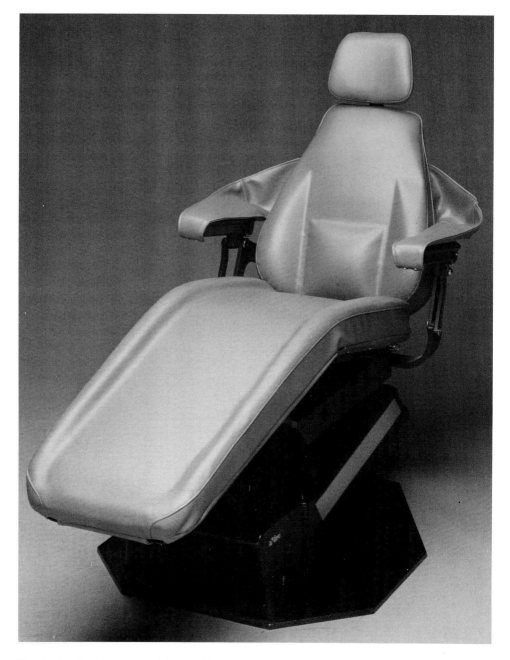

Fig. 11–6.   One-piece, shaped foam cushions with a minimum of seams for asepsis and a fabric center for patient comfort. (Photo courtesy of A-dec, Newberg, OR.)

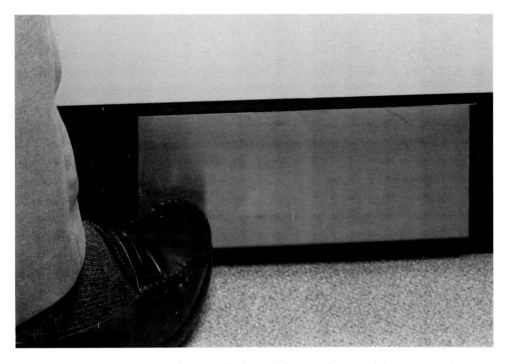

Fig. 11–7. Electronic water controls operated either with foot switches or with faucet mounted sensors. (Photo courtesy of A-dec, Newberg, OR.)

that must be protected, and the exposure button is usually protected with a disposable sleeve. Processors are generally subject to cross-contamination, especially when daylight-type loaders are used. These loaders often accumulate numerous periapical film wrappers, which are potential sources of contamination. For more information on aseptic radiographic procedures, see Chapter 13.

Cabinetry

Cabinetry and work surfaces within the treatment area should be kept to a minimum and as simple in design as possible. Pressure-laminated and molded plastic are normally used as the inner and outer surfaces for modern dental cabinetry. These materials withstand cleaning and disinfection procedures well, especially when constructed with a minimum of seams. Countertops should be seamless from front to back, with a 3 to 4 inch, molded backsplash. Sinks are usually made of stainless steel or porcelain, with foot or electronic faucet controls (Fig. 11–7). Manual faucets are not as good because of the difficulty of keeping water knobs free of contamination.

Drawers and cabinets should also be lined with the same materials as the tops. Storage space should be kept to a minimum in the treatment area in order to reduce the potential for material and debris accumulation. Scheduled periods could be set up in the office routine to make certain that storage areas are cleaned and disinfected at least weekly.

Tubing and Hoses

Suction and delivery hoses deserve special attention because of their proximity to the operating field. Both inside and outside surfaces must be considered here. All surfaces should be smooth and without crevices to prevent buildup of debris. Ideally, tubing should be removed and sterilized with treatment instruments. Recently, manufactured delivery systems have been equipped with removable tubings, thereby minimizing the requirement for cleaning and disinfection.

Suction tubing and connector/flow control assemblies offer examples of items that become readily contaminated. The suction system is routinely exposed to large amounts of saliva and blood. Finger-operated flow control valves are also often covered with fluid and may not be properly cleaned between patients. The end of each hose with its connector assembly should be rinsed in copious amounts of fresh water, carefully scrubbed with a detergent, and disinfected by immersion in an approved disinfectant. The interior of suction tubing should also be cleaned between patient appointments, by flushing them with fresh water, and disinfecting them at the end of the work day with a commercial cleansing solution.

Handpiece and air/water syringe tubing pose difficult problems. They should be straight, not coiled, and should not be used in enclosed retraction devices. Most older retraction systems pull the tubings into closed areas, which are potential sources for microbial accumulation. Fabric-covered tubing further potentiates this buildup and should not be utilized. Smooth plastic outer surfaces allow efficient cleaning. Coiled tubings are more difficult to clean and should be replaced with straight ones where possible. A further benefit for the treatment provider, is the reduction of "tug-back" when using straight tubing.

The internal surfaces of water and air tubing are subject to both defects and the accumulation of microbial-contaminated bioburden. Water lines are particularly susceptible to microbial buildup, and must be protected from water retraction, or "suckback." This occurrence was designed into older dental units to prevent water from dripping on the patient. In order to test a practice delivery system for water retraction, a turbine handpiece can be first operated in a dye solution for a few seconds, and then the head of the handpiece immersed for 5 minutes. The handpiece is then removed from the hose and the connector is held over a white paper towel while the foot control is activated. If any color is expressed in the water from the connector, water retraction is present. A one-way valve can be easily and inexpensively installed in the tubing water line. If any doubt exists that water retraction is occurring, the valves may still be installed as a safety measure. Although most current delivery systems contain antiretraction valves as standard features, all units should be checked for water retraction, regardless of their age.

It is also recommended that all water lines be flushed for 3 to 5 minutes if the system has not been used for a few hours. Flushing lines for several minutes each morning, for a minute after lunch or prolonged breaks in patient treatment, and for several seconds between patient appointments will ensure fresh water from the source and removal of any debris from the lines. Be certain handpieces are disconnected from hoses during flushing, because free running could damage the bearings. Installing sterilized handpieces and syringe tips after line flushing will ensure a clean water stream for each patient. If sterile water is required for treatment, the use of heat-sterilized bulb syringes with sterile water is recommended.

Handpieces

A modern dental handpiece is heat/pressure sterilizable up to 275°F, does not require the use of a tool for changing burs, contains internal fiber optic elements, and can have the turbine cartridge and/or chuck replaced by the operator. Handpieces in use also contain a number of edges that make effective disinfection difficult. Debris, saliva, blood, and other fluids are often drawn into the internal working mechanism. Fortunately, most of the quality handpieces manufactured in the last several years are heat-sterilizable, and as described in an earlier chapter, sterilization of this important piece of equipment has become an attainable goal. A compromise for those units that are unable to withstand heat sterilization involves a thorough cleaning, followed by disinfection with an EPA-approved, tuberculocidal disinfectant. It must be emphasized that disinfection of handpieces is *not* a substitute for sterilization.

Preparation of a handpiece for heat sterilization is also important. The unit should be scrubbed and rinsed with soap and water to remove gross debris. All water should be removed prior to lubrication and bagging for sterilization. Most manufacturers recommend lubrication before sterilization, but some also call for lubrication afterwards. One must carefully follow the manufacturer's instructions, otherwise the product warranty may be voided if damage occurs. All other "powered" instruments, such as scalers and curing lights, should also be sterilized between patients. Practically every type of instrument is available in sterilizable form, and this feature should be considered when new equipment is purchased.

STAFF RESPONSIBILITIES

It is the responsibility of the dentist and the staff to develop an infection control plan for patient and health professional protection. This plan must include specific procedures for maintaining the treatment equipment in the most aseptic condition possible. All instructions and documents pertaining to equipment should be safely filed, and excerpts copied of items pertaining to infection control. This information should be assembled in a manual that describes specific tasks for each individual, as well as time sequences for accomplishing each procedure. A written log should be kept to document infection control activities. Periodic meetings could serve to review and update infection control procedures.

It is important that new employees are trained in their duties and responsibilities regarding infection control. Periodic checks should be carried out by a designated individual to ensure compliance with established procedures, and the results of such checks written into the log and discussed in staff meetings.

Graphic illustrations of the spread of contamination are always valuable. The use of marker dyes or finger paints to illustrate the potential spread of saliva is an excellent teaching aid (see Chapters 4 and 13). One staff "team" goes through a mock treatment procedure with their hands covered with a water soluble dye or finger paint. The next group uses their normal materials, time, and sequence to clean the area prior to the next appointment. Following the clean up, both teams carefully examine all equipment and instruments used. The amount of marker material left in crevices, on cavity varnish and base metal containers, under edges, around seams, on switches, etc., can serve as a vivid reminder of the importance of the use of barriers and careful cleaning procedures.

FUTURE DEVELOPMENTS

Manufacturers are constantly working to improve the sterilization and asepsis properties of their equipment. Ornamental trims, decorative seams, and bulk storage bins are rapidly disappearing from currently marketed items. Molded, seamless components are being designed and manufactured for all types of treatment equipment, including cabinetry and sinks. Noncontact controls are coming into wider use for dispensing hand cleansing agents and controlling water flow. Better materials are also more resistant to the destructive effects of many cleaning and disinfectant preparations.

Equipment controls will probably also undergo significant changes. Common push button and rocker style switches are already being replaced with seamless "membrane" switches, which are easy to clean and disinfect without harming the electrical circuitry. Toggle switches now have long flexible stems, which are operated with the back of the hand or the forearm. There will be an increased use of remote control modules in order to remove unnecessary items from the vicinity where treatment is occurring. These modules will be individually removable and replaceable by the user. Self-diagnostic systems will also be commonplace, thereby reducing down-time for the dentist. There is little reason to have the basic components for handpieces, electrosurgical units, ultrasonic scalers, and curing lights in an area prone to contamination. These units will be remotely controlled, primarily with membrane and noncontact elements, such as laminar air and energy beam switches. The use of foot controls for task seating, as well as patient chairs and dynamic instrumentation, will be expanded as the use of hand controls decreases.

Hoses or cords for many treatment instruments will most likely remain necessary for the immediate future. Extremely lightweight and flexible hose materials will be commonplace, thus reducing "tug-back" and improving the dexterity of the operator. These items will, however, become removable and be sterilized with the item they serve. This will allow only those items necessary for a particular procedure to be placed in service, thereby preventing possible contamination of unused equipment. Storage of handpieces and other dynamic items on a treatment unit will become a thing of the past. The internal passages and exterior surfaces of fluid and air hoses will also be smooth and defect-free to discourage accumulation of microbial debris. Finally, there will be a substantial increase in the use of fitted barrier materials, both for existing and future equipment.

SUMMARY

In the past, dental equipment was designed for function and esthetics, with little concern for the potential of cross-contamination. Recent advances in equipment technology are making all forms of treatment equipment much easier to clean and disinfect. The use of barrier materials and effective cleaning and disinfection agents has further enhanced the capability of dental professionals to provide aseptic conditions during patient treatment.

Practicality and cost will continue to be major factors for equipment asepsis. Protection procedures cannot completely overshadow delivery of quality patient care. Costs to the patient must be kept in check, while still providing optimum service. Recommendations based on sound scientific data, common sense, and experience will therefore dictate practical standards, and the profession must use all available means to make certain those standards are followed.

REFERENCES

ADA Council on Dental Therapeutics, ADA Council on Prosthetic Services and Dental Laboratory Relations: Guidelines for infection control in the dental office and the commercial dental laboratory. J. Am. Dent. Assoc., 110:969–974, 1985.

ADA Council on Dental Therapeutics: Facts about AIDS for dental professionals, 1986.

ADA, CDC, and NIDR.: Proceedings: National Conference on Infection Control in Dentistry. US Department of Health and Human Services, Atlanta, 1986.

Autio, K.L., Rosen, S., Reynolds, N.J., and Bright, J.S.: Studies on cross-contamination in the dental clinic. J. Am. Dent. Assoc., 100:358–361, 1980.

Bagga, B.S.R., Murphy, R.A., Anderson, A.W., and Punwani, I.: Contamination of dental unit cooling water with oral microorganisms and its prevention. J. Am. Dent. Assoc., 109:712–716, 1984.

Centers for Disease Control: Recommended infection control practices in dentistry. MMWR, 35:237–242, 1986.

Crawford, J.J.: State-of-the-art: Practical infection control in dentistry. J. Am. Dent. Assoc., 110:629–633, 1985.

Davis, L.: Don't share the air. Sci. News, 129:216, 1986.

Infection control is DMA/DDA seminar topic. Proofs, 69:24–25, 1986.

Matis, B.A., and Young, J.M.: Infection Control in Air Force Dental Clinics. Brooks AFB, USAF Dental Investigation Service, 1980.

Runnells, R.R.: Infection Control in the Wet Finger Environment. Salt Lake City, Publishers Press, 1984.

Runnells, R.R.: Infection Control in the Dental Laboratory. Salt Lake City, Publishers Press, 1984.

Runnells, R.R.: Dental Infection Control, Wet Finger Update—'86. North Salt Lake, Infection Control Publications, 1986.

Sildve, P.O.: The Dentronix disinfecting study—Part 1. Dentronix Quarterly, 3:1–4, 1986.

section five

Aseptic Technique

Chapter 12

Proper Operatory Preparation and Instrument Recirculation

A practical program to control harmful microorganisms must consist of those sterilization and disinfection methods that kill or inhibit even the most resistant pathogens. Effective operatory preparation and instrument recirculation are an imperative part of this program. Practical infection control in the operatory is a multistep process. The protocol should be constantly updated to meet or exceed government and professional regulations, and to utilize the most advanced technology. This chapter will concentrate on some of the steps in operatory preparation and instrument recirculation. Equipment procedures will be mentioned in passing, but are more thoroughly discussed in Chapter 11, Aseptic Considerations in Dental Equipment Selection.

OPERATORY PREPARATION

General

All surfaces and items touched by hands contaminated with saliva or blood should be scrupulously cleaned and disinfected with an effective agent before seating each patient. An alternative is to use protective disposable covers because surfaces that will be repeatedly touched or soiled can have covers discarded and quickly replaced between patients. A list of suggested surfaces where covers are useful is in Table 12–1. Covers limit the number of surfaces that must be cleaned and disinfected, save time, and can ultimately be more protective. Impervious backed paper, large food bags, plastic wrap, and aluminum foil are readily available. Large, clear plastic food or waste can liner bags fit over many chair backs and dental units if the operator wants to cover these surfaces. Better fitting, prepackaged bags may cost slightly more, but are more convenient and may offer a better appearance.

When covering a tray, the plastic wrap (or paper or surgical towel) should cover the entire surface including the edges and overlap under the tray, such that when one reaches for the tray, fingers are not exposed to contaminants on the underside of the tray (Fig. 12–1). Discard and replace covers after each appointment. Surfaces protected with barriers should be cleaned and disinfected at least daily *but do not need to be cleaned and disinfected after each patient*. To limit contamination and cleanup, avoid unnecessary touching of operatory surfaces with soiled gloved hands. Use a paper towel, "overglove," or some other barrier to handle items (Fig. 12–2A, B, and C). A tongue blade may be used to operate switches (Fig. 12–3).

Table 12–1.   Items To Be Routinely Covered in a Dental Operatory

Item	Recommended Covering
Laboratory/operatory bench and counter surfaces	Plastic or paper
Chair back (optional)	Plastic
Headrest (only if not covered with chair back)	Plastic or paper
Bracket table including hose supports	Plastic
Side support for auxiliary hoses	Plastic
Air/water syringe handle	Plastic
High volume evacuation control	Plastic
Saliva ejector control	Plastic
X-ray head and control unit	Plastic
Lamp handles	Foil, plastic wrap, or bag

A number of items are attached to the dental unit that are used intraorally, or are handled and touched interchangeably with treatment instruments such as the high-volume evacuator, air-water syringe, and saliva ejector. These items become contaminated with blood and saliva and must be cleaned and disinfected or, preferably, sterilized. If removal for processing is not possible, use disposable covers (plastic, foil, or paper) to protect them until removable items are installed (Fig. 12–4). Removable sterilizable air-water syringe assemblies have recently been introduced. Small flatware bags available from restaurant supply houses also work well as surface covers.

Cleaning of items that are attached to the unit is best accomplished by pulling the item to the nearby sink where it can be cleaned with a disinfectant scrub and rinsed in running water. Then wipe dry with a paper towel. Next, completely wet the item with an EPA registered and ADA accepted surface disinfectant, and leave the solution in contact with the items for the time specified by the disinfectant manufacturer (Fig. 12–5). Follow the manufacturer's directions as to whether rinsing is needed or if the items should be allowed to air dry.

Disinfectants used on operatory items will not kill spores. This is acceptable as evidence indicates that hospital disinfectants that can destroy *Mycobacterium tuberculosis* and lipophilic and hydrophilic viruses are also effective against human immunodeficiency virus (HIV) and hepatitis B virus (HBV) on cleaned surfaces.

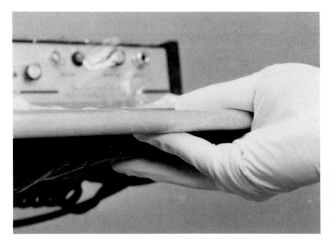

Fig. 12–1. Plastic wrap extending over the front and under the bracket table protecting the operator/auxiliary when grasping the tray.

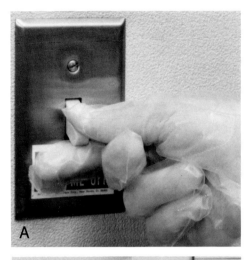

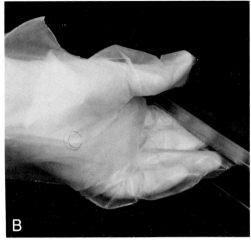

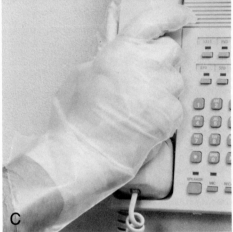

Fig. 12–2. *A–C,* Food handlers glove used as an "overglove" to avoid contaminating items.

Aqueous synthetic dual phenolic, iodophor, and chlorine disinfectants have been approved for this use. Approved iodophor or phenolic disinfectants that contain a detergent are preferred to clean and disinfect items on the dental unit. These are best applied from a pump spray bottle. Some of these disinfectants must be mixed fresh daily in order to ensure their tuberculocidal efficacy. See Chapter 9 for more information on chemical disinfectants.

Paper towels are recommended for cleaning as they are large, fast, economical and are not rendered useless as quickly by bioburden accumulation as 4 × 4 gauze sponges. 2 × 2 sponges should *never* be used for applying disinfectants primarily because of their limited size. Chapter 10 of this text addresses environmental surface disinfection procedures.

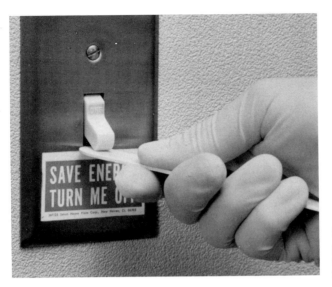

Fig. 12–3. Tongue blades or paper towels can be used to operate switches without contamination.

Disinfecting and Preparing the Operatory

1. Put on heavy-duty utility gloves. Nitrile rubber gloves are more puncture resistant than are other utility gloves (Fig. 12–6). Remove instruments, tip of air/water syringe, and other items to be cleaned and place them into a holding solution if one is used. The holding solution and container should be one that is made of clear plastic so instruments can be checked to ensure they are below the level of the solution. Either a diluted dual synthetic phenol or glutaraldehyde solution can be used.

2. Discard used covers and all cotton and paper debris (masks, gloves, soiled but not *soaked* cotton rolls and gauzes, sponges and paper towels used in cleaning).

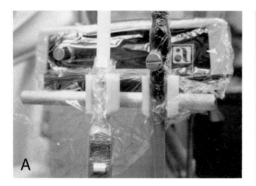

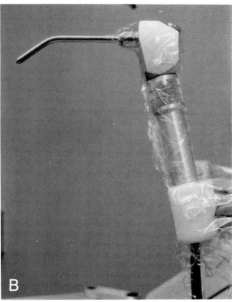

Fig. 12–4. *A, B,* Plastic wrap over the high-volume evacuation control, saliva ejector, and air-water syringe.

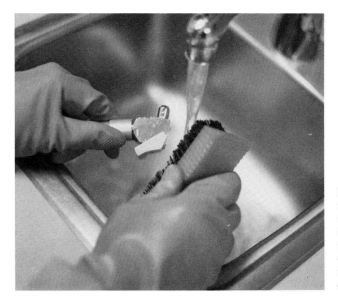

Fig. 12–5. When covers are not used, equipment that will be touched and reused must be scrubbed clean before disinfection. Scrubbing and rinsing is done quickly and thoroughly in the sink with an iodophor or other detergent.

These items should be disposed of with other contaminated waste at the Instrument Recirculation Center (IRC). The operatory receptacle is for handwashing debris only. Blood and saliva *soaked* items are considered "medical waste" (Table 12–2, Waste Definitions, and Table 12–3, Medical Waste Items) and must be contained in a plastic "medical waste" bag taped to the side of the assistant cart during procedures (Fig. 12–7). This medical waste bag is to be discarded in an approved biohazard bag. "Sharps" must be disposed into a puncture-resistant leakproof biohazard container. Wash utility gloves.

3. Smooth environmental surfaces that have not been covered must be sprayed with a cleaner/disinfectant and wiped or scrubbed clean with a paper towel. Most control switches should be covered with barrier materials and not be sprayed directly; excess fluid may cause short circuits and corrosion of electrical compo-

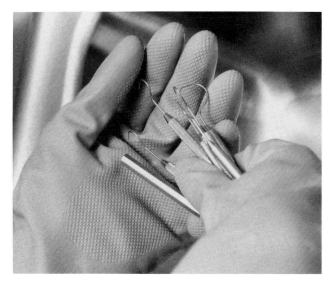

Fig. 12–6. Nitrile latex utility gloves are preferred to handle contaminated sharp equipment and instruments. After use, wash with an iodophor detergent and hang to dry or, preferably, steam autoclave.

Table 12–2.   Waste Definitions

Infectious Waste: *Waste capable of causing an infectious disease*
 For waste to be infectious, it must contain pathogens with sufficient virulence and quantity so that exposure to the waste by a susceptible host could result in infectious disease.*

Contaminated Waste: *Items that have had contact with blood or other body secretions*
 All infectious waste is also considered contaminated waste, but not all contaminated waste is infectious because it may not harbor a sufficient quantity of disease-causing organisms and it may not provide a vector for the infectious agent to infect a susceptible host.*

Hazardous Waste: *Waste posing a risk or peril to humans or the environment**

Toxic Waste: *Waste capable of having a poisonous effect**

Medical Waste: *Any solid waste that is generated in the diagnosis, treatment, or immunization of human beings or animals in research pertaining thereto, or in the production or testing of biologicals. The term does not include any hazardous waste or household waste*
 Waste generated by health care providers in private homes where they provide medical services to individuals would be household waste. Because the household waste stream is excluded, the waste generated by health care providers in private homes is not subject to tracking or management requirements even when removed from the home and transported to the health care worker's place of business.†

*Adapted from Reis-Schmidt, T.: Waste handling and processing standards developing in dentistry: Agencies, associations, and legislators respond to waste management issue. DPR, May, 1989, p. 46.
 †Adapted from Environmental Protection Agency: 40 CFR Parts 22 and 259. Standard for the tracking and management of medical waste. Fed. Reg. *54(56)*:12326, March 24, 1989.

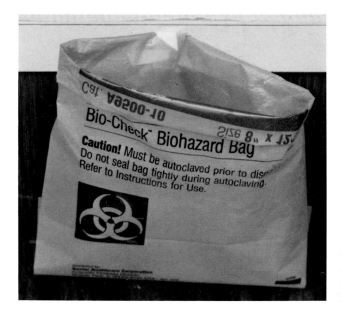

Fig. 12–7. Attach a "medical waste" bag of suitable size to the assistant's cart for saliva and blood soaked items.

Table 12–3.   "Medical Waste" Items in Dentistry

Sharps: *Used and unused needles, scalpel blades, sutures, instruments, burs, and broken glass*
Human tissue removed during surgery: *Teeth and incidental tissue*
Blood-soaked materials: *Soaked cotton rolls, gauze, pellets, and tissue coverings (packs)*

Note: Matrix bands, masks, gloves, patient napkins, impression materials, and x-ray packets are *not* classified as medical waste.

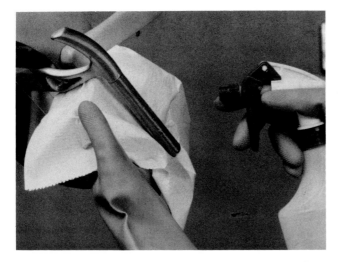

Fig. 12–8. Hold a paper towel behind items that cannot be removed from the unit when spraying them.

nents. A second application of disinfectant is then needed on the clean surface to allow effective disinfectant action. Leave the surface moist so that the disinfectant will continue to act. Use a disinfectant that provides residual activity if possible.

4. For suction hose ends, the air/water syringe handle, and handpieces that cannot be removed and sterilized, hold a paper towel behind the items to catch excess spray (Fig. 12–8). Spray both sides of the items and wipe them clean. Then respray on both sides and allow to air dry. This need only be performed once a day if items are protected adequately with covers that are replaced after each patient.

5. A clean brush can be used to scrub items with irregular surfaces. Brushes should be disposable or autoclavable.

6. If they are not covered, spray support holders for the high volume evacuator (HVE), the saliva ejector, handpieces, and the air/water syringe, then wipe clean with a paper towel. Use a second towel moistened with the disinfectant to wipe each hose end and the attached instrumentation. Wipe each hose back along its most accessible length. Place each back in the support. Hold a paper towel behind the replaced items to catch excess spray and spray the items again. Leave them wet until ready to reuse. Ten minutes is specified on most disinfectant labels. Items still wet can be dried with a paper towel or a 4 × 4 before use, if necessary. "Smooth surface" hoses are now available for vacuum and handpiece lines. These hoses are much easier to clean and maintain.

7. Cleaning a chair with a good detergent is sufficient if the chair surfaces are not spattered and touched during patient treatment. When cleaning a chair, moisten a paper towel with cleaner/disinfectant and clean the unprotected chair and arms where it may have been contaminated. Dry the chair just prior to seating the patient. Do not leave diluted bleach to dry on chairs as the clothing on subsequent patients may develop bleach stains.

8. Clean by spraying the outside, then the inside of the cuspidor. Wash utility gloves, clean and disinfect faucet handles, remove utility gloves, and wash hands. Wash and disinfect utility gloves inside and out and steam sterilize them at the end of the day, following the manufacturer's guidelines.

9. With clean hands, cover surfaces with barriers. The armamentarium (preset tray with instruments, suction tips, and syringe tip) is brought from the IRC. The

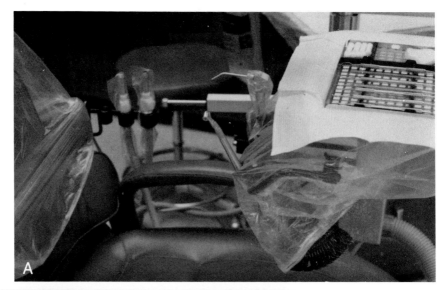

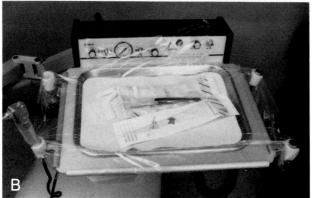

Fig. 12–9. *A & B,* Operatory drapes are used in many private offices and large clinics for care of all patients.

tray is covered with an impervious-backed patient napkin to be placed on the patient when seated. A completed operatory ready for patient care is shown in Figure 12–9.

After each appointment, repeat the appropriate steps to prepare for the next patient. As is evident, changing plastic covers at a cost of a few cents is much faster and economical than cleaning and disinfecting many surfaces between patients according to the authors' unpublished studies.

The time required to leave items wet is often a concern to practitioners as the next patient may be treated sooner than the 10-minute drying time often specified. A product such as iodophor, which offers residual activity, will help remedy this concern. Unpublished evidence indicates that some disinfectants work in approximately 5 minutes on a precleaned surface if the surface is left wet. This can be carefully considered for chemicals that specify a 10-minute wait time if confirmed by calling the manufacturer of the disinfectant in question before decreasing the contact time. Dry items with a paper towel if they are still wet when you need to use them. Time and expense involved in adequate infection control lead many dentists to seat fewer patients at a time and plan longer appointments for each

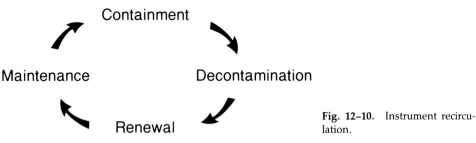

Fig. 12–10. Instrument recirculation.

patient. See also Chapter 7 of this text concerning the use of practical barrier techniques and Chapter 11 concerning aseptic considerations of dental equipment.

INSTRUMENT RECIRCULATION

Instrument recirculation addresses four issues: The CONTAINMENT of contaminated instrumentation, the DECONTAMINATION PROCESS, the RENEWAL process of sterilization and disinfection and the MAINTENANCE of instruments until ready for reuse (Fig. 12–10).

Containment

Policy. During and after each operatory procedure, every effort should be made to confine all instruments, devices, and supplies that have come into contact with the patient to a well-defined and limited area.

Rationale. By containing contaminated instruments, devices, and debris to specific trays, procedure, work, and decontamination areas, microorganisms are not unnecessarily spread. The chances of cross-contamination and infection are greatly reduced, and operatory clean-up can be safely and quickly accomplished.

Recommendations

1. A specific, well-defined area should be designated for initial storage and decontamination of contaminated materials. This area should be identified as a contaminated area and thoroughly scrubbed and decontaminated by gloved personnel after each day's use.

2. Under no circumstances should decontamination be attempted, or contaminated waste be disposed of, in the operatory. Biohazard bags should be utilized in accordance with local, state, and federal regulations.

3. New procedure gloves, face masks, and disinfected protective eyewear should be worn by the practitioner and auxiliary personnel with each patient. Used procedure gloves and face masks should be considered contaminated and thus be removed and placed on the procedure tray prior to its transfer to the decontamination area.

4. All contaminated instruments, devices, and debris should be handled carefully, only by personnel wearing utility gloves.

5. Procedure trays should be covered during transfer from operatory to decontamination area to control airborne microorganisms.

6. Contaminated instruments and devices should remain covered or placed in a holding solution prior to processing in the decontamination area. A holding solution will keep blood, protein, and saliva from drying, can begin to disinfect, and ease the decontamination process.

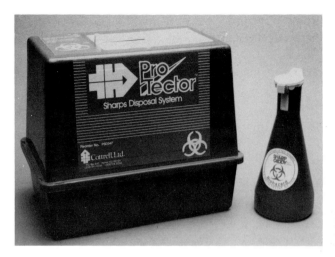

Fig. 12–11. Puncture-resistant, leakproof, and disposable needle containers.

Key CONTAINMENT Points to Remember

1. Contain contaminated materials—from point of origin to termination
2. When you "See Blood—Think HBV"
3. Always wear utility gloves when handling contaminated materials
4. Minimize contact with contaminated materials
5. Dispose of contaminated waste appropriately, using biohazard bags when indicated by government regulations
6. "Good Enough" isn't good enough!

Decontamination (Gross and Ultrasonic)

Policy. Contaminated waste should be separated for processing or disposal in biohazard bags according to government regulations. Single-use materials should be disposed of in a specific location, needles and other sharps should be placed in a puncture-proof container. Begin the process by the removal of gross debris from materials to be decontaminated and reused. Ultrasonic decontamination of all instruments and devices should be performed before the sterilization process is begun when possible.

Rationale. Formal decontamination and waste disposal procedures are major factors in the prevention of cross-contamination and infection. The reduction of the bioburden on instruments and devices to be sterilized is essential to the success of any sterilization process. Modern ultrasonic cleaning units and chemicals are capable of removing contamination from all surface areas of instruments and devices, thereby facilitating the sterilizing process.

Recommendations

1. All contaminated instruments, devices, and debris should be handled carefully only by personnel wearing utility gloves, protective eyewear, and a disposable or washable protective apron.
2. All disposable instruments, devices, and debris should be removed and disposed of in the designated area.
3. All needles, sutures, blades, and other sharp items should be placed in a designated puncture-proof container (Fig. 12–11).

4. Products designated as single-use or disposable should not be reused. They should be disposed of according to government regulations. The time necessary for proper decontamination, the diminished product performance, and the liability risk far outweigh perceived cost savings.

5. All instruments and devices to be recycled should be rinsed in cold water as soon as possible after use if they had not been placed in a holding solution. Cold water will help to remove blood and other debris, however, hot water could coagulate blood and protein and make removal more difficult.

6. Gross debris can now be removed by placing the instruments into an ultrasonic cleaner. Utilize a quality, high-output ultrasonic unit that is properly sized to permit complete immersion of the instruments or devices to be decontaminated. A basket or holder should be used to keep instruments the proper distance from the bottom of the tank. A well-fitting cover should be used at all times during the operation of the cleaner to prevent escape of aerosols into the atmosphere. Follow the manufacturer's operating instructions carefully to ensure maximum decontamination efficiency. Test the ultrasonic unit on a regular basis.

7. Use quality detergents that are specifically formulated to ensure the maximum ultrasonic cleaning action. A nonionic detergent containing a rust inhibitor is recommended. Follow the manufacturer's mixing directions carefully to ensure maximum removal of the widest range of contaminants.

8. Should ultrasonic cleaning not be possible, place instruments into warm water (125°F) with a good quality, low-sudsing, slightly alkaline detergent. Instruments should be scrubbed individually with a stiff-bristle, autoclavable brush, keeping the instruments and brush below the surface of the water to prevent splashing, the release of aerosols and airborne particulates, and the spread of microorganisms. Particular attention should be paid to serrated and crevicular areas. Hinges and joints should be opened and scrubbed thoroughly.

9. Instrument cleaning brushes should be regularly cleaned, inspected, and sterilized.

10. After ultrasonic or manual cleaning, the instruments are rinsed thoroughly in warm water and inspected for any remaining debris or defects. If debris is found, manually clean until removed.

11. Instruments must be completely dried before being packaged for sterilization.

Key DECONTAMINATION Points to Remember

1. It is possible to decontaminate without sterilizing; it is not possible to sterilize without decontaminating

2. "Clean" is not "sterile"

3. Always wear utility gloves and protective eyewear and clothing when handling contaminated materials

4. Use a quality ultrasonic unit and chemicals that are specifically designed for ultrasonic decontamination

5. Follow the manufacturer's operating and chemical mixing instructions carefully for maximum decontamination

6. Always use a well-fitting cover on the ultrasonic unit to prevent the spread of aerosols

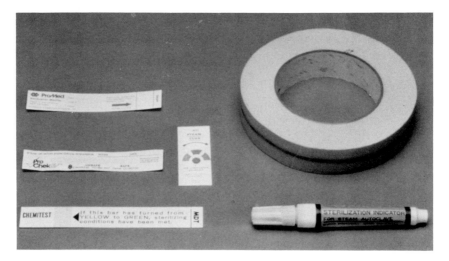

Fig. 12–12.   Color change process indicators.

7. Follow local, state, and federal regulations concerning the disposal of bio-hazardous waste
8. "Good Enough" isn't good enough!

Renew (Heat Sterilization)

Policy. All instruments and devices that can be heat sterilized should be heat sterilized and packaged in quality material that will maintain sterility.

Rationale. Sterile instruments and devices are recognized as the most effective method of preventing cross-contamination and infection.

Recommendations

1. Instruments and devices to be sterilized must be effectively decontaminated and completely dry prior to packaging and processing.
2. Quality packaging material that will maintain sterility should be used to ensure that instruments remain uncontaminated and safe to use. Paper stamped "Made in the United Kingdom" presently must meet the most rigid standards concerning strength of the wet paper, air permeability and resistance, wet and dry seal strength, tear resistance, and peel characteristics. Similarly, packaging that has the ADA acceptance seal also meets those standards.
3. Inspect all instruments and devices prior to packaging to ensure all bioburden has been removed.
4. Open all hinged instruments to permit the sterilizing agent contact with all surfaces.
5. Use the size of package that is appropriate to the size of the device or the number of instruments to be processed. Do not put an excessive number of instruments into the packaging.
6. Have a color change sterilization indicator in each package to ensure that the package has been penetrated by the heat and to detect gross malfunctions or errors (Fig. 12–12). The indicator ink should not come in contact with the instrument surface to prevent false positives.
7. The package must be sealed effectively to ensure that sterility is maintained.

Self-seal or heat-seal paper/poly pouches and tubing provide the highest level of integrity and sterility maintenance. Nylon bags and tubing may be sealed by heat or indicator tape. Paper bags may also be sealed by indicator tape.

8. Under no circumstances should paper clips, staples, or other devices that close the package, but do not totally seal it, be used.

9. Correct loading of the sterilizer chamber is essential to the assurance that conditions necessary to achieve sterility are met. Overloading the chamber will jeopardize the sterilization process. Underloading the chamber could cause damage to instruments by overheating.

10. Packages should be placed in the chamber *on edge*, so that the sterilizing agent contacts every surface of every article to be sterilized.

11. Follow the sterilizer manufacturer's operating instructions carefully to ensure that conditions for sterilization are achieved.

12. A proper sterilization cycle consists of the *Heat-Up Period*; the time necessary for the entire load to reach the selected sterilizing temperature, and the *Exposure Period*; the total time required for sterilization of the load. The exposure period should have a safety factor for maximum protection.

13. Sterilization units should be monitored using a biologic monitor spore test system at least monthly and preferably weekly, or according to governmental recommendations, to ensure that conditions necessary for sterilization are being achieved. Evidence of the results of this monitoring and daily color change indicator strips should be retained to verify that the sterilization unit is operating properly.

14. Allow instruments and devices to cool prior to removal from the sterilization unit.

15. Proper cleaning and maintenance of sterilizers, following manufacturers' instructions, is essential in maintaining reliability.

Key RENEW Points to Remember

1. Use quality packaging to ensure that sterility is maintained
2. Be sure that the package to be sterilized is properly sealed
3. Load the sterilizer chamber properly
4. Follow the manufacturer's operating and maintenance instructions carefully
5. Biologically monitor the performance of the sterilization unit as recommended by governmental agency
6. Retain records of the sterilization unit's performance
7. "Good Enough" is not good enough!

Maintenance

Policy. Instruments and devices that have been packaged in sterility maintenance material and exposed to an effective sterilization procedure must be stored in a manner that will prevent contamination.

Rationale. Proper care and storage of packaged, sterilized instruments will ensure that they will remain sterile until the package integrity is broken at the time of use.

Recommendations

1. Instruments should never be stored unpackaged. Loose instruments are con-

taminated each time the cabinet door or drawer is opened. The major sources of contamination during storage include:

—Airborne microorganisms from environmental dust or from airborne oral microorganisms

—Handling with contaminated hands

2. The simplest and most time-efficient method for preventing instrument contamination during storage is to properly package instruments in quality materials that will maintain sterility prior to use, and to keep the sterile packaged instruments covered until use.

3. Sterile package instruments should be placed on clean shelves or in clean drawers. The shelf or drawer surfaces should be covered or lined with paper or poly-backed patient towels. Cabinets and drawers should be cleaned and disinfected on a regular basis (once a week). However, packaged items need not be resterilized following this process.

4. If packaged sterile items are to be stored for extended time periods, the packs should be sealed inside plastic dust cover pouches.

5. The sterile instrument storage area should be removed as far as possible from the decontamination area. Never store sterile instruments under a sink because a wet package is no longer sterile.

6. The recirculation of air contaminated by office traffic, operatory aerosols, and particulate debris may reduce the sterility life of stored instruments and devices. Closed cabinets, drawers, and plastic dust covers provide maximum protection.

7. Keep instruments and devices wrapped until they are needed during the procedure, thus reducing the chance of contamination.

8. Instrument packaging should be opened in the operatory so that the inside of the package functions as a sterile field on which the instruments are presented.

Key STORAGE Points to Remember

1. Proper storage of sterile instruments and devices is essential to preserve sterility

2. Keep instrument cabinet doors and drawers closed

3. Minimize exposure of sterile instruments to airborne contamination

4. "Good Enough" isn't good enough!

Specific Instruments and Items

Disposable Needles and Anesthesia Cartridges. These items should never be used for more than one patient. Used needles should be placed in a puncture-proof box or metal container for safe disposal. Thick-walled biohazard containers with a one-way valve are a necessity.

Rubber Prophylaxis Cups. Cups accumulate debris in cracks. They tear and cannot be disinfected. They are to be discarded after each patient.

Plastic Suction Tips and Impression Trays. Clean and chemically sterilize items that cannot be heat sterilized in 2 to 3.2% glutaraldehyde or ethylene oxide for the manufacturer's recommended time, according to ADA and EPA recommendations.

Prosthodontic Items, Instruments, and Materials Used Chairside. These items (impression material tubes, bowls, and spatulas) should be thoroughly cleaned and disinfected after each appointment. Before removable or fixed prostheses are returned from a laboratory (office or commercial) to the patient's mouth, such devices should be meticulously cleaned with an iodophor scrub, adequately disinfected in an effective solution and rinsed thoroughly. When using a lathe in the laboratory, protect eyes, nose, and mouth with eyewear and face masks. Disinfectants can also be used to rinse impressions without damage. See Chapter 15 of this text concerning practical infection control in the dental laboratory.

Handpieces and Prophy Angles. Heat sterilizable handpieces and prophy angles are available from most manufacturers. These can be steam autoclaved or chemiclaved in efficient, small, lightweight units. Handpieces and prophy angles that are not heat sterilizable can be surface disinfected using the protocol outlined in Chapter 11 on dental equipment. Disposable prophy angles are readily available, inexpensive and recommended.

PROTECTION WHEN PROVIDING TREATMENT IN THE OPERATORY

Dentists and auxiliaries must protect skin and mucous membranes against spatter and debris. Wear full-protection eyewear, high filtration masks, and quality gloves. The patient's eyes should also be protected against debris by use of protective eyewear. Use rubber cups in place of polishing brushes when possible to avoid spatter. Discard gloves and wash hands thoroughly, lathering and rinsing two or three times when possible before moving from patient to patient. A high-level antimicrobial handwash with residual activity will keep bacteria levels reduced and inhibit dermatitis for continual glove users. Antiseptic foams are available but are not substitutes for washing. Remove all rings when providing dental treatment. Jewelry about the neck and ears will become contaminated with spatter and aerosol and should not be worn during treatment. Hands should be kept away from nose, face, hair, mobile chair, soiled pencils, and charts during treatments. Wear a clean uniform with a protective cover. Keep hair away from face and uniform collar. Wear a hair cover when spray and spatter is anticipated to contaminate the hair. *"Street" clothes should not be worn when providing treatment.*

Patients should use an antimicrobial mouthrinse just prior to treatment. This action has been shown to reduce the number of oral microbes by up to 90%. A mouthrinse with residual antimicrobial action, such as 0.12% chlorhexidine gluconate is appropriate.

SUMMARY

Operatory preparation and instrument recirculation involves many individual steps and decisions. It is important that the entire office become familiar with the rationale behind each step and decision in order to carry out a comprehensive infection control program. Periodic review of the protocols used is necessary to ensure that all necessary steps are accomplished without unplanned redundancy.

ADDITIONAL READING

Cottone, J.A.: Infection control in dentistry. In: Proceedings of the National Symposium on Infection Control in Dentistry. US Department of Health and Human Services, October, 1986, pp. 36–43.

Crawford, J.J.: Sterilization, disinfection and asepsis in dentistry. In: Block, S.S. ed. Disinfection, Sterilization and Preservation. 3rd Ed. Philadelphia, Lea & Febiger, 1983.

Crawford, J.J.: State of the art: Practical infection control in dentistry. J. Am. Dent. Assoc., 110:629–633, 1985.

Environmental Protection Agency. 40 CFR Parts 22 and 259. Standard for the tracking and management of medical waste. Fed. Reg., 54(56):12326, March 24, 1989.

Reis-Schmidt, T.: Waste handling and processing standards developing in dentistry: Agencies, associations, and legislators respond to waste management issue. DPR, May, 1989, p. 46.

Runnells, R.R.: Infection control in the former wet finger environment. Salt Lake City, IC Publications, 1987.

Saunders, M., and Cottone, J.A.: Sterilization and its discontents: What is good enough? Tex. Dent. J., 104:20–29, 1987.

Total Operatory Protection System (TOPS). Englewood, Cottrell Ltd. Education Services, 1985.

Chapter 13

Infection Control in Dental Radiology

THE EXTENT OF CONTAMINATION IN DENTAL RADIOLOGY

Most of the literature in infection control generally applies to all areas of dentistry. Only recently has the literature specifically dealt with problems unique to dental radiology. The radiology area is not routinely associated with needles, sharp instruments, or the spatter of blood and saliva; however, transmission of infectious diseases is possible because of the contamination of equipment and supplies in the making of intraoral radiographs.

The literature addresses infection control primarily from three points of view: (1) the microorganisms that can be isolated from a variety of surfaces, (2) the methods to remove and kill some or most of these microorganisms through proper cleaning and disinfection or sterilization, or (3) ways to prevent microbial spread through personal protection and aseptic technique.

Potential infection control problems in the area of intraoral radiography can be recognized once they are given some thought. Film must be placed in the mouth with precision and speed, the tube head and extension cone must be aligned as quickly as possible, and then the control panel must be touched to make the proper exposure. Once the film is removed from the mouth, it must be placed somewhere while other films of the series are being exposed, again creating a potential for cross-contamination. The chair and headrest often must be repositioned several times while completing a series of films on one patient. And even if the chair and headrest are positioned and settings selected in advance for the particular exposure, the extension cone and control panel, at minimum, must be touched with the same fingers that placed the film into the mouth thereby contaminating surfaces.

The operator must then move into the darkroom, which may include touching the door handle. Once in the darkroom, the exposed film must be placed on a surface as individual film packets are opened and the film is placed in the developing solution. Finally, the film packaging material must be handled as it is discarded.

To determine the full extent of cross-contamination in the radiographic workplace, a demonstration was devised in which dental assistant volunteers were asked to expose twenty film intraoral surveys on a mannequin (Fig. 13–1). The mannequin had a simulated face so that cheeks, lips, and tongue were present. A solution was placed in the floor of the mouth of the mannequin simulating saliva. The fluid solution was a mixture of Shannon Glow 40 Invisible yellow and Shannon Glow 20 Invisible blue (Shannon Luminous Materials Co., Los Angeles, California 90046)

167

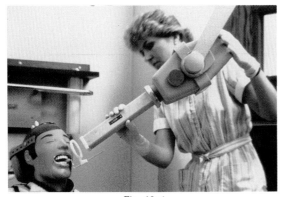

Fig. 13–1

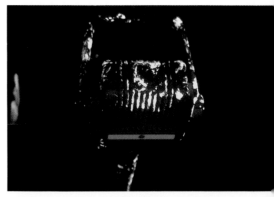

Fig. 13–2

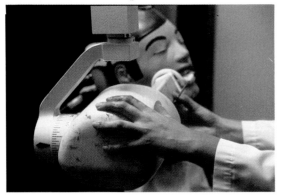

Fig. 13–3

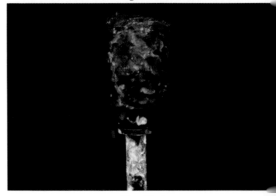

Fig. 13–4

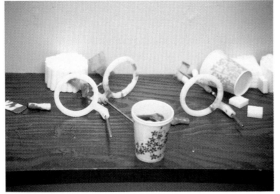

Fig. 13–5

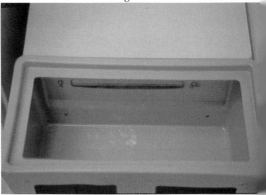

Fig. 13–6A

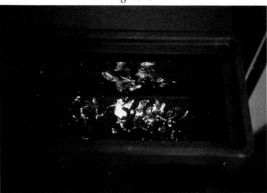

Fig. 13–6B

Fig. 13–1. A dental assistant performing an intraoral diograph survey on a mannequin. **Fig. 13–2.** Ultravic light demonstrates contamination on the intraoral rad graphic unit after one full mouth series of rad graphs. **Fig. 13–3.** Second assistant using red fluoresc dye. **Fig. 13–4.** Ultraviolet light demonstrates conta nation of the tube head and extension cone of a der radiographic unit. **Fig. 13–5.** Red dye demonstrates c tamination on the table below the exposure panel. **13–6.** Contamination of the floor of the daylight loa using room light (A) and ultraviolet light (B).

that were mixed with glycerin to give it the consistency of saliva but would fluoresce under ultraviolet light. It appeared rather unobtrusive to the naked eye so the assistant would not be distracted, and she was asked to take a complete intraoral radiographic survey in the same way she would normally take one. She was told the reason for the fluid was that the film packets were being evaluated for potential leakage. While the assistant made the radiographic exposures, one dental student added fluid periodically and another dental student worked the controls that opened and closed the mouth of the mannequin.

A second demonstration involved another dental assistant who was asked to do the same procedure. This time a red fluorescent dye (Artista II Tempera paint, Binney & Smith Inc., Easton, PA 18042) mixed with glycerin was used.

The first dental assistant, adhering to her normal procedures, wore gloves even though this demonstration occurred before publication of the 1986 CDC infection control guidelines. The light color of the fluid did not appear to distract her. She was asked to develop the films in a normal fashion when she completed the survey. Photographs were made of the contaminated radiographic unit while the assistant processed the films (Fig. 13–2). The assistant was then asked to return to the room and complete her normal cleanup routine. Interestingly, the assistant remained gloved while developing the film yet took them off during her cleanup procedures. Her usual cleanup protocol consisted of wiping clean the headrest, armrests, and extension cone with a 2×2 gauze soaked in alcohol even though this procedure is not recommended.

The second dental assistant did not routinely wear gloves when the demonstration was done (prior to publication of the 1986 CDC infection control guidelines), therefore she did not wear them for this demonstration. Although she was not aware that contamination was being studied, the bright red was distracting and she tried to minimize spreading it by being more careful about what she touched (Fig. 13–3). This self-consciousness seemed less apparent in the later half of the radiographic survey. She was not asked to cleanup in the usual way because it would not have been possible for her to remove all the red dye.

In both cases, the extent of the contamination was much greater than anticipated by the authors. Not only was the extension cone contaminated, but also the entire tube head (Fig. 13–4). This part of the machine had not been included in the assistant's usual cleanup routine. Other unexpected areas contaminated included the back of the chair, the headrest controls, the lead apron, and the table below the exposure control panel (Fig. 13–5). The exposed films as well as the different positioning devices used for different areas of the mouth had been laid on this table. The sink handles were also contaminated as they were hand rather than foot, elbow, or electronically controlled.

Both assistants used the daylight loader on the automatic X-ray film processor. Although they removed the film packet debris from the loader when finished, contamination from the packets on the floor of the loader was evident (Fig. 13–6 A and B).

SOLUTION TO THE PROBLEM

One of the most important solutions to any problem is to first become aware of the extent of the problem. In the dental radiology unit, personnel must (1) recognize the extent of the contamination that occurs so that the cleaning and disinfecting procedures are not limited to the traditional headrest, armrest, extension cone, and some of the control panel, and (2) be aware that the traditional 2×2 gauze sponges soaked in alcohol are ineffective for cleaning and disinfecting surfaces. As previously mentioned in Chapter 9, alcohol is not an ADA accepted surface disinfectant and a 2×2 gauze sponge is too small to do much more than spread debris.

Recommended Cleanup Procedures

Surface Cleaning and Disinfecting. Cleaning and disinfecting of environmental surfaces and equipment between patients should include the following areas of the dental radiology unit if they are touched or not protected by impervious barriers:

1. The entire tube head, including the swivel arms that are used to turn the tube head
2. The entire length and extension of the extension cone
3. The chair, including headrest, headrest adjustment apparatus, armrest, back support (which is often used to turn the chair), controls that adjust the position of the back support, and any other manual controls for vertically moving the chair
4. Control panel including all knobs, buttons, or levers that are altered between films on the same patient
5. Any surfaces onto which exposed films or positioning devices are placed between films taken on the same patient
6. Aprons and thyroid shields
7. Light switches, sink, faucet, soap dispenser, if manually controlled
8. Darkroom doorknob and all surfaces on which exposed films and used intraoral devices are placed
9. Interior of a daylight loader

The cleaning and disinfecting procedure most often recommended for environmental surfaces and equipment involves a "spray-wipe-spray" technique using an EPA registered and ADA accepted hospital disinfectant that is tuberculocidal and will kill hydrophilic and lipophilic viruses. The area to be disinfected is sprayed liberally using a pump spray container. A standard-size disposable towel or sponge is used to wipe down the surfaces. In general, the larger the towel, the quicker this procedure will be accomplished. The areas are then sprayed again leaving a film of solution on the surfaces to air dry.

Instrument Sterilization. All nondisposable instruments used for positioning the film should be cleaned with soap and water or an ultrasonic cleaner to remove debris prior to heat sterilization. All items that are damaged by heat sterilization may be sterilized by use of a 2 to 3.2% glutaraldehyde mixed to manufacturer's specification for sterilization (see Chapter 8). There is no longer an excuse to use intraoral items that cannot be heat sterilized or discarded between patients because instruments that can be sterilized are increasingly available for dental radiographic procedures.

Preventive Measures

Patient Screening. As discussed in Chapter 2, even a good medical history will not always identify the high-risk person; therefore, each patient should be

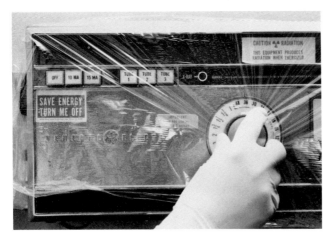

Fig. 13-7. Covered control panel appropriately prepared for use.

considered to be high risk so that one standard infection control protocol can be devised and used for every patient.

Personal Protection. The use of appropriate gloves is still the best preventive measure for personal protection against infections to which one is not immune. Disposable latex gloves should be worn throughout the entire radiographic procedure. Prior to leaving the radiology area, latex gloves should be removed and properly disposed of so that subsequent doors and other surfaces touched are not contaminated on the way to the darkroom. An "over glove" is a reasonable alternative to changing gloves in some offices. Once in the darkroom, clean disposable gloves should be used. Puncture-resistant nitrile rubber utility gloves are recommended for cleanup procedures. Masks and eyewear are not necessary unless it is suspected that either patient or clinician has an upper respiratory infection or an aerosol spray will be generated.

Prevention of Contamination. A totally aseptic technique is impossible if one person is taking the films; however, there are measures that can be taken in advance to reduce the number and size of surfaces that will need to be cleaned and disinfected after patient treatment. These include the following:

1. *A disposable cover, placed in advance, on which the films and positioning instruments are laid.* A paper cup is a good way to keep the films together. If a tray is used it can also be carried into the darkroom and discarded or resterilized if a disposable cover was not used.

2. *Plastic wrap over the control panel.* The control panel can be covered with single or multiple layers of plastic wrap (Fig. 13-7). If multiple layers are used, the topmost contaminated layer can be torn off when finished leaving a clean plastic cover below. One would need to be careful not to use too many layers as changing the dials would become difficult. Note that paper covers cannot be used in multiple layers because of seepage of fluids. Also, paper or other nontransparent covers over the dials and switches will make adjustments impossible. Another alternative would be the use of a foot switch, in which case, cleaning and disinfection between patients is not necessary (Fig. 13-8).

3. *Plastic wrap for the tube head and extension cone.*

4. *Removable headrest covers.*

5. *A two-person technique.* One person places the radiographic films into the mouth, the other adjusts the chair, extension cone, control panel, and makes

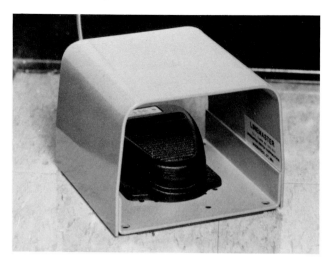

Fig. 13–8. Foot switch used to make exposures in place of a hand-held switch.

the exposure (Fig. 13–9). The person placing the films would be the only one capable of cross-contamination. No surfaces would be contaminated if that person wore gloves, did not touch any items or surfaces except the radiographic film, and discarded the gloves upon leaving the room.

6. *Disposable cover (plastic-backed paper towel or plastic wrap) over a designated area in the darkroom, on which films should be set.* The person developing the films should be wearing clean latex gloves. All film packets can be opened, gloves discarded and hands washed, before the films are picked up for placement into the developer. Alternately, as film packets are unwrapped with gloved hands, the film can be handled solely by the edge and fed into an automatic processor (Fig. 13–10). Studies have confirmed that developer and fixer are incapable of sustaining bacterial growth under normal use conditions.

7. *Film packets may also be cleaned and disinfected with a spray-wipe technique prior to being opened.* Alternately, film can be placed or wrapped in plastic protective covers prior to placement in the mouth. This wrapping is disposed of prior to development. Commercially made protective covers for dental radiography film are now available.

8. *Plastic covers for the bite pieces used in panoramic units.* Several manufacturers

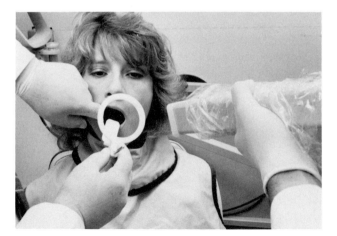

Fig. 13–8. Foot switch used to make exposures in place of a hand-held switch.

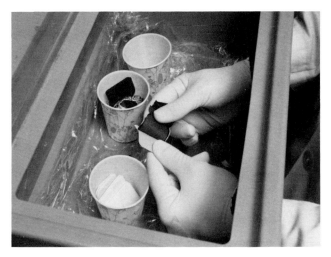

Fig. 13–10. Correct use of daylight loader with the operator wearing gloves, contaminated film packets in one cup, extra cups for debris, and plastic lining the loader floor.

currently make disposable plastic covers for their panoramic machines (Fig. 13–11). If covers are not used, proper cleaning and disinfection of the bite blocks between patients is required. Heat sterilizable bite blocks are preferable.

SPAULDING CLASSIFICATION OF INANIMATE OBJECTS

Dr. E.H. Spaulding's classification of germicidal chemicals is related to three types of surfaces categorized according to proximity of contact with a patient. These categories are as follows:
1. *Critical items: Surfaces that commonly penetrate or touch **broken** skin or mucous membranes.* In radiology, probes used in sialography would fall into this category.
2. *Semicritical items: Surfaces that commonly touch **intact** mucous membranes but do not usually enter normally sterile areas of the body.* In radiology, this would include

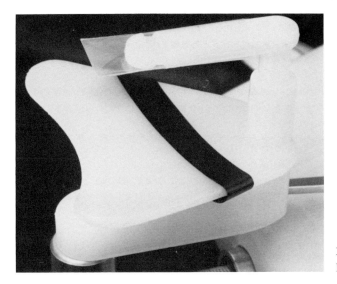

Fig. 13–11. Plastic cover for panoramic bite pieces.

any position indicator devices used intraorally and the bite blocks of panoramic machines.
3. *Noncritical items: Surfaces that do not commonly touch mucous membranes.* In radiology, this would include all the surfaces mentioned under environmental surface disinfection.

All critical items from this classification system **must** be cleaned and sterilized; semicritical items should be cleaned and sterilized (chemicals may be used if heat sterilization cannot be performed); and noncritical items must be cleaned and disinfected between patients.

SUMMARY

There are multiple opportunities for cross-contamination in the dental radiology unit, many of which are not recognized by dental personnel. Once the extent of cross-contamination is fully recognized and manufacturers become aware of the clinician's desires to minimize these occurrences, changes in equipment and supplies used in dental radiology will help to reduce and possibly eliminate the problem. Some of these changes may include the following:
1. More foot controls for changes in exposure setting, chair, and headrest position.
2. Foot or other "no-touch" controls for soap and water dispensors.
3. Exposure panels that are flat and have touch-sensitive capability so that proper surface cleaning and disinfecting procedures would not damage controls and there would be no openings for solution seepage. Touching could also be done with the elbow on these types of controls. Foot controls would eliminate this problem totally.
4. The plastic sleeves for intraoral film produced by Kodak have the potential for eliminating all contamination in the darkroom. Currently, the sleeves are marketed for use with known high-risk patients, which is contrary to universal precautions. Additionally, x-ray film must be manually placed into the sleeves, one at a time. Ideally, intraoral x-ray film could be sold by the manufacturer with the plastic sleeve already in place. Once the film is exposed, the outer sleeve would be removed without touching the inner packet with contaminated gloves. Then, using washed ungloved hands, the uncontaminated exposed film packets would be taken into the darkroom or to the daylight loader for processing.
5. An extension cone that automatically finds its position (demonstrated by J. Morita, Inc. at the 1985 Congress of the International Association of Dento-Maxillo-Facial Radiology in London).

As more attention is focused onto this area, creative thinking will result in other innovative changes that should occur. It is anticipated that the reader will look for these improvements when selecting new equipment.

SELECTED READINGS

ADA Councils on Dental Materials, Instruments and Equipment; Dental Practice; and Dental Therapeutics: Infection control recommendations for the dental office and the dental laboratory. J. Am. Dent. Assoc., *116*:241–248, 1988.

Clinical Affairs Subcommittee on Infection Control and Safety (CASICS), The University of Texas Dental School at San Antonio. Manual: Infection control procedures at The University of Texas Dental School at San Antonio Clinics, 1989.

Katz, J.O., Cottone, J.A., Hardman, P.K., and Taylor, T.S.: Infection control in dental school radiology. J. Dent. Educ., 53:222–225, 1989.

Katz, J.O., Cottone, J.A., Hardman, P.K., and Taylor, T.S.: Infection control protocol for dental radiology. Gen. Dent. (In press).

Katz, J.O., et al.: Potential for bacterial and mycotic growth in developer and fixer solutions. Dentomaxillofac. Radiol., 17(Suppl. 10):52, 1988.

Material Safety Data Sheet, Kodak RP X-OMAT Developer and Replenisher, Part C, Rochester, Eastman Kodak Company, November, 1986.

White, S.C., and Glaze, S.: Interpatient microbiological cross-contamination after dental radiographic examination. J. Am. Dent. Assoc., 96:801–804, 1978.

Chapter 14

Infection Control: A Consideration in Office Design

Historically, dental offices have been designed around concepts that support production with little or no regard to infection control. Although the number of treatment rooms still remains an important element, the amount of work space and the design layout have proven to be even more important in terms of function, safety, and long-term practice development.

The success of an effective infection control program depends, in part, on proper office design. The following areas should be addressed with consideration to aesthetics, patient appeal, and effect on productivity:

1. Floor Plan and Traffic Flow
2. Materials
3. Fixtures
4. Operatory Design
5. Instrument Recirculation Center (IRC)

Additionally, these five areas must be evaluated as they relate to treatment, non-treatment, and treatment support functions.

Treatment areas are defined as any area where *direct intraoral mucosal contact occurs*. Examples of areas where direct mucosal contact occurs are operatories, radiographic processing areas, and oral hygiene instruction areas.

Treatment support areas are where *indirect patient contact occurs through directly handling contaminated procedure support items such as impressions, instruments, and exposed film*. Examples of these areas are the laboratory, IRC, and radiograph processing room.

Nontreatment areas usually require no direct patient contact. The business office, reception room, patient lavatory, staff lavatory, staff lounge, and private offices are generally considered nontreatment areas.

FLOOR PLAN AND TRAFFIC FLOW

Most design errors begin when work space requirements have been either overlooked or mismanaged. Work space is the amount of area necessary to carry out operational tasks or functions required for production. Insufficient work space forces workers to function inefficiently. Furthermore, exposed items and surrounding surfaces become contaminated from splash and spatter. Considering most office schedules and practical time management principles, decontamination procedures continue to be a frustrating challenge.

Patient treatment areas generate the highest level of microbial-laden spatter. These areas must be separated from the treatment support area as well as the nontreatment areas in an attempt to confine the population of pathogens to where it can be quickly and easily reduced. One must be aware, however, that microbes are inevitably transported from one area to another via air handling systems, patients, personnel, and visitors. Thus the goal in this area must be to reduce **excess** cross-contamination beyond that normally seen in any shared human environment. Careful office planning in design and remodeling can maximize this reduction.

Patient and visitor traffic flow must avoid passage through the laboratory, IRC, or other treatment and support areas (Figs. 14–1 and 14–2). Direct access should be available from the reception area to the scheduled operatory. Consultation areas should be located closest to the administrative and reception areas, followed by the hygiene/patient education room(s) and full treatment operatories. Longer appointments should be scheduled in the most distant operatory with short visits scheduled in the first treatment rooms. This directs the heaviest flow of patient/visitor traffic away from extensive treatment and treatment support areas.

If a central radiographic exposure room is used, access is needed from the hygiene and full treatment rooms. Processing rooms are best supported when located adjacent to the exposure area.

The IRC should be convenient to the treatment areas. The laboratory should be accessible to the treatment areas that require laboratory support. Patient traffic areas should not include the laboratory and IRC. A utility room containing the central vacuum and air compressor is best located adjacent to the laboratory to provide access for cleaning of filters and traps. A private entrance for staff is desirable and should be located with the staff lounge and lavatory in a remote yet accessible area. The private office should be located away from treatment and support areas unless it will be used for patient consultations.

MATERIALS

Though patient appeal and aesthetics are a consideration, our primary concern must be with protection. All floors, walls, surfaces, cabinets, drawers, and equipment must be capable of being quickly and easily cleaned and disinfected. The use of wood surfaces, textured wall coverings, stuffed animals and fabrics for decoration should be minimized. Smooth and seamless nonporous materials will inhibit the collection and protection of microbes.

Carpet should not be used in treatment or treatment support areas. Continuous roll hard vinyl floor covering has been recommended for several years. Tile squares create cracks and crevices that harbor debris. Where carpeting is used, it should be low pile, tightly woven synthetic fiber with no pad and glued directly to the subflooring. Wool or high pile carpets are difficult to clean and may attract large numbers of pathogens. Some carpeting is now available with an antimicrobial agent but as yet is relatively untested.

Vinyl, glass, resin laminates, stainless steel, or processed resins may be used for cabinets and counters. Dimethyl methylacrylate (Corian-Dupont) is a nonporous, nonstaining material that will not chip, discolor, or crack, according to the manufacturer. It may be used for back splash, counters, cabinet fronts, dental cart top surfaces, or sinks. It is also available as a "coating" for existing structures.

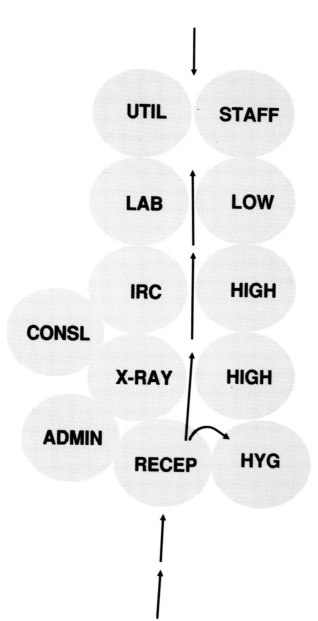

Fig. 14–1. "Bubble diagram" indicating patient traffic flow from reception to hygiene and other high-traffic rooms. Low-traffic treatment and support areas are located away from the busiest areas. Note separate but central location of the Instrument Recirculation Center.

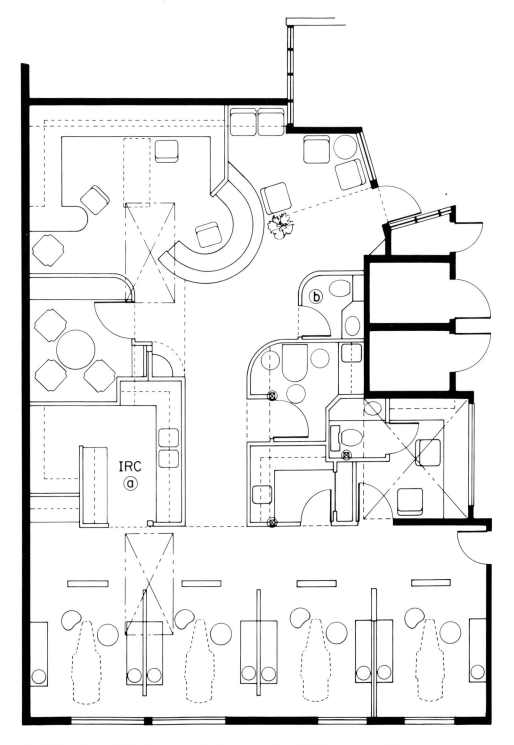

Fig. 14–2.   Sample Office Design. *A*, Sterilization center (IRC) illustrates an ''L''-shaped counter and a large double sink with designated space for precleaning, drying, sorting, and bagging of items. IRC is separate from laboratory and accessible to all operatories. *B*, Patient restroom in view of business area. *C*, Dual entrance to all treatment rooms to provide easy access for doctor and primary and secondary auxiliaries. (Courtesy of Cowan Design Company and Associates, Mill Valley, CA.)

Extremely white surfaces should be avoided, as some surface disinfectants may discolor certain materials over a period of time. Aluminum should also be avoided on drawer handles, pulls, or switches as it can also be affected by some chemical agents.

FIXTURES

Sink Faucets, Liquid Dispensers, and Waste Receptacles

Carefully choosing fixtures that require minimal hand contact will maximize the effectiveness of your infection-control program. Sink faucets and soap or lotion dispensers should be foot or arm operated. Hand contact should be avoided. Dispensers should be mounted on the wall to reduce handling and eliminate microbial contamination. Electric "eye" sink faucets and dispensers are available and may be an attractive alternative. Paper towel dispensers also pose a contamination dilemma. "No touch" wall mounted towel dispensers are preferred. Hand-controlled sink faucets, if present, should be turned off using a paper towel after handwashing and drying. Cloth towels should *never* be used, as they retain a high number of microbes and serve as a source of cross-contamination.

Waste receptacles in the treatment and support areas should be recessed into counter tops or cabinet fronts. Openings should be large enough to dispose of debris with ease. Treatment room receptacles should be used for handwashing waste only. "Medical waste" items taken from the mouth and *soaked* with blood or saliva (e.g., cotton rolls, gauze, pellets, and tissue "packs" from treatment procedures) should be disposed into biohazard containers in accordance with governmental regulations. Puncture resistant leakproof biohazard containers must be used for "sharps."

OPERATORY DESIGN

The objective of incorporating infection control considerations in a office design plan goes beyond aesthetics and numbers. It involves function. Form must follow function; therefore, all form should be designed around required tasks. Each task should be walked through so that space requirements are determined accurately. If it takes 3 feet of counter space to perform a task, then 3 feet should be provided in that area. Assumptions and lack of information will automatically guarantee problems. Information should be gathered early in the design planning stages to avoid costly errors. Last minute "change orders" can increase costs considerably.

The main objective during treatment is to treat the patient in the least amount of time possible without compromising quality. This is accomplished by keeping the operator's hands and eyes on the treatment site throughout the procedure. The assistant must also be "set-up" so movements can be minimized as well as the size of the zone of contamination. Time and motion studies show that an operator leaves the operating field an average of 10 times during one procedure. Not only is this a time management problem, but it is the number one source of cross-contamination. Imagine contaminated hands leaving the oral cavity, touching the side counter, touching a drawer handle or two and then proceeding to retrieve a bur by handling several others before returning to the treatment site. Now, multiply that by 10, the average number of patients treated daily in one room and the potential for cross-contamination is more easily understood.

Historically, dental manufacturers designed equipment and support cabinetry for the doctor in a two-handed dentistry situation. An overabundant supply of cabinetry and equipment, positioned for doctor-only access, encouraged the doctor to "reach out and touch something" with contaminated hands.

Furthermore, chair-mounted auxiliary equipment (suction and 3-way syringe) encourage the assistant to lay the aspirator on the lap when freeing the hands to exchange instruments or mix materials. Chair-mounted auxiliary equipment is often awkward and time consuming because a twisting motion is required to retrieve and replace support equipment.

Poorly positioned equipment leads to poorly positioned operating teams working in unbalanced positions. Therefore, proper balance is also an important issue. When operators are off balance they need to stabilize themselves on nearby surfaces such as sterile trays or contaminated cart tops. Poor balance can also challenge coordination, thereby increasing the chances of injury.

The operatory is the treatment area that produces the highest level of pathogens. Choice and placement of equipment should address ease of use, comfort, durability and performance, but first and foremost, it must be easily cleaned, disinfected, and covered with disposable barriers. Chapter 11 addresses aseptic considerations of dental equipment.

The operatory should be designed with adequate work surface to accommodate preset procedure trays and support armamentarium. Drawers should be deep enough to accommodate sterile packages of extra instruments, burs, and disposables. Minimize the number of drawers to promote the "less is more" concept. Drawers should be made of impervious materials and be easily removable for cleaning and disinfection.

All instrumentation should be retrieved from the IRC and returned at the conclusion of the treatment. Cabinetry must also support small auxiliary equipment such as amalgamators, curing lights, electrosurgical devices, and other support items that are impractical to remove from the operatory after each appointment. Be sure to protect these items from aerosol and spatter.

Decorations such as posters, an overabundance of plants, stuffed animals, and fabrics should be avoided. The operatory should maintain a smooth, simple, aseptic, clean look. Chapter 12 addresses other aspects of proper aseptic technique, particularly operatory preparation and instrument recirculation.

TREATMENT ROOM MANAGEMENT

If the main objective is to keep the doctor's hands in the patient's mouth throughout the procedure, then all equipment should be primarily accessible to the assistant. The unit and instrument tray is most effective when positioned directly in front of the chairside auxiliary.

A treatment room is in all respects an operating room (Fig. 14–3). It is not an area to stock supplies or sterilize instruments. Cabinetry must be minimized to reduce temptations to leave the work site and handle other nonsterile items. Storage in the treatment room should be limited to only what must be immediately accessible for patient treatment.

As an example of one style of office design, a "bread board" shelf can offer a

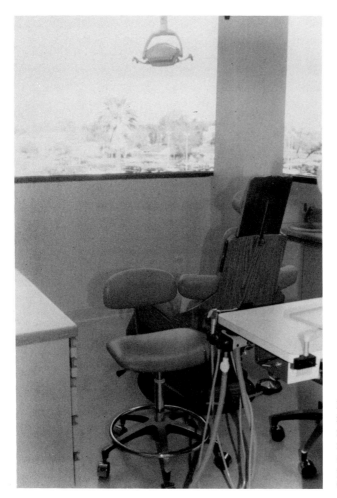

Fig. 14–3. Operatory with minimal chair-mounted equipment, roll hard vinyl floor covering, and minimal extra ornamentation. (Courtesy of Cowan Design Company and Associates, Mill Valley, CA.)

clean surface when the patient record must be handled. The top drawer underneath the bread board should be shallow, approximately 3″ deep. This drawer can contain extra sterile packages of instruments, burs and small support items such as rubber dam clamps.

The second and third drawer should be approximately 5″ deep to support disposable items and extra materials. The fourth drawer can house gloves, masks, and tissues and should be approximately 7″ deep (Fig. 14–4). The amalgamator can be positioned on the cart, in a deeper drawer or side cabinet shelf that slides out to the treatment area, or on the counter if the cart or side cabinetry alternatives are not available. Ideally, drawers should be positioned on both sides of the treatment room, mirror images of each other (Fig. 14–5), to accommodate both right- and left-handed operators. Placement of amalgamator, curing lights, and electro-surgical unit are highly individual decisions for each operator and staff member.

Side cabinetry should be approximately 30″ high and positioned approximately 26″ from the patient chair side arm to stay within comfortable reaching distance. This distance also allows walk-through access for patients and personnel.

Sinks may, if desired, be positioned more toward the foot of the patient chair to provide additional countertop work space adjacent to the operating team. Ideally,

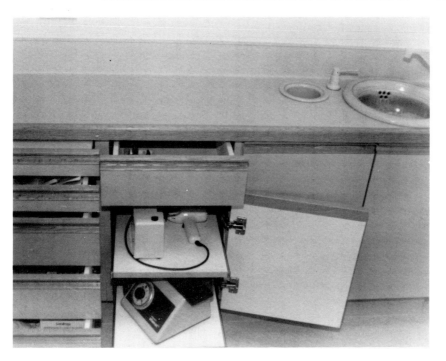

Fig. 14–4. Counter unit with "bread-board" shelf, shallow top drawer, and several deep drawers next to sliding shelves. Waste receptacle and sink can be recessed to eliminate "lip." (Courtesy of Cowan Design Company and Associates, Mill Valley, CA.)

sinks should be operated by either a foot control, electronic eye, or single lever that can be activated by an arm or elbow to avoid contamination. Trash chutes can be positioned in the counter top nearest the sink for paper towel disposal. Small contaminated items are best disposed of in a paper cup positioned on the tray and carried over to the patient's mouth to avoid spillage. A small biohazard bag can be taped to the side of the mobile cart and used to dispose of medical waste directly from the patient's mouth. Biohazard bags should be available and used in accordance with governmental agency recommendations.

RADIOGRAPHIC EQUIPMENT AND NITROUS OXIDE

The radiographic unit has proved to be most flexible and stable when positioned at 12:00, directly behind the patient. One does not need to excessively handle the x-ray head when it can be directed with ease. Pass-through radiographic units positioned between operatories have created problems with "drifting," often experienced after final positioning, because of added strain on the unit arm. In addition, if two people need the machine at the same time, it has been found that proper cleaning and disinfection procedures do not take place because of time restraints between each patient.

Nitrous oxide hoses and masks may contribute to added contamination. Protection from spatter and aerosols generated during treatment can be enhanced by positioning the unit in the rear utility wall and running the hoses through the floor

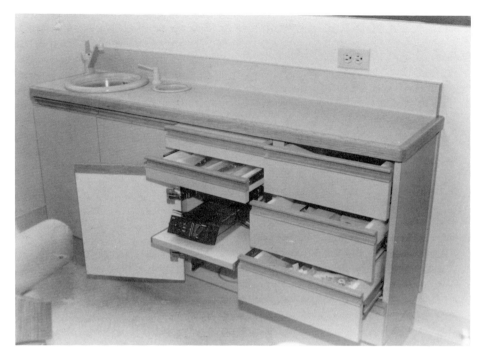

Fig. 14–5. Opposite counter to that pictured in Figure 14–3 has same features to accommodate both right- and left-handed operators. (Courtesy of Cowan Design Company and Associates, Mill Valley, CA.)

and back up the base of the patient chair. Sterilizable or disposable nitrous oxide masks and hoses are available and recommended.

INSTRUMENT RECIRCULATION CENTER (IRC)

The Instrument Recirculation Center has been the most overlooked and underestimated space in dental office design. For years, supply houses and architects designed sterilization areas as one straight counter with a sink at one end. Unfortunately, the functional needs required of an Instrument Recirculation Center have not been well understood. Often times this area is located in a hallway or worse, combined with a laboratory, resulting in an extremely difficult area to maintain asepsis. Consequently, clutter and confusion invariably lead to frustration, poor time management, and severe cross-contamination.

The IRC serves as the nucleus of the office infection control program and therefore must be conveniently located to all treatment areas. The IRC must also be designed in an area that avoids direct patient traffic pathways.

The IRC serves the following needs:
a. Precleaning of all contaminated instrumentation
b. Drying, sorting, and packaging items
c. Sterilization (heat and chemical)
d. Storage

Construction of the cabinetry should be of smooth, nonporous material such as metal, resin laminates, or processed resins. Storage areas should be covered with clear glass cabinet doors. Shelves and drawers should be removable for frequent cleaning and disinfection. Sinks should be spacious to allow for scrubbing of trays and containers and should contain sloping drains. The area must also have positive ventilation to control noxious vapors from various chemicals and sterilization procedures. The IRC should be limited to instrument recycling and tray preparation *only* and should not be used as a "lab" or a bulk storage area just as the laboratory should not be used as the IRC.

The IRC must accommodate these phases of activity: Containment, Decontamination (precleaning and packaging), Renewal (sterilization), and Maintenance (storage). See Chapter 12 for more details on these phases of activity.

Preparation of instruments prior to sterilization begins with a cleaning process that is more effectively accomplished with a predisinfectant bath and an ultrasonic cleaner. A sink for washing and rinsing instruments must also be available. A chemical disinfectant solution tub must be available for processing heat-sensitive items.

Given that both the ultrasonic and the chemical disinfectant solution require a nearby sink, special attention should be given to their positioning on the counter to avoid cross-contamination. The sink can be used to separate zones of activity by viewing it as a boundary between the break-down zone and the processing zone. Establishing work zones will standardize procedures and help ensure consistency among staff members.

Ideally the processing room cabinetry should include 16 to 21 linear feet. Two separate sections of cabinetry, positioned parallel to one another (Fig. 14–6), or in an "L" shape design, will facilitate adequate processing space, and simplify procedural flow.

SPECIAL CONSIDERATIONS

Recessing the ultrasonic unit into the countertop adjacent to the sink can ease access and simplify instrument transfers for rinsing (Fig. 14–6). One possible problem with recessed units is access for repair and maintenance. Countertop trash chutes should be used to eliminate the need to open cabinet doors for receptacle access. Positioning the trash chute to the furtherest corner will prevent accidental disposal of instruments when drying and packaging. The shape of the trash chute should be rectangular rather than circular. This will provide easy "insertion" of disposables from tray to chute and reduce handling by eliminating the need to compact paper products into smaller masses. Trash compactors can also be helpful in reducing the handling and transferring of contaminates from one receptacle to another. Special bags for contaminated items should be available in this area.

Providing a drawer to store sterilization bags, sterile wrap, and autoclavable disposables within this section of cabinetry will enhance procedural flow. The use of a dryer or heat lamp could expedite the drying process considerably, however there is no such item available to the dental market at this time.

Auxiliary sink attachments can also be helpful. "Spray guns" improve rinsing by allowing one to direct the flow of spray more effectively.

The central processing sink should be at least 32″ wide. A double sink provides sufficient work space, however loss of counter space should be taken into consideration. Water activation should either be operated by foot or by electronic eye.

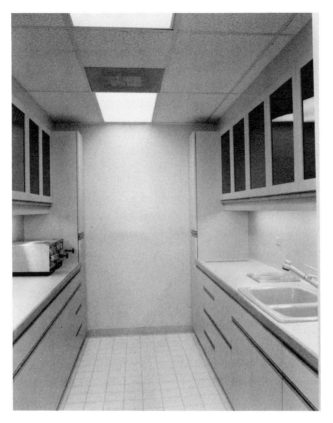

Fig. 14–6. Two separate parallel sections of cabinetry with the sink in the middle of the decontamination zone in the Instrument Recirculation Center (IRC). Note recessed ultrasonic cleaner adjacent to sink. (Courtesy of Cowan Design Company and Associates, Mill Valley, CA.)

Soap dispensers should be recessed into the sink or mounted on the wall above the sink along with paper towel holder for quick and easy access.

PROCESSING COUNTER

The section of cabinetry on the opposite side of the sink is designated for chemical processing. Chemical solutions can be either on the countertop or recessed. A hygienic dishwasher with high temperature settings and sanitizing cycles, positioned in the base cabinetry, can help simplify the cleaning and drying of instrument trays, cassettes, and other items that are too large to heat process.

The opposite side of cabinetry or continuation of cabinetry in an "L" shaped format is designated for sterilizing, cooling, and storage. A drawer positioned underneath the sterilizer can be used for hot instrument storage (also known as the "cool-down drawer") if proper ventilation is provided to exhaust heat from the drawer. Cycles will not be backed up if hot items can be transferred to a drawer immediately following processing.

Top drawers should be approximately 18″ W × 24″ L × 5″ D and are used to store nonsterilizable and disposable tray accessories. Impression trays can also be stored in drawers or base cabinetry "slide outs" (Fig. 14–7). They should be individually packaged prior to sterilization to maintain sterility after packaging. Sectioned drawers can assist in separating individual groups of trays.

After instrument packages are cool enough to handle, they are selected from the cool-down drawer and matched with the appropriate coordinating tray. Pack-

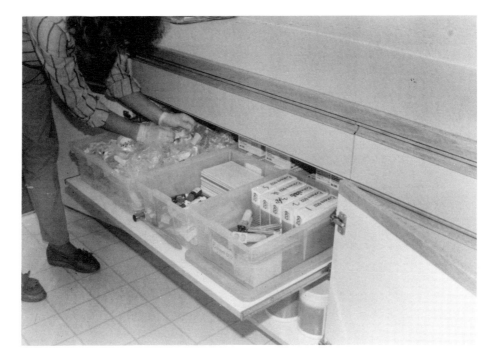

Fig. 14–7. "Slide out" shelf for storage of bulky items such as packaged impression trays. (Courtesy of Cowan Design Company and Associates, Mill Valley, CA.)

ages are left sealed on each tray and cassettes should remain wrapped until used. Trays and cassettes are then replaced in upper cabinets until needed.

Base cabinetry storage can be easily managed when "slide out" shelves are provided. Slide out shelves improve access. Traditional shelving can require a staff member to be on "hands and knees" for visual access, whereas a slide out shelf can eliminate this need all together. In addition, fewer items are lost or misplaced.

Patient set-ups should be "customized" for specific patients before appointments to save time between patients. The customization process involves adding appropriate nonsterilizable items not included in the sterile packages and/or cassettes as noted on the day sheet underneath the patient's name. For example, if the 8:00 patient is scheduled for an MO on #30, a long needle might be retrieved along with articulating paper, a wedge and a new matrix retainer. If the use of a rubber dam is anticipated, the dam is punched and a clamp is selected. The customized tray is then stored on a specific numbered shelf. The corresponding number is then noted next to the patient's name on the day sheet. This process will assist other staff members when setting up for specific patients.

Providing individual storage areas for customized trays and contaminated trays expedite turn around time considerably in between patient appointments. For example, the assistant can enter the central processing area with a contaminated tray, immerse instruments into the predisinfectant bath, store the contaminated tray, wash hands, retrieve the next customized patient tray, and proceed to the designated treatment room, which has been properly prepared for the next patient.

Production can be maximized, stress minimized, and procedures simplified when instrument processing and preparation procedures are organized in this centralized fashion. Adequate work space and strategic design principles must be incorporated to ensure proper technique. Consistency allows each operating team member the ability to provide quality patient care with maximum infection control protection.

SELECTED READINGS

Pollack, R.: Form follows function. CDAJ, *17*:18, 1989.

Young, J.: Dilemma in dentistry: Implementing infection and hazard control in dentistry. Dent. Sch. Quart, *4*:1–8, 1988.

Young, J.: Hang out a shingle: Tips on office design. Dentist, *63*:32–36, July/August, 1985.

Young, J.: Infection control in dentistry. Dent. Advisor, *3*:1–8, 1986.

Young, J.: Interview: Infection Control Report—Operatory and office design and equipment selection. Dent. Prod. Rep., *20*:63, 1986.

Young, J.: Special equipment issue. Dent. Advisor, *2*:1–7, 1985.

Young, J.: The health of the dental professional. J. Am. Dent. Assoc., *114*:515–518, 1987.

Chapter 15

Practical Infection Control in the Dental Laboratory

Most dental personnel prefer to preplan more carefully when providing care for a patient who has been diagnosed with an infectious disease. Items chosen to be used in treatment are disposable or more readily cleaned and disinfected than customary.

These same alternatives in choice of materials and procedures occur in the commercial laboratory when working on a case involving a patient with a known infectious disease. The office and laboratory that preplans for these occasions will be less confused, more relaxed, and adept in providing care for these patients and ultimately *all* patients.

Given the limitations of routine health history information, it is not possible for dental practitioners or laboratories to know the infectious disease status of most patients because:

1. Many infected patients are unaware of their infected status and that their blood or saliva is capable of transmitting an infectious disease.
2. Some patients will not reveal known infectious diseases to health care providers.
3. Health care providers cannot interpret negative findings to mean that the patient is presently "infectious-disease-free" or will remain so upon subsequent clinical visits.

The prudent dental office and dental laboratory considers *all* blood and saliva to be infectious, and routinely manages each patient's treatment and laboratory work as if the patient's body fluids were infected with transmissible infectious microorganisms. Furthermore, prudent dental offices and laboratories use infection control measures proven to be effective in minimizing hepatitis B cross-contamination between patients and personnel because these measures are also effective for controlling all other known infectious agents.

DENTAL OFFICE PROCEDURES

Microorganisms present on or inside impressions can easily be transferred to

1. The skin or hair of the operator
2. Instruments and larger pieces of equipment
3. Stone casts and the general environment

The chance of cross-infection from an impression is much higher without special handling and treatment.

Table 15–1.   Disinfection of Prosthesis

Disinfectant	Problem(s)	Incompatible With
Chlorine solutions (10 to 30 minutes)	Corrosive	Metals
Glutaraldehyde and Phenols (10 to 30 minutes)	1. Incomplete removal with water rinse 2. Tissue irritation	Acrylic
Iodophors (10 minutes)	None documented	—

Adapted from Merchant, V. and Molinari, J.A.: Infection control in prosthodontics: A choice no longer. Gen. Dent., *37*:30, 1989.

The following dental office procedures are suggested before any material is sent to the dental laboratory:

Prosthesis. Complete and partial dentures, whether removable or fixed, that have been in a patient's mouth should be rinsed under running water to remove excess blood and saliva. This is the *precleaning* step of the disinfection procedure. Be careful not to splash water excessively as droplet spatter can carry microorganisms. Prostheses can be placed in an ultrasonic cleaner with a good detergent for the manufacturer's recommended time.

The item should then be *disinfected* by soaking in the EPA registered and ADA accepted hospital level tuberculocidal disinfectant that will kill lipophilic and hydrophilic viruses, for the time specified by the manufacturer. See Table 15–1 for a list of disinfectants available for this use.

Diluted household bleach may be used as a disinfectant solution (¼ cup bleach to 1 gallon of water) mixed fresh daily. If diluted bleach is used, soak the *nonmetal* prosthesis (bleach can corrode metals) for a minimum of 10 minutes and rinse thoroughly. Alternately, full-strength bleach can be used for a prosthesis if it is soaked for only 5 minutes. The prosthesis should then be wrapped in plastic or put into a plastic bag to prevent contaminating the shipping container before being sent to the laboratory. Do *not* add disinfectant in the plastic bag because of the possibility of adverse reactions (see page 196).

Impressions. All impressions should be rinsed under running water to remove excess blood and saliva. Be careful not to splash the water for the same reasons previously mentioned.

Silicone or rubber-based impressions can be disinfected by immersion in any ADA-accepted product except neutral glutaraldehyde (Table 15–2). Rinse again and pour the cast or send to the laboratory for pouring.

Alginate impressions may be rinsed, immersed in iodophor, wrapped in plastic, and allowed to sit for 10 minutes and rinsed again before pouring the cast. Other methods are given in Table 15–3. Unfortunately, there is yet to be universal agreements concerning which disinfectant is best for reversible and nonreversible hydrocolloid. Recommendations for disinfection of reversible hydrocolloid are given in Table 15–4.

The dental office should inform the laboratory if the impression has been disinfected because some dental impression materials are sensitive to multiple immersion procedures.

Cleaning and Disinfecting of Prosthodontics Items. Items that are contaminated only by handling or that have minimal contact with oral fluids do not require sterilization for routine reuse but should be cleaned and disinfected with an EPA-

Table 15–2.   Immersion Disinfection of Elastomeric Impressions

Materials	Disinfectants	Method
Addition silicone	Acid glutaraldehyde, 1%, 2%	Water rinse
Polysulfide rubber	Alkaline glutaraldehyde, 2% Phenolic glutaraldehyde (1:16) Iodophor (1:213) Synthetic phenolic (1:32)	Immersion for time recommended by manufacturer for TB disinfection
	5.25% sodium hypochlorite (1:10) Chlorine dioxide (diluted)	Water rinse Pour as per directions
Polyether	Chlorine dioxide (diluted) Glutaraldehyde, 2% or	Same as above (10-minute maximum)
	5.25% sodium hypochlorite (1:10) Iodophor (1:213)	Same as above except spray or dunk in disinfectant; keep moist for exposure time

Merchant, V.A., 1990. Based on results of published research and manufacturers' recommendations.

registered and ADA accepted disinfectant. These items include torches, facebows (minus the facebow fork), articulators, rulers, mixing spatulas, knives, rubber bowls, shade guides, and mold guides. However, any item (i.e., impression trays and facebow forks) placed in the mouth should be heat sterilized (Table 15–5).

For Known Infectious Patients. The laboratory prescription sometimes indicates that the case is from a patient suspected to be at increased risk for an infectious disease or who has a medical history of an infectious disease that could be transmitted by blood or saliva. The laboratory prescription should be placed in a plastic bag to avoid contamination.

Some dental laboratories recommend the use of an "Alert Label" of conspicuous color that can be placed on the outside of the package to indicate that special handling of the contents may be desirable (Fig. 15–1). Dental offices practicing appropriate infection control procedures for all patients may not use Alert Labels; therefore, the absence of an Alert Label does *not* mean that the case is from a

Table 15–3.   Disinfection of Alginate Impressions

Disinfectants	Sodium hypochlorite (1:5) 2% Acid glutaraldehyde Sodium hypochlorite (1:10)
Method	Water rinse-immerse/dunk-bag (10 minutes)-rinse-pour
Results	Insignificant distortion (0.1 mm) for study casts but not for master casts Surface quality not adversely effected: Acid glutaraldehyde improved quality for some Not all alginates react the same

Adapted from Durr, D.P., et al.: Dimensional stability of alginate impressions immersed in disinfecting solutions. J. Dent. Child., 54:45, 1987, and Polenick, C.: IUSD, Personal communication, 1988.

Table 15–4.   Disinfection of Reversible Hydrocolloid Impressions

Disinfectants	Iodophor (1:213), bleach (1:10), 2% acid glutaraldehyde (1:4)
Method	10 minute immersion-rinse-pour or 10 minute immersion-rinse-K_2PO_4 (20 minute maximum) and shake excess-pour or 10 minute immersion-rinse-humidor (4 hour maximum)-K_2PO_4 (20 minute maximum) and shake excess-pour

Adapted from Van, R., and Merchant, V.A.: Personal communications.

Table 15–5. Common Dental Laboratory Items to be Disinfected or Sterilized

Clean and Heat Sterilize	Clean and Chemically Disinfect
All burs including acrylic	Articulator
Bristle brushes	Casts
Central bearing plates for articulator	Compound heater
Compound heater tray	Facebow (minus fork)
Facebow fork	Knives
Metal handle mixing spatulas	Mixing bowl
#7 Wax spatula	Mixing spatulas
Rag wheels	Mold guides
Stock impression trays	Rulers
	Shade guides
	Torch
	Trial bases

noninfectious patient. Alternatively, some individuals are concerned that Alert Labels may cause concerns with couriers. Whether an Alert Label is or is not used, be careful not to contaminate the outside of the container.

Notice that the use of alert labels is contrary to "universal precautions" although it is sometimes used in addition to universal precautions.

Emergency Procedures. Develop and practice emergency procedures for a contamination accident before it happens. This will usually involve a puncture wound (see Appendix D, Needlestick Protocol). Familiarity with emergency procedures will lessen confusion and instills confidence in the staff when it becomes necessary to implement these procedures.

COMMERCIAL DENTAL LABORATORY PROCEDURES

A large commercial laboratory, analogous to a large dental practice, receives a large number of items, the volume of which magnifies the problem of infection control.

Infection control in the commercial dental laboratory consists of three components:

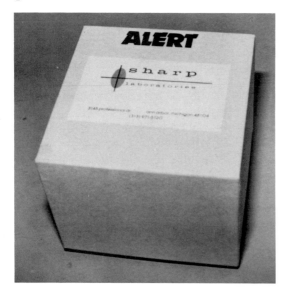

Fig. 15–1. Example of an "Alert Label" used by some dental offices and laboratories.

1. Immunization
2. Barrier techniques
3. Aseptic techniques

All three components must be implemented to have the program be as effective as possible. A consistent series of infection control procedures is followed on *all* work that comes into the dental laboratory in order to ensure full program implementation.

Immunization

All dental personnel should be immunized against hepatitis B as well as receive the other immunizations recommended in Chapter 6.

Barrier Techniques

1. Personnel opening containers as they arrive at the laboratory must wear rubber utility gloves.
2. Work gowns should be worn over street clothes. These gowns should be changed when they become soiled, or at least daily.
3. Protective eyewear and a mask must be worn when splash or spatter may result such as during cast trimming and during any grinding or polishing procedures. Note that a mask and eyewear is not necessary to simply open a container as it comes into the dental laboratory.

Aseptic Techniques

1. Note any package labeling that indicates special precautions in handling when opening cases.
2. After the package is opened, the bag containing the prosthesis or impression that has been in the patient's mouth should be handled carefully to avoid spilling any of the contained disinfectant.
3. Discard all packing material that has been in direct contact with any prosthesis or impression that has been in the patient's mouth.
4. Rinse all prostheses and rubber or silicone impressions before placing them into a disinfectant solution (Fig. 15–2) if they have not already been disinfected at the dental office. Some laboratories keep a list of offices that disinfect impressions to try to omit duplication. Rinse the prosthesis or the impression again before sending the impression to the proper department for work.
       Disinfection solutions suggested are as follows: (see Tables 15–1 to 15–4):
   a. Household bleach (¼ cup to 1 gallon of water) mixed and discarded daily; 10 minute immersion (nonmetallic items)
   b. Iodophor (1 part to 213 parts water according to manufacturer's instructions) mixed and discarded daily; 10 minute immersion
   c. Glutaraldehyde (prepared and used accordingly to manufacturer's instructions). Pay close attention to use and reuse life (see Chapter 9).
       As alginate impressions cannot be disinfected prior to some procedures requiring great accuracy without causing slight distortion, the cast should be disinfected after it is set using an iodophor spray for stone or a glutaraldehyde

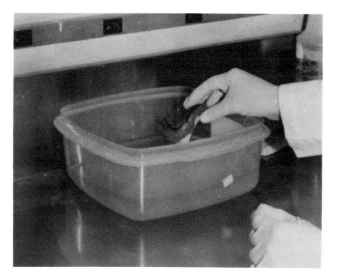

Fig. 15–2. An elastomeric impression being immersed into a disinfectant after rinsing with water. Notice the gloves on the practitioner. A lid should be placed on the disinfectant container after immersion of the impression.

soak for plaster. Note that caution is advised as some disinfectants may damage the surface of the cast. Dental stones with antibacterial properties are beginning to appear on the market. These stones may be appropriate if clinical testing verifies their properties.

Choosing a disinfectant can be confusing if laboratory personnel are not familiar with them. Unfortunately there is no single disinfectant that will do all the jobs necessary in the laboratory, so choose cleaners and disinfectants according to the task you wish them to perform. More information about the selection and use of disinfectants can be found in Chapters 9 and 10.

After items have been cleaned and disinfected, they should not be handled with the same gloves used to open the package or they will be recontaminated. Plastic tongs are recommended for this step.

All impression trays should be cleaned, packaged, and heat sterilized.

5. Protective eyewear and a mask must be worn when the cast is being trimmed as well as during other grinding or polishing procedures (Fig. 15–3). Laboratory personnel must wear disposable gloves during these procedures taking care not to have the glove material "catch" into a lathe. Wearing gloves is not necessary if the impression or cast has been adequately disinfected. The sink and cast trimmer must then be cleaned and disinfected.

6. The shipping bench should be cleaned and disinfected immediately after it is cleared of incoming work so as not to contaminate outgoing work. Utility gloves should be worn during these procedures.

7. Work pans should be cleaned and disinfected after each use. All work benches should be cleaned and disinfected at least daily.

8. An antimicrobial handwash with residual action should be used to clean hands in the laboratory (see Chapter 7).

9. Iodophor solutions can be mixed with 1 part green soap to wet pumice. Separate pans of pumice for new (clean) work versus contaminated repairs should be used. A separate lathe should be set up to divide clean from contaminated work. Repair pan pumice should be discarded after *each* case. Premeasured amounts of pumice in plastic bags will facilitate this rapid turnover of pumice. Pumice for new work should be discarded at least weekly.

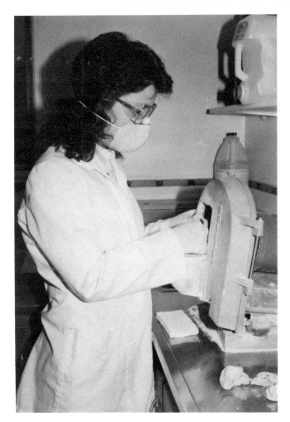

Fig. 15–3. Protective eyewear and a mask must be worn when trimming a cast as well as when performing other grinding or polishing procedures.

10. Personnel should not be allowed to eat or drink at the work bench.
11. Bleach should never be mixed with any solution that contains alcohol or ammonia as a deadly gas will be generated.
12. Conscientious housekeeping procedures should be observed in all nonwork areas of the laboratory.
13. Laboratory personnel with patient contact for the purpose of shade verification for fixed or removable prostheses must ensure that the consultation room is properly cleaned and disinfected after each patient appointment. Shade tabs must be properly cleaned and disinfected after use. Disposable latex examination gloves must be worn if personnel come in contact with a patient's saliva (Fig. 15–4).

    In states where denturism is legal, the Licensed Denturist should follow the same precautions as a dentist contacting patient secretions.
14. All mailing or shipping labels and envelopes should be of the self-adhesive type. Do not lick closed any envelopes and do not lick postage stamps in the laboratory because of possible contamination of these items. Instead, a wet sponge or other available moistening device should be used.
15. All prostheses should be disinfected and rinsed for a final time in the laboratory before they are returned to the dentist's office in a plastic bag (Fig. 15–5).
16. A label is affixed to the bag containing the prosthesis that states: *"This prosthesis has been DISINFECTED for protection of your staff and patients as part of our LABORATORY INFECTION CONTROL PROGRAM."*

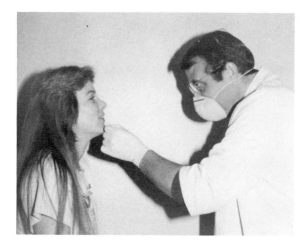

Fig. 15–4. Shade verification *requires* the use of gloves. Masks and eyewear are optional and only necessary if splash or spatter are generated.

In the case of complete or removable denture with resin bases that must be kept wet on the return to the dental office, it is *not* recommended that a disinfectant be placed in the plastic bag for two reasons:

1. The exposure time to the disinfectant will be excessive and may damage the prosthesis or denture.
2. A chemical burn may result if the prosthesis or denture is not properly rinsed before it is placed into the patient's mouth.

Instead, place a 50/50 dilution of a pleasant mouthwash in the plastic bag. A mouthwash will not damage the prosthesis or denture and no harm will be done if it is not thoroughly rinsed before being placed into the patient's mouth.

SUMMARY

It is the dentist's responsibility to notify the laboratory when packages are

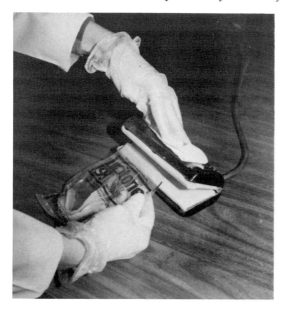

Fig. 15–5. Heat sealing a denture in a plastic bag after disinfection for transportation back to the dental office.

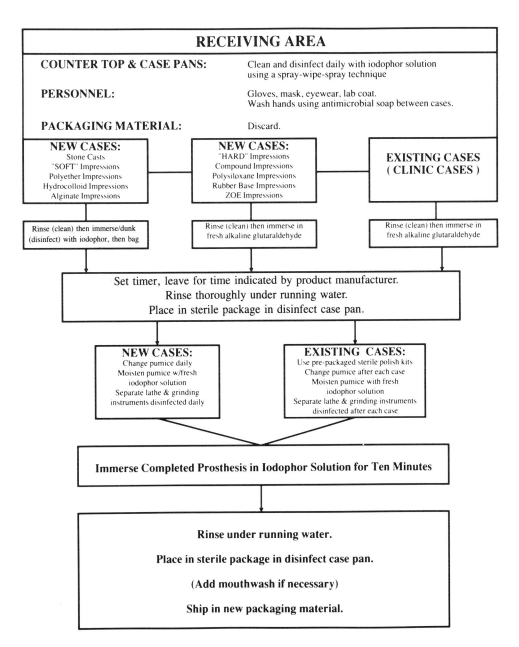

Fig. 15–6. A flowsheet for use in the dental laboratory regarding appropriate infection control procedures (courtesy of Sarah Dirks, DDS).

being sent containing items from known infectious patients and also to avoid sending laboratory cases that are contaminated without taking precautions to avoid cross-contamination. Generally speaking, most items should be cleaned and disinfected only once because of the risk of distortion of impressions or corrosion of prostheses. This reinforces the need for good communication between the dental office and the laboratory regarding disinfection procedures.

It is the responsibility of the dental laboratory personnel to *clean* and *disinfect* all materials coming into the laboratory that have been in the patient's mouth to protect both themselves and their employees, and to clean and disinfect every item returning to the dental office to avoid possible cross-contamination (Fig. 15–6).

The dentist, assistant, hygienist, patient, laboratory owner, manager, department heads, technicians, and delivery persons all have the responsibility to inform and protect each other against infectious diseases in dental practice. The potential for contamination is staggering if a complete infection control program is not implemented.

SELECTED READINGS

ADA Councils on Dental Materials, Instruments and Equipment; Dental Practice; and Dental Therapeutics: Infection control recommendations for the dental office and the dental laboratory. J. Am. Dent. Assoc., *116*:241–248, 1988.

Durr, D.P., and Novak, E.V.: Dimensional stability of alginate impressions immersed in disinfecting solutions. J. Dent. Child., *54*:45, 1987.

Johnson, G.H., Drennon, D.G., and Powell, G.L.: Accuracy of elastomeric impressions disinfected by immersion. J. Am. Dent. Assoc., *11*:525, 1988.

Merchant, V., and Molinari, J.A.: Infection control in prosthodontics: A choice no longer. Gen. Dent., *37*:29–32, 1989.

Tullner, J.B., et al.: Linear dimensional changes in dental impressions after immersion in disinfectant solutions. J. Prosthet. Dent., *60*:725, 1988.

Medical-Legal Issues

Chapter 16

Legal Implications for the Dental Profession of OSHA's Proposed Standard on Bloodborne Pathogens

Constance H. Baker

The most significant legal development in infection control in dentistry is the proposal by the federal Occupational Safety and Health Administration (OSHA) of its Standard to reduce occupational exposure to HIV, hepatitis B, and other bloodborne pathogens. OSHA published the long-awaited Proposed Standard for Occupational Exposure to Bloodborne Pathogens in the May 30, 1989, issue of the *Federal Register*. The proposed standard, if adopted in final form, will require all health-care employers, *including all dental employers who employ at least one employee*, to adopt specific measures designed to protect employees from occupational exposure to human immunodeficiency virus (HIV), the virus associated with acquired immune deficiency syndrome (AIDS), the hepatitis B virus (HBV), and other blood-borne disease-causing agents.

The Proposed Standard does not differ substantially from the Draft Standard released by OSHA on January 9, 1989. OSHA's consistent stance with regard to protecting health-care workers from bloodborne pathogens, coupled with its current policy of inspecting health-care facilities to determine compliance with prior OSHA directives concerning bloodborne pathogens, make it incumbent upon dental employers to pay careful attention to, and begin to implement, the detailed requirements of the Proposed Standard.

The document issued by OSHA consists of 97 pages; the Proposed Standard is only 6½ of these 97 pages. The rest of the document provides a wealth of information on the biology, epidemiology, transmission, testing and control of HIV, HBV, and other bloodborne pathogens. Of particular interest to employers are a list of questions inviting comments that indicate areas where OSHA may be

---

This chapter is based in part upon an article entitled "OSHA Issues Proposed Standard to Reduce Occupational Exposure to HIV, Hepatitis B and Other Bloodborne Pathogens," which appeared in *The AIDS Manual* (National Health Publishing, Fall, 1989).

This chapter is not for the purpose of providing specific legal advice, but attempts only to summarize general principles of law. An attorney should be consulted for specific legal advice.

open to change; summaries of compliance costs for each aspect of the Proposed Standard; and a summary and explanation of the Proposed Standard that provide helpful clues about OSHA's intent in developing the Standard.

OSHA is currently investigating health-care facilities for compliance with Instructions it issued in February of 1990. The Instruction is similar to the Proposed Standard—the basic difference being the Standard's application outside the health-care field. OSHA is currently citing health-care facilities for noncompliance. The majority of citations and fines thus far are for failure to train employees about procedures for avoiding infection, and for failure to properly dispose of waste materials, especially sharps that are not disposed of in puncture-resistant containers.

THE PROPOSED STANDARD

The Proposed Standard provides that all dental employers who can reasonably anticipate that their employees may have skin, eye, mucous membrane, or parenteral contact with blood or other potentially infectious materials,[1] must first *document all tasks and procedures* that could reasonably be anticipated to involve exposure to blood, body fluids, or other potentially infectious materials. Using this documentation, the dental employer must then *identify and document all job positions* with occupational exposure "without regard to the use of personal protective equipment."

Finally, the dental employer must *establish and implement a written infection control plan*. The plan must be "reviewed and updated as necessary to reflect significant changes in tasks or procedures." The infection control plan must address the areas discussed below.

Universal Precautions

Compliance with universal precautions is at the heart of the OSHA Standard. Universal precautions are not new. For a number of years the CDC has published recommendations that all blood and body fluids in the dental workplace be treated as if they were potentially infectious. Numerous dental professional associations have joined the CDC in urging health-care employers to adopt universal precautions. Dental employers who are not currently enforcing universal precautions are exposing themselves to the risk of legal liability.

Employers must enforce employee observance of universal precautions. That is, dental employers must ensure that employees take precautions to prevent all contact with blood and saliva in dental procedures, or any body fluid that is visibly contaminated with blood.

Qualification on Universal Precautions Incorporated

OSHA has included a significant qualification that did not appear in the January, 1989 Draft Standard. The Proposed Standard now states that universal precautions must be taken, *unless* such precautions "would interfere with the proper delivery of health care or public safety services in a particular circumstance, or would create a significant risk to the personal safety of the worker." This qualification reflects OSHA's recognition that "extraordinary situations" may arise that are unexpected and may threaten the life or safety of a dental patient or worker. Under no circumstances should a dental employer interpret this qualification as permission to avoid the general use of universal precautions. This qualification does *not* excuse noncompliance because the dental employer believes that he or she can be more efficient, accurate, or productive without gloves, masks, or other protective equipment, or because he or she was not trained with the now-required equipment, or if the dental employer has a sincere and genuine belief in the lack of wisdom of the new proposed Standard. On the contrary, this exemption is not intended to excuse general nonadherence to the concept of universal precautions. Examples of "extraordinary situations" include: a tear in a surgeon's glove in the midst of critical surgery; a patient's sudden unexpected profuse hemorrhaging; a rescue victim needing CPR when a firefighter has lost or damaged resuscitation equipment in a fire; and a police officer unexpectedly attacked with a knife by a bleeding suspect. The qualification is limited to the extent and time necessary to stabilize these sorts of life-threatening situations.

Engineering and Work Practice Controls

Dental employers must regularly examine and maintain (or replace) effective systems that enable employees to wash their hands immediately after removal of protective gloves, to remove personal protective equipment immediately in appropriately designated areas or containers, and to minimize splashing, spraying, and aerosolizing blood and other potential infectious materials.

Dental employers must maintain effective systems to prevent employees from shearing, bending, breaking, recapping, or resheathing used needles by hand; removing used needles from disposable syringes; eating, drinking, smoking, or applying cosmetics or lip balm, and handling contact lenses in work areas with a potential for occupational exposure; storing food or drink in refrigerators, freezers, or cabinets where blood or other potentially infectious materials are stored; and pipetting or suctioning, by mouth. The new enforcement instruction (February 1990) does stipulate that if needles are resheathed, a resheathing device must be used.

Personal Protective Equipment

Dental employers must provide and assure appropriate use of gloves, gowns, fluid-proof aprons, laboratory coats, head and foot coverings, face shields or masks, eye protection, mouthpieces, resuscitation bags and pocket masks, or other ventilation devices.

The Standard specifies circumstances under which each of the above must be worn.

Dental employers must assure that appropriate sizes of the required equipment are readily accessible.

Dental employers must assure that protective equipment is cleaned, laundered, disposed of, repaired, or replaced as needed.

Housekeeping

Dental employers must determine the appropriate written schedule for cleaning and disinfecting work areas based on location, type of surfaces, type of soil, and procedures being performed. Work surfaces must be cleaned and disinfected after each procedure, after any contamination, and at the end of each work shift. Contaminated reusable items must be decontaminated prior to washing and/or reprocessing. Infectious waste must be placed in closable, leakproof containers or bags, color coded, and labeled. Used sharps must be disposed of in closable, puncture-resistant, disposable, leakproof containers, color coded, and labeled. Disposal containers must be easily accessible and routinely replaced. Laundry soiled with blood or other potentially infectious materials must be treated as contaminated, bagged in leakproof bags at the location where used, color coded, and labeled. Laundry workers must wear gloves and other appropriate protective equipment.

HBV Vaccination and Post-HBV/HIV Exposure Follow-up

Dental employers must make HBV vaccination and antibody testing available at the employer's expense, under the supervision of a licensed physician, to all dental employees who have a risk of occupational exposure on average of one or more times per month, unless the employee has had a previous HBV vaccination or is immune.

Following a report of occupational exposure to HBV or HIV, medical evaluation and monitoring must be made available to the exposed dental employee. The employee may request that his or her blood be tested for antibodies immediately or at a later date. The dental employer must comply with this request. If the source patient is known, the dental employer must request the source patient's consent to perform an HIV-antibody test. Further follow-up of the exposed dental employee includes testing, counseling, illness reporting, and prophylaxis.

The dental employer must provide the postexposure evaluating physician with a copy of the Standard and a description of the dental employee's duties as they relate to occupational exposure.

For each postexposure medical evaluation, the dental employer must obtain the evaluating physician's written opinion. The dental employer must be sure the employee receives a copy of the written opinion within 15 days of the evaluation.

Educational Requirements

The Proposed Standard imposes significant educational requirements on dental employers. *The key to compliance with the OSHA Standard is to develop an employee education program consistent with all of the Standard's other requirements.* Employee education is a prerequisite to enforcing universal precautions. Dental employers who are currently implementing programs related to universal precautions, therefore, may already have a head start in complying with at least some of the Proposed Standard's educational requirements.

The Proposed Standard, if adopted, will impose a number of educational obligations. The dental employer must require all employees with a risk of occupational exposure to participate in a training program at the time of initial employment or within 90 days after the effective date of the Final Standard and at least annually thereafter. Materials for the training program must be appropriate to the employees' educational, literacy, and language background.

The training program must include a copy and explanation of the Standard and of the epidemiology and symptoms of bloodborne diseases; an explanation of modes of transmission and the dental employer's infection control program and methods for recognizing tasks and activities that may involve exposure; information about practices to reduce exposure; information on the proper use and disposal of personal protective equipment; information on the benefits of HBV vaccination; and emergency procedures for handling exposure, reporting exposure and post-exposure medical follow-up.

Record-Keeping

The Proposed Standard imposes significant record-keeping obligations on dental employers. Dental employers are required to maintain two types of records—medical records and training records.

Medical Records. Dental employers must maintain a record for each dental employee with a risk of occupational exposure including HBV vaccination records, the physician's written opinion, and any postexposure follow-up. Medical records must be kept confidential for the duration of employment plus 30 years.

Training Records. Dental employers must record the dates of training sessions and include a summary of the training. Training records must be maintained for 5 years. All records must be made available upon request to OSHA. Records should be transferred only in accordance with law.

State Worker's Compensation Laws

In addition to potential liability for citations and fines under the Occupational Safety and Health Administration laws, a dental employee who is injured in the workplace may also file a worker's compensation claim. In most cases, this will be the sole method of recovery by the injured employee.

State worker's compensation laws set fixed amounts for recovery by injured employees and prohibit the employees from filing law suits against their employers. In the area of dentistry, where an employee of the dentist contracts an infectious disease while performing "on the job" duties, he or she may file a worker's compensation claim and obtain recovery if certain requirements are met.

First, an injured dental employee must prove that the disease contracted is an "occupational disease."[2] Alternatively, he or she may demonstrate that an accidental injury occurred. Second, he or she must demonstrate that infection occurred in the dental workplace while on the job.[3] The incidence of hepatitis B is higher among dental professionals than the general background population and therefore may be likely to be considered an occupational disease. Whether HIV infection and AIDS may be considered as such is difficult to predict at this time. However, claims by employees alleging contamination with HIV in the dental workplace are a virtual certainty.

Generally, worker's compensation laws limit the amount of an injured employee's recovery. However, there is an exception to these laws which may afford injured employees additional recovery. In several states, employees may be able to demonstrate that the act of the employer which resulted in the injury was deliberate and intentional.[4] This would require a showing that the employer specifically intended to harm the employee. In such situations, an employee would allege and would have to prove that the dentist had committed some type of intentional tort or wrongdoing which resulted in the injury. Proof of negligence or even reckless behavior would not be sufficient to invoke the exception. This is a most unusual situation, is generally unavailable and the degree of proof required is high.

Furthermore, a worker compensation statute may not bar an employee from pursuing an employment discrimination action for damages under federal or state civil rights statutes.[5] The Supreme Court of Michigan has held that the exclusive remedy provision of that state's worker compensation statute does not bar an action to recover damages for physical, mental or emotional injuries under the civil rights statutes.[6] The plaintiff who succeeds on an employment discrimination claim is entitled to damages under applicable federal and state statutes (generally, reinstatement and back wages).

CONCLUSION

The Proposed Standard will not become final until OSHA considers the public comments made at public hearings held in a variety of locations across the country. The *Federal Register* will note when the Final Standard is effective. Mandatory compliance will be phased-in over a 150-day period. Dental employers must complete their exposure determinations within 90 days of the effective date of the Final Standard. Dental employers must complete the Infection Control Plan within 120 days of the effective date, and the remaining requirements must be in place within 150 days. Publication of the Final Standard, however, is unlikely until mid-1991.

Until then, dental employers should familiarize themselves with the Proposed Standard and establish and implement programs to comply with the February 1990 compliance instruction which does mandate that employers offer hepatitis B vaccine free of charge to all employees. Postexposure follow-up for HIV/HBV exposure is also necessary. Although the Proposed Standard is not yet being enforced, OSHA is conducting unannounced on-site inspections, is interviewing health-care employees about their understanding of the risks and prevention methods of infectious bloodborne diseases, and is imposing fines on individual health-care providers and health-care institutions it finds to be out of compliance.

Noncompliance with the Proposed Standard could cost a dental employer much more than the fines assessed by OSHA. Noncompliance, especially noncompliance with the core requirements of enforcing universal precautions and providing employee education, could also expose dental employers to adverse publicity and further deterioration in employer-employee relations. Fortunately, dental employers can avoid this by educating themselves, and ultimately their employees, as to the requirements of the Proposed Standard.

FOOTNOTES

1. In a Preliminary Regulatory Impact study described in the Proposed Standard, OSHA identified 16 industry sectors that will be affected by the Standard because workers in those sectors come in contact with or handle blood and other potentially infectious materials. In addition to dentists' offices, these industry sectors include private physicians' offices, nursing homes, hospitals, HMOs, medical and dental laboratories, funeral homes, research labs, blood banks, prisons, police, fire and rescue agencies, industrial clinics, residential care facilities and medical equipment repair companies.
2. *Booker v. Duke Medical Center*, 297 N.C. 458,256 S.E. 2d 189 (1979).

3. *Id.*

4. *Blankenship v. Cincinnati Milacron Chemicals, Inc.*, 433 N.E. 2d 572 (Ohio), *cert. denied*, 459 U.S. 857 (1982).

5. *Alexander v. Gardner-Denver Co.*, 415 U.S. 36, 48 (1974) ("[T]he legislative history of Title VII manifests a congressional intent to allow an individual to pursue independently his rights under both Title VII and other applicable state and federal statutes." (footnote omitted)).

6. *Boscaglia v. Michigan Bell Tel. Co.*, 420 Mich. 308, 362 N.W. 2d 642 (1984) (supply foreman at telephone company demoted after refusing transfer; recovery under worker compensation statute no bar to sex discrimination suit).

The "Commandments" of Practical Infection Control

Chapter 17

Today's Minimum Requirements for a Practical Dental Office Infection Control System

Information indicating that the individuals who are at greatest risk of cross-infection in dental practices are the health professionals themselves continues to accumulate. Repeated exposure to blood and saliva during intraoral, often invasive procedures, challenges the health care workers' immune defenses with a variety of microbial pathogens.

The recognized risks of hepatitis B virus (HBV), *Mycobacterium tuberculosis*, and herpes simplex virus infection are well documented. There is a much smaller risk of exposure to human immunodeficiency virus (HIV).

It is important to remember the difference in virulence and numbers of viral particles per milliliter of blood between HIV infection and hepatitis B. The December, 1985 issue of *Discover* magazine illustrated this point by stating that 1 milliliter of blood from a hepatitis B carrier diluted in a 24,000-gallon swimming pool could still result in infection if 1 milliliter of that swimming pool water were injected into a susceptible individual. In contrast, 1 milliliter of blood from a patient with AIDS diluted in 1 quart of water would result in a viral concentration which, if injected into another susceptible individual, would not transmit HIV infection. The difference in the number of viruses per milliliter of blood is dramatic. In hepatitis B there are over 100,000,000 viral particles per milliliter of blood, whereas in diagnosed AIDS, there are 1,000 to 10,000 viruses per milliliter of blood. Thus it is understandable that, by 1990, there has been only one case of a dentist becoming anti-HIV positive possibly associated solely with occupational exposure.

The routine exposure of practitioners and auxiliaries to a multitude of bacterial, viral, and other microbial pathogens led to the development of recommended infection control protocols initially directed at preventing HBV transmission. The same basic protocols were later recommended for situations in which patients who were diagnosed HIV seropositive and those with diagnosed AIDS are provided treatment in dental clinics and offices. Statements included with the guidelines reinforced the positions of the American Dental Association and the Centers for Disease Control that infection control procedures be used with *ALL* patients to routinely minimize the transmission of all infectious diseases. Notice that the word "minimize" is used because all risk cannot be eliminated nor can it be avoided. The development of infection control standards by the Occupational Safety and

Table 17–1.   The Commandments of Infection Control

1. Hepatitis B vaccine*
2. Comprehensive medical history and patient examination
3. Antiseptic mouthrinse
4. Antiseptic handwash*
5. Disposable face mask*
6. Disposable latex gloves*
7. Protective eyewear*
8. Appropriate clinic attire*
9. Rubber dam
10. Sharps disposal system*
11. Sterilizable handpieces
12. Ultrasonic cleaner
13. Instrument packaging
14. Heat sterilizer*
15. Sterilization monitoring
16. Glutaraldehyde solution
17. Surface cleaner*
18. Surface disinfectant*
19. Surface covers
20. Medical waste disposal system*
21. OSHA poster*

*Mandatory according to OSHA standards

Health Administration (OSHA) has made the use of routine precautions even more important.

The purpose of this textbook, "Practical Infection Control in Dentistry," is to outline what federal and professional agencies, the authors, and contributors consider to be appropriate procedures, equipment, and materials for an effective yet practical infection control program in dental practice. For ease in understanding, infection control was divided into the five following areas in this text:

1. Patient assessment
2. Personal protection
3. Sterilization and chemical disinfection
4. Environmental surface and equipment disinfection
5. Aseptic technique

A list of "commandments" (see Table 17–1) that constitute a minimum yet effective infection control system can be enumerated. Each of these items must be appropriately implemented in order to provide optimum protection against transmission of infection in the dental office. Those items with an asterisk should be considered mandatory according to OSHA standards. The others are considered necessary by the authors to meet the ADA recommendations and CDC guidelines. The earlier chapters of the text fully explain the details of each listed commandment.

This protocol is sufficient for hepatitis B carriers, HIV seropositive patients, patients with diagnosed AIDS, patients with other known infectious diseases, and for routine daily use. The use of additional materials and procedures is not necessary and will only increase the cost of infection control both in direct purchase price and time utilized by the dentist and staff.

Unfortunately, there is no one answer for all the infection control needs in a dental office. What is acceptable this year will need to be re-evaluated next year as new products, techniques, and equipment are brought onto the market by innovative manufacturers responding to this new interest in the dental profession.

SUMMARY

Dentists must utilize effective infection control procedures in their practices. A positive step-by-step approach should be employed. Determine your practice's infection control strengths and build upon them by adding new procedures to the office routine.

Occasionally, objections are raised regarding the price of additional infection control supplies and procedures in a dental office. Cost is relative in that the cost of a lifetime infection control system in an average dental practice will be less than one malpractice suit. Implementation of a comprehensive program can be cost effective and can be used to promote dental asepsis. It can serve as a practice builder. Staff, patients, and family members of providers will appreciate the efforts.

The current climate in today's society regarding infectious diseases in general, and herpes, hepatitis, HIV infection and AIDS in particular, dictates that all dental practices must close the door on the way they once practiced dentistry and make a permanent change to incorporate accepted infection control techniques. The choice of whether or not to comply with these recommendations has been removed as more states implement regulations and OSHA continues to inspect, cite, and fine health care facilities. An increasing number of patients are scrutinizing the dental and medical professions' approach to asepsis as a result of extensive media coverage. Questions are being asked. Fortunately, the dental profession is showing a willingness to respond in a positive fashion.

SELECTED READINGS

ADA Council on Dental Materials, Instruments and Equipment; Dental Practice; and Dental Therapeutics: Infection control recommendations for the dental office and the dental laboratory. J. Am. Dent. Assoc., 116:241–248, 1988.

Centers for Disease Control: Recommended infection control practices for dentistry. MMWR, 35:237–241, 1986.

Centers for Disease Control: Recommendations for prevention of HIV transmission in health-care settings. MMWR, 36(2S):1S–18S, 1987.

Coombs, R.W., Collier, A.C., Allain, J.P., et al.: Plasma viremia in human immunodeficiency virus infection. N. Engl. J. Med., 321:1626–1630, 1989.

Cottone, J.A.: Hepatitis B virus infection in the dental profession. J. Am. Dent. Assoc., 110:617–621, 1985.

Appendix A

American Dental Association: Infection Control Recommendations for the Dental Office and the Dental Laboratory

Dental professionals are exposed to a wide variety of microorganisms in the blood and saliva of patients. These microorganisms may cause infectious diseases such as the common cold, pneumonia, tuberculosis, herpes, hepatitis B, and acquired immune deficiency syndrome (AIDS). The use of effective infection control procedures in the dental office and the dental laboratory will prevent cross-contamination that may extend to dentists, dental office staff, dental technicians, and patients.

The American Dental Association has advocated the use of infection control procedures in dental practice for several years.[1-3] As new information has become available, the Association has disseminated it to the profession and will continue to do so. Currently available Association publications that provide detailed information about infection control and treatment of patients with infectious diseases are: *Facts about AIDS for the Dental Team*[4] and *Proceedings of the National Symposium on Hepatitis B and the Dental Profession.*[5]

This report is based on the recommendations of the Centers for Disease Control (CDC)[7,8] and other publications in the medical and dental literature. Although the recommendations in this document have been formally accepted by the Council on Dental Materials, Instruments, and Equipment; the Council on Dental Practice; and the Council on Dental Therapeutics, they are not the official policy of the American Dental Association. Additional specific recommendations for the dental specialties are included in the *Proceedings of the National Conference for Infection Control in Dentistry* (available for a small charge).[6] The councils urge practitioners and dental laboratories to adapt these recommendations to their specific needs and then to routinely practice the infection control procedures. To ensure an effective and safe infection control program, dentists and dental laboratories should discuss their infection control programs with each other.

PREVENTION OF TRANSMISSION OF INFECTIOUS DISEASES

Although much attention is currently focused on AIDS, the dental health team is far more at risk to the hepatitis B virus (HBV) than to the human immunodeficiency virus (HIV) that causes AIDS. HBV is more common in the general population and 0.3% of the US population are HBV carriers.[9]

Experience has shown that patients with hepatitis B or who are HBV carriers can be treated without transmission of disease in a dental office when recommended infection control procedures are used. As HIV appears to be much more difficult to transmit than HBV, it is believed that the same procedures will prevent the transmission of HIV in the dental office.

VACCINATION AGAINST HEPATITIS B

Dental health care personnel have long been recognized to be at high risk for acquiring hepatitis B through contact with patients. A survey conducted from 1983 to 1985 found that 14% of the dentists tested for HBV serum markers showed evidence of natural immunity as a result of HBV exposure. The chronic carrier rate was 0.94%, which was consistent with earlier findings.[10] In June 1982, the Council on Dental Therapeutics adopted a resolution recommending that all dental personnel having patient contact—including dentists, dental students, and dental auxiliary personnel, and all dental laboratory personnel—receive the hepatitis B vaccine.[11] This recommendation was reinforced by the Immunization Practices Advisory Committee, CDC, in June 1985.[9,12]

INFECTION CONTROL PRACTICES FOR THE DENTAL OFFICE

Medical History

A thorough medical history should be obtained and reviewed. The medical history should be updated at subsequent visits. Specific questions should be asked regarding medications, current and recurrent illnesses, unintentional weight loss, lymphadenopathy, oral soft tissue lesions, other infections, and history of hepatitis. Medical consultation may be indicated when a history of active infection or systemic disease is elicited.

Not all patients with infectious diseases can be identified by medical history, physical examination, or readily available laboratory tests. Each patient must be considered as potentially infectious and the same infection control procedures should be used for all patients.

Barrier Techniques

Gloves. Gloves must be worn to prevent skin contact with blood, saliva, or mucous membranes. Gloves should also be worn when touching items or surfaces that may be contaminated with blood, body fluids, or secretions. The gloves should cover the cuffs of long-sleeved gowns. After contact with each patient, hands must be washed and regloved with new gloves before treating another patient. Repeated use of a single pair of gloves by disinfecting them between patients is not acceptable. Exposure to disinfectants often causes defects in the glove material, thereby diminishing its value as an effective barrier, and this method of disinfection may not be adequate to prevent cross-contamination between patients. A second pair of gloves, such as examining gloves, may be placed over a first pair of gloves when

Table A–1.   Infection Control for the Dental Office: A Checklist

Immunization
- Health care workers should have appropriate immunizations such as that for hepatitis B virus

Before Patient Treatment
- Obtain a thorough medical history
- Disinfect prostheses and appliances received from the laboratory
- Place disposable coverings to prevent contamination of surfaces, or disinfect surfaces after treatment

During Patient Treatment
- Treat all patients as potentially infectious
- Use protective attire and barrier techniques when contact with body fluids or mucous membranes is anticipated
  - Wear gloves
  - Wear mask
  - Wear protective eyewear
  - Wear uniforms, laboratory coats, or gowns
- Open intraorally contaminated X-ray film packets in the dark room with disposable gloves without touching the films
- Minimize formation of droplets, spatters, and aerosols
- Use a rubber dam to isolate the tooth and field when appropriate
- Use high volume-vacuum evacuation
- Protect hands
  - Wash hands before gloving and after gloves are removed
  - Change gloves between each patient
  - Discard gloves that are torn, cut, or punctured
  - Avoid hand injuries
- Avoid injury with sharp instruments and needles
  - Handle sharp items carefully
  - Do not bend or break disposable needles
  - If needles are not recapped, place in separate field. If recapping is necessary, use a method that protects hands from injury such as a holder for the cap
  - Place sharp items in appropriate containers

After Patient Treatment
- Wear heavy duty rubber gloves
- Clean instruments thoroughly
- Sterilize instruments
  - Sterilize instruments that penetrate soft tissue or bone
  - Sterilize, whenever possible, all instruments that come in contact with oral mucous membranes, body fluids, or those that have been contaminated with secretions of patients. Otherwise, use appropriate disinfection
  - Monitor the sterilizer with biological monitors
- Clean handpieces, dental units, and ultrasonic scalers
  - Flush handpieces, dental units, ultrasonic scalers, and air/water syringes between patients
  - Clean and sterilize air/water syringes and ultrasonic scalers if possible; otherwise, disinfect them
  - Clean and sterilize handpieces if possible; otherwise, disinfect them
- Handle sharp instruments with caution
  - Place disposable needles, scalpels, and other sharp items intact into puncture-resistant containers before disposal
- Decontaminate environmental surfaces
  - Wipe work surfaces with absorbent toweling to remove debris, and dispose of this toweling appropriately
  - Disinfect with suitable chemical disinfectant
  - Change protective coverings on light handles, X-ray unit head, and other items
- Decontaminate supplies and materials
  - Rinse and disinfect impressions, bite registrations, and appliances to be sent to the laboratory
- Communicate infection control program to dental laboratory
- Dispense a small amount of pumice in a disposable container for individual use on each case and discard any excess
- Remove contaminated wastes appropriately
  - Pour blood, suctioned fluids, and other liquid waste into drain connected to a sanitary sewer system
  - Place solid waste contaminated with blood or saliva in sealed, sturdy impervious bags; dispose according to local government regulations
- Remove gloves and wash hands

it is necessary to briefly examine a second patient. The second pair of gloves should be removed before returning to the first patient.

Gowns. All dental health care workers should routinely wear appropriate attire to prevent skin and mucous-membrane exposure when contact with blood or other body fluids is anticipated. Reusable or disposable gowns, laboratory coats, or uniforms with long sleeves and high collars that protect the user from the spatter of body fluids and cover street clothing provide greater coverage. Head covers that provide an effective barrier are recommended during invasive procedures that are likely to result in the splashing of blood or other body fluids. Gowns should be changed at least daily or more often if they are visibly soiled. After use, protective attire should be removed and placed in laundry or disposal bags before leaving the dental treatment facility.

Masks. Surgical masks or chin-length plastic face shields must be worn to protect the face, the oral mucosa, and the nasal mucosa from spatter of blood and saliva.

Protective Eyewear. Protective eyewear must be worn to protect the eyes from spatter and aerosols of blood and saliva if a face shield is not chosen.

Protecting Environmental Surfaces. Surfaces that may be contaminated by blood or saliva, for example, light handles or X-ray unit heads, may be wrapped with impervious-backed paper, aluminum foil, or clear plastic wrap. Gloves should be used to remove and discard the covering. After ungloving and washing hands, the covering should be replaced with clean material. Alternatively, these surfaces may be decontaminated with chemical disinfectants (Table A–2).

Surfaces and equipment that cannot be covered or removed for cleaning and sterilization should be thoroughly cleaned (rough surfaces scrubbed) and disinfected. A disinfectant should then be applied and left moist on the surface for the amount of time specified on the disinfectant's label.

Limiting Contamination

All procedures should be performed in a way that minimizes the formation of droplets, spatter, and aerosols. This can be accomplished by using high-speed evacuation, proper patient positioning, and the use of a rubber dam, whenever appropriate. Dental personnel should limit the field contamination by avoiding contact with objects such as charts, telephones, and cabinets during patient treatment procedures. A second pair of disposable gloves, such as examining gloves or food handling gloves, may be placed over a first pair of gloves when it is necessary to prevent contamination of these objects.

Hands

Handwashing. Hands should be washed thoroughly with an antimicrobial handwash solution at the beginning of the day and before gloving. A listing of accepted antimicrobial hand cleaners is available from the Council on Dental Therapeutics.[13] Gloves should be removed and hands washed between patients and after touching inanimate objects likely to be contaminated by blood or saliva.

Care of Hands. Precautions should be taken to avoid hand injuries during procedures. If an injury, such as a needlestick, occurs or gloves are torn, cut, or punctured, gloves should be removed as soon as is compatible with the patient's

Table A–2.   Guide to Chemical Agents for Disinfection and/or Sterilization

Chemical[1] Classification Accepted Products	Disinfectant[2,3]			Sterilant[2]
	Dilution	Time	Temperature (20C = 68F) (25C = 77F)	
	Surface/Immersion			
Chlorine compounds				
Alcide	10:1:1	3 minutes	20°C	NA[5]
Exspore	4:1:1	2 minutes	20°C	4:1:1, 6 hours, 20°C
Bleach (5.25% sodium hypochlorite)	1:10	10 minutes	20°C	NA

Iodophors
  Biocide
  Surf-A-Cide
  ProMedyne-D
	1:213	10 minutes	—[4]	NA

Combination synthetic phenolics
  Dentaseptic
  Multicide
  Omni II
	1:32	10 minutes	20°C	NA

	Immersion			
2% Glutaraldehyde with phenolic buffer Sporicidin	1:16	10 minutes	20°C	Full strength, 6¾ hours, 20°C
2% Glutaraldehyde[6] acidic Banicide concentrate	1:40	30 minutes	20°C	1:10, 10 hours, 25°C
Banicide Sterall Wavicide-01	1:4	30 minutes	20°C	Full strength, 10 hours, 25°C
2% Glutaraldehyde[6] neutral Glutarex	Full strength	—	—[4]	Full strength, 10 hours, 20°C
2% Glutaraldehyde alkaline[6] Cidex activated dialdehyde	Full strength	45 minutes	25°C	Full strength, 10 hours, 25°C
Cidex 7	Full strength	90 minutes	25°C	Full strength, 10 hours, 25°C
CoeCide Germ-X Glutall	Full strength	—	—[4]	Full strength, 10 hours, 20°C
Omnicide Orthicide Sporex Vitacide	Full strength	45 minutes	20°C	Full strength, 10 hours, 20°C
Steril-Ize	Full strength	45 minutes	25°C	Full strength, 10 hours, 20°C
Centra 28 K-Cide 10 Maxicide Procide 14 Procide 30 Protec-top Saslow solution	Full strength	10 minutes	25°C	Full strength, 10 hours, 20°C

1. ADA Accepted Products as of 9/1/87; a list of currently accepted products may be obtained by contacting the office of the Council on Dental Therapeutics

2. Always use disinfectant/sterilant products according to the instructions specified on the product label

3. The conditions listed reflect the time required for tuberculocidal activity for reused solution, if such use is possible, at the minimum temperature and maximal dilution specified on the Environmental Protection Agency (EPA) approved product label. Tuberculocidal test methodologies may vary, consult label or manufacturer for specifics

4. Data not available at time of publication

5. Not approved for use as sterilants

6. Alternate conditions, such as increased temperature or fresh solution as opposed to reused solution, may decrease disinfection time, consult label instructions for alternate uses

safety. Hands should be washed thoroughly and regloved before completing the dental procedure. Dentists, dental hygienists, and dental assistants who have exudative lesions or weeping dermatitis should refrain from all direct patient contact and from handling patient care equipment until the condition is resolved.

Sharp Instruments and Needles

A sterile syringe, a new disposable needle, and new solution should be used for each patient. Needles, scalpel blades, and other sharp instruments should be handled carefully to prevent unintentional injuries. As an individual patient may require multiple injections of anesthetic or other medications from a single syringe, a number of techniques can be used to minimize the likelihood of injury: the unsheathed needle can be placed in a "sterile field" during the procedure rather than recapping the needle with the unprotected hand, (exposed needles should not be left on dental trays where they are more likely to cause injury); the needle can be recapped by laying the cap on the tray or placing the cap in a holder so that the needle can be guided into it without injury; or the needle can be recapped by holding the cap with forceps.

Disposable needles should not be bent or broken after use. Needles should not be removed manually from disposable syringes or otherwise handled manually. Hemostats or pliers may be used to handle sharp items. Disposable syringes, needles, scalpel blades, and other sharp items should be discarded into puncture-resistant containers located as close as is practical to the area in which they have been used.

STERILIZATION AND DISINFECTION

Sterilization is the process by which all forms of microorganisms are destroyed, including viruses, bacteria, fungi, and spores. Methods of sterilization include the use of steam under pressure (autoclave), prolonged dry heat, chemical vapor, ethylene oxide gas, or immersion in chemical sterilants.[14] Disinfection is generally a less lethal process than sterilization. It eliminates virtually all recognized pathogenic microorganisms, but not necessarily all microbial forms (bacterial endospores), on inanimate objects.[15] Disinfection may be accomplished by using a chemical disinfectant according to the directions specified for use on the product label. A chemical agent for disinfection in dental settings must be registered by the Environmental Protection Agency (EPA) as a hospital disinfectant and must be tuberculocidal. Virucidal efficacy must include, as a minimum, both lipophilic and hydrophilic viruses. Chemical disinfectants/sterilants accepted by the Council on Dental Therapeutics for use in dentistry are listed in Table A–2.

Debris must be removed from the instruments and surfaces before sterilization or disinfection. This may be done by scrubbing the instruments with hot water and soap or detergent, or by using a device such as an ultrasonic cleaner with an appropriate cleaning solution. Guides for disinfecting impressions are summarized in Table A–4. Dental personnel responsible for handling instruments should wear heavy-duty rubber gloves to prevent hand injuries.

Table A–3.   Infection Control for the Dental Laboratory: A Checklist

Incoming Cases
- Wear laboratory coats and gloves
- Open a receiving center separate from the production area
- Disinfect cases as required when they are received. (If an impression cannot be disinfected without distortion, disinfect the model after it is poured)
- Disinfect or sterilize case containers
- Disinfect work surfaces
    —Wipe work surfaces with absorbent toweling to remove debris
    —Disinfect with suitable chemical germicide
- Place solid waste contaminated with blood or saliva in impervious bags and dispose properly

Production Area
- Wear safety glasses and masks
- Decontaminate work surfaces
    —Wipe work surfaces with absorbent toweling to remove debris
    —Disinfect with a suitable chemical germicide daily
- Use separate sets of instruments, attachments, and materials for new prostheses and cases that have been in the mouth
- Change pumice after every case
- Clean and disinfect brushes and other equipment that have been used with prostheses that have been in the mouth
- Autoclave ragwheels

Outgoing Case
- Disinfect each case before returning to dental office
- Communicate infection control program to dentists

Dental Materials, Instruments, and Equipment

Table A–5 summarizes appropriate sterilization and disinfection methods for dental instruments, materials, and other commonly used items. Consideration should be given to the effect of sterilization on materials. Manufacturers should be consulted on appropriate sterilization/disinfection of specific products.

Instruments. Surgical and other instruments that normally penetrate soft tissue or bone (forceps, scalpels, bone chisels, scalers, and surgical burs) must be sterilized after each use.

Instruments that are not intended to penetrate oral soft tissues or bone (amalgam condensers, burs, and plastic instruments) but that may come into contact with oral tissues should also be sterilized after each use. However, if sterilization is not feasible, these instruments should be immersed in a chemical disinfectant.

Metal or heat-stable dental instruments should be sterilized between use by steam under pressure (autoclave), dry heat, or chemical vapor. The instruments should be wrapped or bagged before sterilizing, using a suitable wrap material such as muslin, clear pouches, or paper as recommended by the manufacturer of the sterilizer. The wrap or bag should be sealed with appropriate tape. Pins, staples,

Table A–4.   Disinfection of Impressions

Polysulfides	Use immersion in accepted products listed in Table A–2
Silicones	Use immersion in accepted products listed in Table A–2
Polyethers	Spray, or use products with short disinfection time, for example, chlorine compounds
Alginates	Use spray and then leave impression in sealed bag for the recommended disinfection time
Agar	Insufficient information on effect of disinfectants in agar impressions
Stone casts	Insufficient information on effect of disinfectants on stone casts

Table A–5.   Sterilization and Disinfection of Dental Instruments, Materials, and Some Commonly Used Items

	Steam Autoclave	Dry Heat Oven	Chemical Vapor	Ethylene Oxide	Chemical Disinfection/ Sterilization	Other Methods/Comments
Angle attachments*	+	+	+	+ +	+	
Burs						
Carbon steel	−	+ +	+ +	+ +	−	
Steel	+	+ +	+ +	+ +	+	
Tungsten-carbide	+	+ +	+	+ +	+	
Condensers	+ +	+ +	+ +	+ +	+	
Dapen dishes	+ +	+	+	+ +	+	
Endodontic instruments (broaches, files, reamers)						Hot salt/glass bead sterilizer 10 to 15 seconds, 218°C (425°F)
Stainless steel handles	+	+ +	+ +	+ +	+	
Stainless with plastic handles	+ +	+ +	−	+ +	−	
Fluoride gel trays						
Heat-resistant plastic	+ +	− −	−	+ +	−	
Nonheat-resistant plastic	− −	− −	−	+ +	−	Discard (+ +)
Glass slabs	+ +	+ +	+ +	+ +	+	
Hand instruments						
Carbon steel	−	+ +	+ +	+ +	−	
	[Steam autoclave with chemical protection (1% sodium nitrite)]					
Stainless steel	+ +	+ +	+ +	+ +	+	
Handpieces*						Sterilizable preferably
Sterilizable*	(+ +)*	−	(+)*	+ +	− −	
Contra-angles*	−	−	−	+ +	+	} Combination synthetic phenolics or iodophors (−)
Nonsterilizable*	−	−	−	+ +	+	
Prophylaxis angles*	+	+	+	+	+	
Impression materials						Table A–4
Impression trays						
Aluminum metal	+ +	+	+ +	+ +	−	
Chrome-plated	+ +	+ +	+ +	+ +	+	
Custom acrylic resin	− −	− −	− −	+ +	+	
Plastic	− −	− −	− −	+ +	+	Discard (+ +); preferred
Instruments in packs	+ +	+ Small packs	+ +	+ + Small packs	− −	
Instrument tray setups						
Restorative or surgical	+ Size limit	+	+ Size limit	+ + Size limit	− −	
Mirrors	−	+ +	+ +	+ +	+	
Needles						
Disposable	− −	− −	− −	− −	− −	Discard (+ +) Do not reuse

Table A–5. Sterilization and Disinfection of Dental Instruments, Materials, and Some Commonly Used Items *(continued)*

	Steam Autoclave	Dry Heat Oven	Chemical Vapor	Ethylene Oxide	Chemical Disinfection/ Sterilization	Other Methods/Comments
Nitrous oxide						
Nose piece	$(++)^*$	$--$	$(++)^*$	$++$	$(+)^*$	
Hoses	$(++)^*$	$--$	$(++)^*$	$++$	$(+)^*$	
Orthodontic pliers						
High quality stainless	$++$	$++$	$++$	$++$	$+$	
Low quality stainless	$-$	$++$	$++$	$++$	$-$	
With plastic parts	$--$	$--$	$--$	$++$	$+$	
Pluggers	$++$	$++$	$++$	$++$	$+$	
Polishing wheels and disks						
Garnet and cuttle	$--$	$-$	$-$	$++$	$--$	
Rag	$++$	$-$	$+$	$++$	$--$	
Rubber	$+$	$-$	$-$	$++$	$+$	
Prostheses, removable	$-$	$-$	$-$	$+$	$+$	
Rubber dam equipment						
Carbon steel clamps	$-$	$++$	$++$	$++$	$-$	
Metal frames	$++$	$++$	$++$	$++$	$+$	
Plastic frames	$-$	$-$	$-$	$++$	$+$	
Punches	$-$	$++$	$++$	$++$	$+$	
Stainless steel clamps	$++$	$++$	$++$	$++$	$+$	
Rubber items						
Prophylaxis cups	$-$	$-$	$-$	$++$	$-$	Discard $(++)$
Saliva evacuators, ejectors						
Low-melting plastic	$-$	$-$	$-$	$++$	$+$	Discard $(++)$
High-melting plastic	$++$	$+$	$+$	$++$	$+$	
Stones						
Diamond	$+$	$++$	$++$	$++$	$+$	
Polishing	$++$	$+$	$++$	$++$	$-$	
Sharpening	$++$	$++$	$++$	$-$		
Surgical instruments						
Stainless steel	$++$	$++$	$++$	$++$	$+$	
Ultrasonic scaling tips	$+$	$--$	$--$	$++$	$+$	
Water-air syringe tips	$++$	$++$	$++$	$++$	$+$	
X-ray equipment						
Plastic film holders	$(++)^*$	$--$	$(+)^*$	$++$	$+$	
Collimating devices	$-$	$--$	$--$	$++$	$+$	

The table is adapted from *Accepted Dental Therapeutics* and *Dentists' Desk Reference Materials, Instruments, and Equipment.*

*As manufacturers use a variety of alloys and materials in these products, confirmation with the equipment manufacturers is recommended, especially for handpieces and the attachments.

$++$ Effective and preferred method.

$+$ Effective and acceptable method.

$-$ Effective method, but risk of damage to materials.

$--$ Ineffective method with risk of damage to materials.

or paper clips make holes in the wrap that permit entry of microorganisms. After sterilization, the instruments should be stored in the sealed packages until they are used. Biological monitors should be used routinely to verify the adequacy of sterilization cycles. According to the CDC, weekly verification should be adequate for most dental practices.[7]

Handpieces. Sterilization of handpieces between patients is recommended when possible. Although not all handpieces can be sterilized, an increasing number of sterilizable handpieces are currently available, and this is an important factor to be considered in the selection of equipment. The first step, whether the handpiece can be sterilized or only disinfected, is to flush it by running the handpiece for 20 to 30 seconds, discharging the water into a sink or container. The manufacturer's recommendations should be followed for proper flushing of handpieces, and for the use and maintenance of waterlines and check valves. The handpiece should then be scrubbed thoroughly with a detergent and hot water to remove any adherent material. The handpiece should be sterilized according to manufacturer's instructions. If the handpiece cannot be sterilized, a chemical germicide that is registered with the Environmental Protection Agency as a "hospital disinfectant" and is tuberculocidal at use-dilution should be applied (combination synthetic phenolics, iodophors). The disinfecting solution should remain in contact with the handpiece for the time specified on the disinfectant's label. Any chemical residue should be removed by rinsing with sterile water or wiping with alcohol-soaked gauze.

Air/Water Syringes and Ultrasonic Scalers. Units should be flushed as described for handpieces. These attachments should be sterilized or, if not possible, disinfected in the same manner as the handpieces—scrubbing thoroughly, wiping with a disinfecting solution, and removing any residue by rinsing with sterile water or wiping with alcohol. If possible, removable tips should be used.

X-Ray Equipment and Films. Protective covering or disinfectants should be used to prevent microbial contamination of collimating tubes. Intraorally contaminated film packets should be handled in a manner to prevent cross-contamination. Contaminated packets should be opened in the darkroom, using disposable gloves. The films should be dropped out of the packets without touching the films. The contaminated packets should be accumulated in a disposable towel. After all packets have been opened, they should be discarded and the gloves removed. The films can then be processed without contaminating darkroom equipment with microorganisms from the patient.[16]

Countertops and Surfaces. Countertops and surfaces that may have become contaminated with blood or saliva should be precleaned to remove extraneous organic matter and then disinfected with a suitable chemical germicide. These include combination synthetic phenolics, iodophors, and chlorine compounds. A solution of sodium hypochlorite (household bleach) prepared fresh daily is an inexpensive and effective germicide. A concentration of sodium hypochlorite ranging from 5,000 ppm to 500 ppm, achieved by diluting household bleach in a ratio ranging from 1:10 to 1:100 is effective, depending on the amount of organic matter (blood and mucus) present on the surface to be cleaned and disinfected. Sodium hypochlorite should be used with caution because it is corrosive to some metals, especially aluminum; corrosiveness is less of a problem with combination synthetic phenolics.

IMPRESSIONS

Impressions should be rinsed to remove saliva, blood, and debris and then disinfected before being cast in die stone or sent to a dental laboratory. The procedures differ depending on whether alginate or elastomeric impressions are to be disinfected.

Several studies have been conducted dealing with disinfection of elastomeric impressions.[17–27] Results indicate that polysulfide and addition silicone impressions can be disinfected by immersion with any of the accepted products (Table A–4) without affecting accuracy and detail reproduction. Surface detail has been shown to be enhanced with 2% acidic glutaraldehyde solutions.[27,28] Times for disinfection vary so information supplied with the disinfectant should be consulted to determine the proper time.

Polyether impressions may be adversely affected with disinfection by immersion.[21,27] To minimize dimensional change with polyether impressions, a chlorine compound product with a short disinfection time (2 to 3 minutes) should be selected or the impressions should be disinfected with a spray.[27]

Disinfection of alginate impressions has been investigated as well.[25,28–32] Results showed differences based on selection of alginate product[30,32] and disinfectant.[25,28,29] Differences noted were generally not clinically significant for most applications of casts retrieved from alginate impressions.[25,28,31,32] The most accurate casts were associated with disinfection of alginate impressions by spray rather than immersion.[30,31]

Recommended clinical procedures are first to remove saliva, blood, and debris with tap water and gently shake the alginate impression to remove excess water. The surface of the alginate impression should then be coated with a disinfectant that has been accepted for use as a surface disinfectant. The impression should then be sealed in a plastic bag for the recommended disinfection time, immediately after which the impression should be cast in stone.

Information on the disinfection of reversible hydrocolloid impressions (agar) is limited; thus, recommendations for their disinfection must await further study. An alternate method would be to disinfect the casts recovered from agar impressions, but effects of disinfectant solutions on gypsum casts are not known at this time.

Disinfection times will vary with the chemical agent used, and may change as information on disinfectants is updated. A longer immersion time than that used in the previously cited studies on impression materials may become necessary. The effect of increased immersion time on impression materials is unknown.

DISPOSAL OF WASTE MATERIALS

Disposable materials such as gloves, masks, wipes, paper drapes, and surface covers that are contaminated with blood or body fluids should be carefully handled and discarded in sturdy, impervious plastic bags to minimize human contact. Blood, suctioned fluids, or other liquid waste may be carefully poured into a drain connected to a sanitary sewer system. Care should be taken to ensure compliance with applicable local regulations. Sharp items, such as needles and scalpel blades, should be placed intact into puncture-resistant containers before disposal in plastic bags. Human tissue may be handled in the same manner as sharp items. Such contaminated solid wastes and sharp items should be disposed of according to the requirements established by local or state environmental regulatory agencies and published recommendations. Infectious medical waste, including tissues and culture media, should be handled in a manner consistent with local regulations before disposal.[33]

Liquid chemicals should be carefully poured into a drain connected to a sewer while flushing with copious amounts of water unless labeling or local, state, or federal regulations prohibit such a practice. Disposable methods for solid chemicals will vary with the type of chemical and regulations governing waste management practices.

PRACTICES FOR THE DENTAL LABORATORY

Dental laboratories should practice appropriate infection control programs.[34,35]

Receiving Area. A receiving area should be established separate from the production area. Countertops and work surfaces should be precleaned and the area should be disinfected daily with a chlorine compound, a combination synthetic phenolic, or an iodophor solution that has been diluted according to the manufacturer's directions.

Incoming Cases. Unless the laboratory employee knows that the case has been disinfected by the dental office, all cases should be disinfected as they are received. Case containers should be disinfected or sterilized after each use. Packing materials should be discarded to avoid cross-contamination.

Use of Protective Attire and Barrier Techniques. Persons working in the receiving area should wear a clean uniform or laboratory coat, a face mask, protective eyewear, and disposable gloves.

Disposal of Waste Materials. Solid waste that is contaminated with blood or other body fluids should be placed in sealed, sturdy impervious bags to prevent leakage of the waste materials. The bag should be disposed, following regulations established by local or state environmental agencies.

Production Area. Work surfaces and equipment should be kept free of debris and disinfected daily. Any instruments, attachments, and materials to be used with new protheses/appliances should be maintained separately from those to be used with protheses/appliances that have already been inserted in the mouth. Ragwheels can be washed and autoclaved after each case. Brushes and other equipment should be disinfected at least daily. A small amount of pumice should be dispensed in small disposable containers for individual use on each case. The excess should be discarded. A liquid disinfectant (5 parts sodium hypochlorite to 100 parts distilled water) can serve as a mixing medium for pumice. Adding three parts green soap in the disinfectant solution will keep the pumice suspended.

Outgoing Cases. Each case should be disinfected before it is returned to the dental office. Dentists should be informed about infection control procedures that are used in the dental laboratory.

REFERENCES

1. Council on Dental Materials and Devices and Council on Dental Therapeutics: Infection control in the dental office. JADA, 97(4):673–677, 1978.

This report was approved by the councils in November 1987. Address requests for reprints to the Council on Dental Therapeutics.

2. Council on Dental Therapeutics and Council on Prosthetic Services and Dental Laboratory Relations: Guidelines for infection control in the dental office and the commercial dental laboratory. JADA, *110(6)*:969–972, 1985.

3. Council on Dental Materials, Instruments, and Equipment: Dentists' desk reference, 1983, and Council on Dental Therapeutics. Accepted dental therapeutics, 1984. Chicago, American Dental Association.

4. Division of Scientific Affairs: Facts about AIDS for the dental team, rev ed. Chicago, American Dental Association, 1987.

5. Proceedings of the National Symposium on Hepatitis B and the Dental Profession. JADA, *110(4)*:613–650, 1985.

6. American Dental Association, Centers for Disease Control, and National Institute of Dental Research: Proceedings, National Conference on Infection Control in Dentistry, 1986.

7. Centers for Disease Control: Recommended infection-control practices for dentistry. MMWR, *35*:237–242, 1986.

8. Centers for Disease Control: Recommendations for prevention of HIV transmission in health care settings. MMWR, *36*:Suppl no. 2S, 1987.

9. Centers for Disease Control: Recommendations for protection against viral hepatitis. MMWR, *34*:313–335, 1985.

10. Siew, C., et al.: Survey of hepatitis B exposure and vaccination in volunteer dentists. JADA, *114(4)*:457–459, 1987.

11. Council on Dental Therapeutics: ADA council recommends hepatitis vaccine for dentists, students, and auxiliary personnel. ADA News, *13(17)*:4, 1982.

12. Centers for Disease Control: Update on hepatitis B prevention. MMWR, *36(23)*:353–360, 366, 1987.

13. Council on Dental Therapeutics: Accepted therapeutic products. JADA, *113(6)*:1018–1023, 1986.

14. Council on Dental Materials, Instruments, and Equipment: Current status of sterilization instruments, devices, and methods for the dental office. JADA, *102(5)*:683–689, 1981.

15. Block, S.S.: Disinfection, sterilization and preservation, ed. 3. Philadelphia, Lea & Febiger, 1983.

16. Council on Dental Materials, Instruments, and Equipment: Recommendations for radiographic darkrooms and darkroom practices. JADA, *104(6)*:886–887, 1982.

17. Rowe, A.H., and Forrest, J.O.: Dental impressions: the probability of contamination and a method of disinfection. Br. Dent. J., *145(6)*:184–186, 1978.

18. Bergman, M., Olsson, S., and Bergman, B.: Elastomeric impression materials. Dimensional stability and surface detail sharpness following treatment with disinfectant solutions. Swed. Dent. J., *4*:161–167, 1980.

19. Merchant, V.A., et al.: Preliminary investigation of a method for disinfection of dental impressions. J. Prosthet. Dent., *52(6)*:877–879, 1984.

20. Rhodes, C.J., et al.: Effect of commercial glutaraldehyde solutions on elastomeric impression materials. J. Dent. Res. (Special Issue), *64*:243, abstract no. 619, 1985.

21. Setcos, J.C., et al.: Disinfection of polyether dental impression materials. J. Dent. Res. (Special Issue), *64*:244, abstract no. 620, 1985.

22. Setcos, J.C., et al.: The effects of disinfectants on a polysulfide impression material. J. Dent. Res., *65*:260, abstract no. 815, 1986.

23. Toh, C.G., et al.: Influence of disinfectants on a vinyl polysiloxane impression material. J. Dent. Res., *66*:133, abstract no. 212, 1987.

24. Minagi, S., et al.: Disinfection method for impression materials: freedom from fear of hepatitis B and acquired immunodeficiency syndrome. J. Prosthet. Dent., *56(4)*:451–454, 1986.

25. Herrera, S.P., and Merchant, V.A.: Dimensional stability of dental impression after immersion disinfection. JADA, *113(3)*:419–422, 1986.

26. Johansen, R.E., and Stackhouse, J.A.: Dimensional changes of elastomers during cold sterilization. J. Prosthet. Dent., *57(2)*:233–234, 1987.

27. Johnson, G.H., Drennon, D.G., and Powell, G.L.: Accuracy of elastomeric impressions disinfected by immersion. JADA, *116*:525–530, 1988.

28. Durr, D.P., and Novak, E.V.: Dimensional stability of alginate impressions immersed in disinfecting solutions. ASDC J. Dent. Child., *54(1)*:45–48, 1987.

29. Setcos, J.C., Peng, L., and Palenik, C.J.: The effects of disinfection procedures on the alginate impression material. J. Dent. Res., *63*:235, abstract no. 582, 1984.

30. Bergman, B., Bergman, M., and Olsson, S.: Alginate impression materials, dimensional stability

and surface detail sharpness following treatment with disinfectant solutions. Swed. Dent. J., 9:255–262, 1985.

31. Matyas, J., et al.: Effects of disinfectants on dimensional accuracy of impression materials. J. Dent. Res. (Special Issue), 65:764, abstract no. 344, 1986.

32. Minagi, S., et al.: Prevention of acquired immunodeficiency syndrome and hepatitis B. II: Disinfection method for hydrophilic impression materials. J. Prosthet. Dent., 58(4):462–465, 1987.

33. United States Environmental Protection Agency: EPA guide for infectious waste management. EPA/530-SW-86-014, May 1986.

34. Dental Laboratory Infection Control Council: DLICC infection control procedures. Manchester, NH, H&O Dental Laboratory, Inc., 1986.

35. National Board for Certification of Dental Laboratories: Infection control requirements for certified dental laboratories. Alexandria, VA, National Association of Dental Laboratories, 1986.

36. Crigger, L.P., Matis, B.A., and Young, J.M.: Infection control in Air Force dental clinics, ed. 2. Brooks Air Force Base, TX, USAF School of Aerospace Medicine, 1983.

From Council on Dental Materials, Instruments, and Equipment; Council on Dental Practice; Council on Dental Therapeutics: Infection control recommendations for the dental office and the dental laboratory. J. Am. Dent. Assoc., 116:241–248, 1988. Reprinted with permission from ADA Council on Dental Therapeutics.

Appendix B

Department of Labor, Occupational Safety and Health Administration: Occupational Exposure to Bloodborne Pathogens

XI. THE STANDARD

General Industry

Part 1910 of title 29 of the Code of Federal Regulations is amended as follows:

PART 1910–(AMENDED)

SUBPART Z–(AMENDED)

1. The general authority citation for subpart Z of 29 CFR part 1910 continues to read as follows and a new citation for § 1910.1030 is added:

Authority: Secs. 6 and 8, Occupational Safety and Health Act, 29 U.S.C. 655, 657, Secretary of Labor's Orders Nos. 12–71 (36 FR 8754), 8–76 (41 FR 25059), or 9–83 (48 FR 35736), as applicable; and 29 CFR part 1911.

*   *   *   *   *

Section 1910.1030 also issued under 29 U.S.C. 653.

*   *   *   *   *

2. Section 1910.1030 is added to read as follows:

§ 1910.1030   Bloodborne Pathogens.

(a) *Scope and Application.* This section applies to all occupational exposure to blood or other potentially infectious materials as defined by paragraph (b) of this section.

(b) *Definitions.* For purposes of this section, the following shall apply:

Assistant Secretary means the Assistant Secretary of Labor for Occupational Safety and Health, or designated representative.

Blood means human blood, human blood components and products made from human blood.

Bloodborne Pathogens means pathogenic microorganisms that are present in human blood and can cause disease in humans. These pathogens include, but are not limited to, hepatitis B virus (HBV) and human immunodeficiency virus (HIV).

Clinical Laboratory means a workplace where diagnostic or other screening procedures are performed on blood or other potentially infectious materials.

Contaminated means the presence or the reasonably anticipated presence of blood or other potentially infectious materials on an item or surface.

Contaminated Laundry means laundry which has been soiled with blood or other potentially infectious materials or may contain sharps.

Contaminated Sharps means any contaminated object that can penetrate the skin including, but not limited to, needles, scalpels, broken glass, broken capillary tubes, and exposed ends of dental wires.

Decontamination means the use of physical or chemical means to remove, inactivate, or destroy bloodborne pathogens on a surface or item to the point where they are no longer capable of transmitting infectious particles and the surface or item is rendered safe for handling, use, or disposal.

Director means the Director of the National Institute for Occupational Safety and Health, U.S. Department of Health and Human Services, or designated representative.

Engineering Controls means controls (e.g., sharps disposal containers, self-sheathing needles) that isolate or remove the bloodborne pathogens hazard from the workplace.

Exposure Incident means a specific eye, mouth, other mucous membrane, nonintact skin, or parenteral contact with blood or other potentially infectious materials that results from the performance of an employee's duties.

Handwashing Facilities means a facility providing an adequate supply of running potable water, soap and single use towels or hot air drying machines.

Licensed Healthcare Professional is a person whose legally permitted scope of practice allows him or her to independently perform the activities required by paragraph (f) Hepatitis B Vaccination and Post-exposure Evaluation and Follow-up.

HBV means hepatitis B virus.

HIV means human immunodeficiency virus.

Occupational Exposure means reasonably anticipated skin, eye, mucous membrane, or parenteral contact with blood or other potentially infectious materials that may result from the performance of an employee's duties.

Other Potentially Infectious Materials means

(1) The following body fluids: semen, vaginal secretions, cerebrospinal fluid, synovial fluid, pleural fluid, pericardial fluid, peritoneal fluid, amniotic fluid, saliva in dental procedures, any body fluid that is visibly contaminated with blood, and all body fluids in situations where it is difficult or impossible to differentiate between body fluids.

(2) Any unfixed tissue or organ (other than intact skin) from a human (living or dead) and

(3) HIV-containing cell or tissue cultures, organ cultures, and HIV- or HBV-containing culture medium or other solutions; and blood, organs or other tissues from experimental animals infected with HIV or HBV.

Parenteral means piercing mucous membranes or the skin barrier through such events as needlesticks, human bites, cuts and abrasions.

Personal Protective Equipment is specialized clothing or equipment worn by an employee for protection against a hazard. General work clothes (e.g., uniform pants, shirts or blouses) not intended to function as protection against a hazard are not considered to be personal protective equipment.

Production Facility means a facility engaged in industrial-scale, large-volume production of HIV or HBV or in high concentration production of HIV or HBV.

Regulated Waste means liquid or semi-liquid blood or other potentially infectious materials; contaminated items that would release blood or other potentially infectious materials in a liquid or semi-liquid state if compressed; items that are caked with dried blood or other potentially infectious materials and are capable of releasing these materials during handling; contaminated sharps; and pathological and microbiological wastes containing blood or other potentially infectious materials.

Research Laboratory means a laboratory producing research-laboratory-scale amounts of HIV or HBV. Research laboratories may produce high concentrations of HIV or HBV but not in the volume found in production facilities.

Source Individual means any individual, living or dead, whose blood or other potentially infectious materials may be a source of occupational exposure to the employee. Examples include, but are not limited to, hospital and clinic patients; clients in institutions for the developmentally disabled; trauma victims; clients of drug and alcohol treatment facilities; residents of hospices and nursing homes; human remains; and individuals who donate or sell blood or blood components.

Sterilize means the use of a physical or chemical procedure to destroy all microbial life including highly resistant bacterial endospores.

Universal precautions is an approach to infection control. According to the concept of Universal Precautions, all human blood and certain human body fluids are treated as if known to be infectious for HIV, HBV, and other bloodborne pathogens.

Work Practice Controls means controls that reduce the likelihood of exposure by altering the manner in which a task is performed (e.g., prohibiting recapping of needles by a two-handed technique).

(c) *Exposure control—(1) Exposure Control Plan.* (i) Each employer having an employee(s) with occupational exposure as defined by paragraph (b) of this section shall establish a written Exposure Control Plan designed to eliminate or minimize employee exposure.

(ii) The Exposure Control Plan shall contain at least the following elements:

(A) The exposure determination required by paragraph (c)(2).

(B) The schedule and method of implementation for paragraphs (d) Methods of Compliance, (e) HIV and HBV Research Laboratories and Production Facilities, (f) Hepatitis B Vaccination and Post-Exposure Evaluation and Follow-up, (g) Communication of Hazards to Employees, and (h) Recordkeeping of this standard, and

(C) The procedure for the evaluation of circumstances surrounding exposure incidents as required by paragraph (f)(3)(i) of this standard.

(iii) Each employer shall ensure that a copy of the Exposure Control Plan is accessible to employees in accordance with 29 CFR 1910.20(e).

(iv) The Exposure Control Plan shall be reviewed and updated at least annually and whenever necessary to reflect new or modified tasks and procedures which affect occupational exposure and to reflect new or revised employee positions with occupational exposure.

(v) The Exposure Control Plan shall be made available to the Assistant Secretary and the Director upon request for examination and copying.

(2) *Exposure determination.* (i) Each employer who has an employee(s) with occupational exposure as defined by paragraph (b) of this section shall prepare an exposure determination. This exposure determination shall contain the following:

(A) A list of all job classifications in which all employees in those job classifications have occupational exposure;

(B) A list of job classifications in which some employees have occupational exposure, and

(C) A list of all tasks and procedures or groups of closely related task and procedures in which occupational exposure occurs and that are performed by employees in job classifications listed in accordance with the provisions of paragraph (c)(2)(i)(B) of this standard.

(ii) This exposure determination shall be made without regard to the use of personal protective equipment.

(d) *Methods of compliance–(1) General*—Universal precautions shall be observed to prevent contact with blood and other potentially infectious materials. Under circumstances in which differentiation between body fluid types is difficult or impossible, all body fluids shall be considered potentially infectious materials.

(2) *Engineering and work practice controls.* (i) Engineering and work practice controls shall be used to eliminate or minimize employee exposure. Where occupational exposure remains after institution of these controls, personal protective equipment shall also be used.

(ii) Engineering controls shall be examined and maintained or replaced on a regular schedule to ensure their effectiveness.

(iii) Employers shall provide handwashing facilities which are readily accessible to employees.

(iv) When provision of handwashing facilities is not feasible, the employer shall provide either an appropriate antiseptic hand cleanser in conjunction with clean cloth/paper towels or antiseptic towelettes. When antiseptic hand cleansers or towelettes are used, hands shall be washed with soap and running water as soon as feasible.

(v) Employers shall ensure that employees wash their hands immediately or as soon as feasible after removal of gloves or other personal protective equipment.

(vi) Employers shall ensure that employees wash hands and any other skin with soap and water, or flush mucous membranes with water immediately or as soon as feasible following contact of such body areas with blood or other potentially infectious materials.

(vii) Contaminated needles and other contaminated sharps shall not be bent, recapped, or removed except as noted in paragraphs (d)(2)(vii)(A) and (d)(2)(vii)(B) below. Shearing or breaking of contaminated needles is prohibited.

(A) Contaminated needles and other contaminated sharps shall not be recapped or removed unless the employer can demonstrate that no alternative is feasible or that such action is required by a specific medical procedure.

(B) Such recapping or needle removal must be accomplished through the use of a mechanical device or a one-handed technique.

(viii) Immediately or as soon as possible after use, contaminated reusable sharps shall be placed in appropriate containers until properly reprocessed. These containers shall be:

(A) Puncture resistant;

(B) Labeled or color-coded in accordance with this standard;

(C) Leakproof on the sides and bottom; and

(D) In accordance with the requirements set forth in paragraph (d)(4)(ii)(E) for reusable sharps.

(ix) Eating, drinking, smoking, applying cosmetics or lip balm, and handling contact lenses are prohibited in work areas where there is a reasonable likelihood of occupational exposure.

(x) Food and drink shall not be kept in refrigerators, freezers, cabinets, or on countertops or benchtops where blood or other potentially infectious materials are present.

(xi) All procedures involving blood or other potentially infectious materials shall be performed in such a manner as to minimize splashing, spraying, spattering, and generation of droplets of these substances.

(xii) Mouth pipetting/suctioning of blood or other potentially infectious materials is prohibited.

(xiii) Specimens of blood or other potentially infectious materials shall be placed in a container which prevents leakage during collection, handling, processing, storage, transport, or shipping.

(A) The container for storage, transport, or shipping shall be labeled or color-coded according to paragraph (g)(1)(i) and closed prior to being stored, transported, or shipped. When a facility utilizes Universal Precautions in the handling of all specimens, the labeling/color-coding of specimens is not necessary provided containers are recognizable as containing specimens. This exemption only applies while such specimens/containers remain within the facility. Labeling or color-coding in accordance with paragraph (g)(1)(i) is required when such specimens/containers leave the facility.

(B) If outside contamination of the primary container occurs, the primary container shall be placed within a second container which prevents leakage during handling, processing, storage, transport, or shipping and is labeled or color-coded according to the requirements of this standard.

(C) If the specimen could puncture the primary container, the primary container shall be placed within a secondary container which is puncture-resistant in addition to the above characteristics.

(xiv) Equipment which may become contaminated with blood or other potentially infectious materials shall be examined prior to servicing or shipping and shall be decontaminated as necessary, unless the employer can demonstrate that decontamination of such equipment or portions of such equipment is not feasible.

(A) A readily observable label in accordance with paragraph (g)(1)(i)(H) shall be attached to the equipment stating which portions remain contaminated.

(B) The employer shall ensure that this information is conveyed to all affected employees, the servicing representative, and/or the manufacturer, as appropriate, prior to handling, servicing, or shipping so that appropriate precautions will be taken.

(3) Personal protective equipment—(i) Provision. When there is occupational exposure, the employer shall provide, at no cost to the employee, appropriate personal protective equipment such as, but not limited to, gloves, gowns, labo-

ratory coats, face shields or masks and eye protection, and mouthpieces, resuscitation bags, pocket masks, or other ventilation devices. Personal protective equipment will be considered "appropriate" only if it does not permit blood or other potentially infectious materials to pass through to or reach the employee's work clothes, street clothes, undergarments, skin, eyes, mouth, or other mucous membranes under normal conditions of use and for the duration of time which the protective equipment will be used.

(ii) Use. The employer shall ensure that the employee uses appropriate personal protective equipment unless the employer shows that the employee temporarily and briefly declined to use personal protective equipment when, under rare and extraordinary circumstances, it was the employee's professional judgment that in the specific instance its use would have prevented the delivery of health care or public safety services or would have posed an increased hazard to the safety of the worker or co-worker. When the employee makes this judgment, the circumstances shall be investigated and documented in order to determine whether changes can be instituted to prevent such occurrences in the future.

(iii) Accessibility. The employer shall ensure that appropriate personal protective equipment in the appropriate sizes is readily accessible at the worksite or is issued to employees. Hypoallergenic gloves, glove liners, powderless gloves, or other similar alternatives shall be readily accessible to those employees who are allergic to the gloves normally provided.

(iv) Cleaning, Laundering, and Disposal. The employer shall clean, launder, and dispose of personal protective equipment required by paragraphs (d) and (e) of this standard, at no cost to the employee.

(v) Repair and Replacement. The employer shall repair or replace personal protective equipment as needed to maintain its effectiveness, at no cost to the employee.

(vi) If a garment(s) is penetrated by blood or other potentially infectious materials, the garment(s) shall be removed immediately or as soon as feasible.

(vii) All personal protective equipment shall be removed prior to leaving the work area.

(viii) When personal protective equipment is removed it shall be placed in an appropriately designated area or container for storage, washing, decontamination or disposal.

(ix) Gloves. Gloves shall be worn when it can be reasonably anticipated that the employee may have hand contact with blood, other potentially infectious materials, mucous membranes, and non-intact skin; when performing vascular access procedures except as specified in paragraph (d)(3)(ix)(D); and when handling or touching contaminated items or surfaces.

(A) Disposable (single use) gloves such as surgical or examination gloves, shall be replaced as soon as practical when contaminated or as soon as feasible if they are torn, punctured, or when their ability to function as a barrier is compromised.

(B) Disposable (single use) gloves shall not be washed or decontaminated for re-use.

(C) Utility gloves may be decontaminated for re-use if the integrity of the glove is not compromised. However, they must be discarded if they are cracked, peeling, torn, punctured, or exhibit other signs of deterioration or when their ability to function as a barrier is compromised.

(D) If an employer in a volunteer blood donation center judges that routine gloving for all phlebotomies is not necessary then the employer shall:

(1) Periodically reevaluate this policy;

(2) Make gloves available to all employees who wish to use them for phlebotomy;

(3) Not discourage the use of gloves for phlebotomy; and

(4) Require that gloves be used for phlebotomy in the following circumstances:

(i) When the employee has cuts, scratches, or other breaks in his or her skin:

(ii) When the employee judges that hand contamination with blood may occur, for example, when performing phlebotomy on an uncooperative source individual; and

(iii) When the employee is receiving training in phlebotomy.

(x) Masks, Eye Protection, and Face Shields. Masks in combination with eye protection devices, such as goggles or glasses with solid side shields, or chin-length face shields, shall be worn whenever splashes, spray, spatter, or droplets of blood or other potentially infectious materials may be generated and eye, nose, or mouth contamination can be reasonably anticipated.

(xi) Gowns, Aprons, and Other Protective Body Clothing. Appropriate protective clothing such as, but not limited to, gowns, aprons, lab coats, clinic jackets, or similar outer garments shall be worn in occupational exposure situations. The type and characteristics will depend upon the task and degree of exposure anticipated.

(xii) Surgical caps or hoods and/or shoe covers or boots shall be worn in instances when gross contamination can reasonably be anticipated (e.g., autopsies, orthopaedic surgery).

(4) *Housekeeping.* (i) General. Employers shall ensure that the worksite is maintained in a clean and sanitary condition. The employer shall determine and implement an appropriate written schedule for cleaning and method of decontamination based upon the location within the facility, type of surface to be cleaned, type of soil present, and tasks or procedures being performed in the area.

(ii) All equipment and environmental and working surfaces shall be cleaned and decontaminated after contact with blood or other potentially infectious materials.

(A) Contaminated work surfaces shall be decontaminated with an appropriate disinfectant after completion of procedures; immediately or as soon as feasible when surfaces are overtly contaminated or after any spill of blood or other potentially infectious materials; and at the end of the work shift if the surface may have become contaminated since the last cleaning.

(B) Protective coverings, such as plastic wrap, aluminum foil, or imperviously-backed absorbent paper used to cover equipment and environmental surfaces, shall be removed and replaced as soon as feasible when they become overtly contaminated or at the end of the workshift if they may have become contaminated during the shift.

(C) All bins, pails, cans, and similar receptacles intended for reuse which have a reasonable likelihood for becoming contaminated with blood or other potentially infectious materials shall be inspected and decontaminated on a regularly scheduled basis and cleaned and decontaminated immediately or as soon as feasible upon visible contamination.

(D) Broken glassware which may be contaminated shall not be picked up directly with the hands. It shall be cleaned up using mechanical means, such as a brush and dust pan, tongs, or forceps.

(E) Reusable sharps that are contaminated with blood or other potentially infectious materials shall not be stored or processed in a manner that requires employees to reach by hand into the containers where these sharps have been placed.

(iii) Regulated Waste.

(A) Contaminated Sharps Discarding and Containment. (1) Contaminated sharps shall be discarded immediately or as soon as feasible in containers that are:

(i) Closable;

(ii) Puncture resistant;

(iii) Leakproof on sides and bottom; and

(iv) Labeled or color-coded in accordance with paragraph (g)(1)(i) of this standard.

(2) During use, containers for contaminated sharps shall be:

(i) Easily accessible to personnel and located as close as is feasible to the immediate area where sharps are used or can be reasonably anticipated to be found (e.g., laundries);

(ii) Maintained upright throughout use; and

(iii) Replaced routinely and not be allowed to overfill.

(3) When moving containers of contaminated sharps from the area of use, the containers shall be:

(i) Closed immediately prior to removal or replacement to prevent spillage or protrusion of contents during handling, storage, transport, or shipping;

(ii) Placed in a secondary container if leakage is possible. The second container shall be:

(A) Closable;

(B) Constructed to contain all contents and prevent leakage during handling, storage, transport, or shipping; and

(C) Labeled or color-coded according to paragraph (g)(1)(i) of this standard.

(4) Reusable containers shall not be opened, emptied, or cleaned manually or in any other manner which would expose employees to the risk of percutaneous injury.

(B) Other Regulated Waste Containment. (1) Regulated waste shall be placed in containers which are:

(i) Closable;

(ii) Constructed to contain all contents and prevent leakage of fluids during handling, storage, transport or shipping;

(iii) Labeled or color-coded in accordance with paragraph (g)(1)(i) this standard; and

(iv) Closed prior to removal to prevent spillage or protrusion of contents during handling, storage, transport, or shipping.

(2) If outside contamination of the regulated waste container occurs, it shall be placed in a second container. The second container shall be:

(i) Closable;

(ii) Constructed to contain all contents and prevent leakage of fluids during handling, storage, transport or shipping;

(iii) Labeled or color-coded in accordance with paragraph (g)(1)(i) of this standard; and *(iv)* Closed prior to removal to prevent spillage or protrusion of contents during handling, storage, transport, or shipping.

(C) Disposal of all regulated waste shall be in accordance with applicable regulations of the United States, States and Territories, and political subdivisions of States and Territories.

(iv) Laundry.

(A) Contaminated laundry shall be handled as little as possible with a minimum of agitation. (1) Contaminated laundry shall be bagged or containerized at the location where it was used and shall not be sorted or rinsed in the location of use.

(2) Contaminated laundry shall be placed and transported in bags or containers labeled or color-coded in accordance with paragraph (g)(1)(i) of this standard. When a facility utilizes Universal Precautions in the handling of all soiled laundry, alternative labeling or color-coding is sufficient if it permits all employees to recognize the containers as requiring compliance with Universal Precautions.

(3) Whenever contaminated laundry is wet and presents a reasonable likelihood of soak-through of or leakage from the bag or container, the laundry shall be placed and transported in bags or containers which prevent soak-through and/or leakage of fluids to the exterior.

(B) The employer shall ensure that employees who have contact with contaminated laundry wear protective gloves and other appropriate personal protective equipment.

(C) When a facility ships contaminated laundry off-site to a second facility which does not utilize Universal Precautions in the handling of all laundry, the facility generating the contaminated laundry must place such laundry in bags or containers which are labeled or color-coded in accordance with paragraph (g)(1)(i).

(e) *HIV and HBV Research Laboratories and Production Facilities.* (1) This paragraph applies to research laboratories and production facilities engaged in the culture, production, concentration, experimentation, and manipulation of HIV and HBV. It does not apply to clinical or diagnostic laboratories engaged solely in the analysis of blood, tissues, or organs. These requirements apply in addition to the other requirements of the standard.

(2) Research laboratories and production facilities shall meet the following criteria:

(i) Standard microbiological practices. All regulated waste shall either be incinerated or decontaminated by a method such as autoclaving known to effectively destroy bloodborne pathogens.

(ii) Special practices.

(A) Laboratory doors shall be kept closed when work involving HIV or HBV is in progress.

(B) Contaminated materials that are to be decontaminated at a site away from the work area shall be placed in a durable, leakproof, labeled or color-coded container that is closed before being removed from the work area.

(C) Access to the work area shall be limited to authorized persons. Written policies and procedures shall be established whereby only persons who have been advised of the potential biohazard, who meet any specific entry requirements, and who comply with all entry and exit procedures shall be allowed to enter the work areas and animal rooms.

(D) When other potentially infectious materials or infected animals are present in the work area or containment module, a hazard warning sign incorporating the universal biohazard symbol shall be posted on all access doors. The hazard warning sign shall comply with paragraph (g)(1)(ii) of this standard.

(E) All activities involving other potentially infectious materials shall be conducted in biological safety cabinets or other physical-containment devices within the containment module. No work with these other potentially infectious materials shall be conducted on the open bench.

(F) Laboratory coats, gowns, smocks, uniforms, or other appropriate protective clothing shall be used in the work area and animal rooms. Protective clothing shall not be worn outside of the work area and shall be decontaminated before being laundered.

(G) Special care shall be taken to avoid skin contact with other potentially infectious materials. Gloves shall be worn when handling infected animals and when making hand contact with other potentially infectious materials is unavoidable.

(H) Before disposal all waste from work areas and from animal rooms shall be decontaminated by a method such as autoclaving known to effectively destroy bloodborne pathogens.

(I) Vacuum lines shall be protected with liquid disinfectant traps and high-efficiency particulate air (HEPA) filters of equivalent or superior efficiency and which are checked routinely and maintained or replaced as necessary.

(J) Hypodermic needles and syringes shall be used only for parenteral injection and aspiration of fluids from laboratory animals and diaphragm bottles. Only needle-locking syringes or disposable syringe-needle units (i.e., the needle is integral to the syringe) shall be used for the injection or aspiration of other potentially infectious materials. Extreme caution shall be used when handling needles and syringes. A needle shall not be bent, sheared, replaced in the sheath or guard, or removed from the syringe following use. The needle and syringe shall be promptly placed in a puncture-resistant container and autoclaved or decontaminated, before reuse or disposal.

(K) All spills shall be immediately contained and cleaned up by appropriate professional staff or others properly trained and equipped to work with potentially concentrated infectious materials.

(L) A spill or accident that results in an exposure incident shall be immediately reported to the laboratory director or other responsible person.

(M) A biosafety manual shall be prepared or adopted and periodically reviewed and updated at least annually or more often if necessary. Personnel shall be advised of potential hazards, shall be required to read instructions on practices and procedures, and shall be required to follow them.

(iii) *Containment equipment.* (A) Certified biological safety cabinets (Class I, II, or III) or other appropriate combinations of personal protection or physical containment devices, such as special protective clothing, respirators, centrifuge safety cups, sealed centrifuge rotors, and containment caging for animals, shall be used for all activities with other potentially infectious materials that pose a threat of exposure to droplets, splashes, spills, or aerosols.

(B) Biological safety cabinets shall be certified when installed, whenever they are moved and at least annually.

(3) HIV and HBV research laboratories shall meet the following criteria:

(i) Each laboratory shall contain a facility for hand washing and an eye wash.

(ii) An autoclave for decontamination of regulated waste shall be available.

(4) HIV and HBV production facilities shall meet the following criteria:

(i) The work areas shall be separated from areas that are open to unrestricted traffic flow within the building. Passage through two sets of doors shall be the basic requirement for entry into the work area from access corridors or other contiguous areas. Physical separation of the high-containment work area from access corridors or other areas or activities may also be provided by a double-doored clothes-change room (showers may be included), airlock, or other access facility that requires passing through two sets of doors before entering the work area.

(ii) The surfaces of doors, walls, floors and ceilings in the work area shall be water resistant so that they can be easily cleaned. Penetrations in these surfaces shall be sealed or capable of being sealed to facilitate decontamination.

(iii) Each work area shall contain a sink for washing hands and a readily available eye wash facility. The sink shall be foot, elbow, or automatically operated and shall be located near the exit door of the work area.

(iv) Access doors to the work area or containment module shall be self-closing.

(v) An autoclave for decontamination of regulated waste shall be available within or as near as possible to the work area.

(vi) A ducted exhaust-air ventilation system shall be provided. This system shall create directional airflow that draws air into the work area through the entry area. The exhaust air shall not be recirculated to any other areas of the building, shall be discharged to the outside, and shall be dispersed away from occupied areas and air intakes. The proper direction of the airflow shall be verified (i.e., in the work area).

(5) *Training requirements.* Additional training requirements for employees in HIV and HBV research laboratories and HIV and HBV production facilities are specified in paragraph (g)(2)(ix).

(f) *Hepatitis B vaccination and post-exposure evaluation and follow-up—(1) General.* (i) The employer shall make available hepatitis B vaccination and vaccination series to all employees who have occupational exposure and post-exposure evaluation and follow-up to all employees with an exposure incident.

(ii) The employer shall ensure that all medical evaluations and procedures including the hepatitis B vaccine and vaccination series and post-exposure evaluation and follow-up, including prophylaxis, are:

(A) Made available at no cost to the employee;

(B) Made available to the employee at a reasonable time and place;

(C) Performed by or under the supervision of a licensed physician or by or under the supervision of another licensed healthcare professional; and

(D) Provided according to recommendations of the U.S. Public Health Service current at the time these evaluations and procedures take place, except as specified by this paragraph (f).

(iii) The employer shall ensure that all laboratory tests are conducted by an accredited laboratory at no cost to the employee.

(2) *Hepatitis B Vaccination.* (i) Hepatitis B vaccination shall be made available after the employee has received the training required in paragraph (g)(2)(vii)(I) and within 10 working days of initial assignment to all employees who have occupational exposure unless the employee has previously received the complete hepatitis B vaccination series, antibody testing has revealed that the employee is immune, or the vaccine is contraindicated for medical reasons.

(ii) The employer shall not make participation in a prescreening program a prerequisite for receiving hepatitis B vaccination.

(iii) If the employee initially declines hepatitis B vaccination but at a later date while still covered under the standard decides to accept the vaccination, the employer shall make available hepatitis B vaccination at that time.

(iv) The employer shall assure that employees who decline to accept hepatitis B vaccination offered by the employer sign the statement in appendix A.

(v) If a routine booster dose(s) of hepatitis B vaccine is recommended by the U.S. Public Health Service at a future date, such booster dose(s) shall be made available in accordance with section (f)(1)(ii).

(3) *Post exposure Evaluation and Follow-up.* Following a report of an exposure incident, the employer shall make immediately available to the exposed employee a confidential medical evaluation and follow-up, including at least the following elements:

(i) Documentation of the route(s) of exposure and the circumstances under which the exposure occurred.

(ii) Identification and documentation of the source individual, unless the employer can establish that identification is infeasible or prohibited by state or local law;

(A) The source individual's blood shall be tested as soon as feasible and after consent is obtained in order to determine HBV and HIV infectivity. If consent is not obtained, the employer shall establish that legally required consent cannot be obtained. When the source individual's consent is not required by law, the source individual's blood, if available, shall be tested and the results documented.

(B) When the source individual is already known to be infected with HBV or HIV, testing for the source individual's known HBV or HIV status need not be repeated.

(C) Results of the source individual's testing shall be made available to the exposed employee, and the employee shall be informed of applicable laws and regulations concerning disclosure of the identity and infectious status of the source individual.

(iii) Collection and testing of blood for HBV and HIV serological status;

(A) The exposed employee's blood shall be collected as soon as feasible and tested after consent is obtained.

(B) If the employee consents to baseline blood collection, but does not give consent at that time for HIV serologic testing, the sample shall be preserved for at least 90 days. If, within 90 days of the exposure incident, the employee elects to have the baseline sample tested, such testing shall be done as soon as feasible.

(iv) Post-exposure prophylaxis, when medically indicated, as recommended by the U.S. Public Health Service;

(v) Counseling; and

(vi) Evaluation of reported illnesses.

(4) *Information Provided to the Healthcare Professional.* (i) The employer shall ensure that the healthcare professional responsible for the employee's Hepatitis B vaccination is provided a copy of this regulation.

(ii) The employer shall ensure that the healthcare professional evaluating an employee after an exposure incident is provided the following information:

(A) A copy of this regulation;

(B) A description of the exposed employee's duties as they relate to the exposure incident;

(C) Documentation of the route(s) of exposure and circumstances under which exposure occurred;

(D) Results of the source individual's blood testing, if available; and

(E) All medical records relevant to the appropriate treatment of the employee including vaccination status which are the employer's responsibility to maintain.

(5) *Healthcare Professional's Written Opinion.* The employer shall obtain and provide the employee with a copy of the evaluating healthcare professional's written opinion within 15 days of the completion of the evaluation. The written opinion shall be limited to the following information:

(i) The healthcare professional's written opinion for Hepatitis B vaccination shall be limited to whether Hepatitis B vaccination is indicated for an employee, and if the employee has received such vaccination.

(ii) The healthcare professional's written opinion for post-exposure evaluation and follow-up shall be limited to the following information:

(A) That the employee has been informed of the results of the evaluation; and

(B) That the employee has been told about any medical conditions resulting from exposure to blood or other potentially infectious materials which require further evaluation or treatment. (iii) All other findings or diagnoses shall remain confidential and shall not be included in the written report.

(6) *Medical recordkeeping.* Medical records required by this standard shall be maintained in accordance with paragraph (h)(1) of this section.

(g) *Communication of hazards to employees*—(1) *Labels and signs*—(i) *Labels.* (A) Warning labels shall be affixed to containers of regulated waste, refrigerators and freezers containing blood and other potentially infectious materials; and other containers used to store or ship blood or other potentially infectious materials, except as provided in paragraph (g)(1)(i) (E), (F) and (G).

(B) Labels required by this section shall include the following legend:

BIOHAZARD

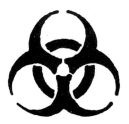

BIOHAZARD

(C) These labels shall be fluorescent orange or orange-red or predominantly so, with lettering or symbols in a contrasting color.

(D) Labels required shall be affixed as close as feasible to the container by string, wire, adhesive, or other method that prevents their loss or unintentional removal.

(E) Red bags or red containers may be substituted for labels.

(F) Containers of blood, blood components, or blood products that are labeled as to their contents and have been released for transfusion or other clinical use are exempted from the labeling requirements of paragraph (g).

(G) Individual containers of blood or other potentially infectious materials that are placed in a labeled container during storage, transport, shipment or disposal are exempted from the labeling requirement.

(H) Labels required for contaminated equipment shall be in accordance with this paragraph and shall also state which portions of the equipment remain contaminated.

(I) Regulated waste that has been decontaminated need not be labeled or color-coded.

(ii) Signs. (A) The employer shall post signs at the entrance to work areas specified in paragraph (e), HIV and HBV Research Laboratory and Production Facilities, which shall bear the following legend:

BIOHAZARD

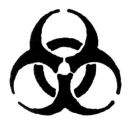

BIOHAZARD

(Name of the Infectious Agent)
(Special requirements for entering the area)
(Name, telephone number of the laboratory director or other responsible person.)

(B) These signs shall be fluorescent orange-red or predominantly so, with lettering or symbols in a contrasting color.

(2) *Information and Training.* (i) Employers shall ensure that all employees with occupational exposure participate in a training program which must be provided at no cost to the employee and during working hours.

(ii) Training shall be provided as follows:

(A) At the time of initial assignment to tasks where occupational exposure may take place;

(B) Within 90 days after the effective date of the standard; and

(C) At least annually thereafter.

(iii) For employees who have received training on bloodborne pathogens in the year preceding the effective date of the standard, only training with respect to the provisions of the standard which were not included need be provided.

(iv) Annual training for all employees shall be provided within one year of their previous training.

(v) Employers shall provide additional training when changes such as modification of tasks or procedures or institution of new tasks or procedures affect the employee's occupational exposure. The additional training may be limited to addressing the new exposures created.

(vi) Material appropriate in content and vocabulary to educational level, literacy, and language of employees shall be used.

(vii) The training program shall contain at a minimum the following elements:

(A) An accessible copy of the regulatory text of this standard and an explanation of its contents;

(B) A general explanation of the epidemiology and symptoms of bloodborne diseases;

(C) An explanation of the modes of transmission of bloodborne pathogens;

(D) An explanation of the employer's exposure control plan and the means by which the employee can obtain a copy of the written plan:

(E) An explanation of the appropriate methods for recognizing tasks and other activities that may involve exposure to blood and other potentially infectious materials;

(F) An explanation of the use and limitations of methods that will prevent or reduce exposure including appropriate engineering controls, work practices, and personal protective equipment;

(G) Information on the types, proper use, location, removal, handling, decontamination and disposal of personal protective equipment;

(H) An explanation of the basis for selection of personal protective equipment;

(I) Information on the hepatitis B vaccine, including information on its efficacy, safety, method of administration, the benefits of being vaccinated, and that the vaccine and vaccination will be offered free of charge;

(J) Information on the appropriate actions to take and persons to contact in an emergency involving blood or other potentially infectious materials;

(K) An explanation of the procedure to follow if an exposure incident occurs, including the method of reporting the incident and the medical follow-up that will be made available;

(L) Information on the post-exposure evaluation and follow-up that the employer is required to provide for the employee following an exposure incident;

(M) An explanation of the signs and labels and/or color-coding required by paragraph (g)(1); and

(N) An opportunity for interactive questions and answers with the person conducting the training session.

(viii) The person conducting the training shall be knowledgeable in the subject matter covered by the elements contained in the training program as it relates to the workplace that the training will address.

(ix) Additional Initial Training for Employees in HIV and HBV Laboratories and Production Facilities. Employees in HIV or HBV research laboratories and HIV or HBV production facilities shall receive the following initial training in addition to the above training requirements.

(A) The employer shall assure that employees demonstrate proficiency in standard microbiological practices and techniques and in the practices and operations specific to the facility before being allowed to work with HIV or HBV.

(B) The employer shall assure that employees have prior experience in the handling of human pathogens or tissue cultures before working with HIV or HBV.

(C) The employer shall provide a training program to employees who have no prior experience in handling human pathogens. Initial work activities shall not include the handling of infectious agents. A progression of work activities shall be assigned as techniques are learned and proficiency is developed. The employer shall assure that employees participate in work activities involving infectious agents only after proficiency has been demonstrated.

(h) *Recordkeeping*—(1) *Medical records.* (i) The employer shall establish and maintain an accurate record for each employee with occupational exposure, in accordance with 29 CFR 1910.20.

(ii) This record shall include:

(A) The name and social security number of the employee;

(B) A copy of the employee's hepatitis B vaccination status including the dates of all the hepatitis B vaccinations and any medical records relative to the employee's ability to receive vaccination as required by paragraph (f)(2);

(C) A copy of all results of examinations, medical testing, and follow-up procedures as required by paragraph (f)(3);

(D) The employer's copy of the healthcare professional's written opinion as required by paragraph (f)(5); and

(E) A copy of the information provided to the healthcare professional as required by paragraphs (f)(4)(ii)(B) (C) and (D).

(iii) Confidentiality. The employer shall ensure that employee medical records required by paragraph (h)(1) are:

(A) Kept confidential; and

(B) Are not disclosed or reported without the employee's express written consent to any person within or outside the workplace except as required by this section or as may be required by law.

(iv) The employer shall maintain the records required by paragraph (h) for at least the duration of employment plus 30 years in accordance with 29 CFR 1910.20.

(2) *Training Records.* (i) *Training records shall include the following information:*

(A) The dates of the training sessions;

(B) The contents or a summary of the training sessions;

(C) The names and qualifications of persons conducting the training; and

(D) The names and job titles of all persons attending the training sessions.

(ii) These records shall be maintained for 3 years from the date on which the training occurred.

(3) *Availability.* (i) The employer shall ensure that all records required to be maintained by this section shall be made available upon request to the Assistant Secretary and the Director for examination and copying.

(ii) Employee training records required by this paragraph shall be provided upon request for examination and copying to employees, to employee representatives, to the Director, and to the Assistant Secretary in accordance with 29 CFR 1910.20.

(iii) Employee medical records required by this paragraph shall be provided upon request for examination and copying to the subject employee, to anyone having written consent of the subject employee, to the Director and to the Assistant Secretary in accordance with 29 CFR 1910.20.

(4) *Transfer of Records.* (i) The employer shall comply with the requirements involving transfer of records set forth in 29 CFR 1910.20(h).

(ii) If the employer ceases to do business and there is no successor employer to receive and retain the records for the prescribed period, the employer shall notify the Director, at least three months prior to their disposal and transmit them to the Director, if required by the Director to do so, within that three month period.

(i) *Dates.*—(1) *Effective Date.* The standard shall become effective on March 6, 1992.

(2) The Exposure Control Plan required by paragraph (c)(2) of this section shall be completed on or before May 5, 1992.

(3) Paragraph (g)(2) Information and Training and (h) Recordkeeping shall take effect on or before June 4, 1992.

(4) Paragraphs (d)(2) Engineering and Work Practice Controls, (d)(3) Personal Protective Equipment, (d)(4) Housekeeping, (e) HIV and HBV Research Laboratories and Production Facilities, (f) Hepatitis B Vaccination and Post-Exposure Evaluation and Follow-up, and (g)(1) Labels and Signs, shall take effect July 6, 1992.

Appendix A to Section 1910.1030—Hepatitis B Vaccine Declination (Mandatory)

I understand that due to my occupational exposure to blood or other potentially infectious materials I may be at risk of acquiring hepatitis B virus (HBV) infection. I have been given the opportunity to be vaccinated with hepatitis B vaccine, at no charge to myself. However, I decline hepatitis B vaccination at this time. I understand that by declining this vaccine, I continue to be at risk of acquiring hepatitis B, a serious disease. If in the future I continue to have occupational exposure to blood or other potentially infectious materials and I want to be vaccinated with hepatitis B vaccine, I can receive the vaccination series at no charge to me.

[FR Doc. 91-28886 Filed 12-2-91; 8:45 am]

BILING CODE 4510-26-M

Appendix C

Environmental Protection Agency: Standards for the Tracking and Management of Medical Waste; Interim Final Rule and Request for Comments

PART 259—STANDARDS FOR THE TRACKING AND MANAGEMENT OF MEDICAL WASTE

Appendix III to 40 CFR Part 259   Transporter Report and Instructions
Appendix IV to 40 CFR Part 259   Recommended Medical Waste Transporter Notification Form and Instructions

Authority: 42 U.S.C. 6912, 6992 *et seq.*

SUBPART A—GENERAL

§ 259.1 Purpose, Scope, and Applicability.

(a) The purpose of this part is to establish a demonstration program for tracking medical waste shipments pursuant to the Medical Waste Tracking Act of 1988.

(b) The regulations in this part apply to regulated medical waste as defined in Subpart D of this part that is generated in a Covered State as defined in Subpart C of this part.

(c) Generators, transporters, and owners or operators of intermediate handling facilities (e.g., treatment or destruction facilities) or destination facilities (e.g., disposal facilities) who transport, offer for transport, or otherwise manage regulated medical waste generated in a Covered State must comply with this part even if such transport or management occurs in a non-Covered State.

(d) *Regulatory presumptions.* The transportation and management of regulated medical waste, as defined in Subpart D of this part, in a Covered State is subject to regulations under this part, unless a person claiming a non-regulated status can demonstrate by a preponderance of the evidence, through shipping papers or other documentation, that the regulated medical waste was generated in a non-Covered State.

§ 259.2 Effective Dates and Duration of the Demonstration Program.

(a) Except for records and reports required to be maintained or submitted under this part, the demonstration program will be effective for the period June 22, 1989, to June 22, 1991.

(b) The length of time parties must keep records required under this part is automatically extended in the case where EPA or a State initiates an enforcement action, for which those records are relevant, until the conclusion of the enforcement action.

SUBPART B—DEFINITIONS

§ 259.10 Definitions.

(a) For the purpose of this part, all of the terms defined in 40 CFR 260.10 are hereby incorporated by reference, except for the following terms, which have been redefined as appropriate to address the management of medical waste specifically:

"Facility" means all contiguous land and structures, other appurtenances, and improvements on the land, used for treating, destroying, storing, or disposing of regulated medical waste. A facility may consist of several treatment, destruction, storage, or disposal operational units.

"Generator" means any person, by site, whose act or process produces regulated medical waste as defined in Subpart D of this part, or whose act first causes a regulated medical waste to become subject to regulation. In the case where more than one person (e.g., doctors with separate medical practices) are located in the same building, each individual business entity is a separate generator for the purposes of this part.

"Landfill" means a disposal facility or part of a facility where regulated medical waste is placed in or on the land and which is not a land treatment facility, a surface impoundment, or an injection well.

"Person" means an individual, trust, firm, joint stock company, corporation (including a government corporation), partnership, association, State, municipality, commission, political subdivision of a State, any interstate body, or any department, agency or instrumentality of the United States.

"Solid waste" means a solid waste defined in Section 1004 (27) of RCRA.

"Storage" means the temporary holding of regulated medical wastes at a designated accumulation area before treatment, disposal, or transport to another location.

"Transfer facility" means any transportation-related facility including loading docks, parking areas, storage areas and other similar areas where shipments of regulated medical waste are held (come to rest or are managed) during the course of transportation. For example, a location at which regulated medical waste is transferred directly between two vehicles is considered a transfer facility. A transfer facility is a "transporter."

"Transportation" means the shipment or conveyance of regulated medical waste by air, rail, highway, or water.

"Transporter" means a person engaged in the off-site transportation of regulated medical waste by air, rail, highway, or water.

"Treatment" when used in the context of medical waste management means any method, technique or process designed to change the biological character or composition of any regulated medical waste so as to reduce or eliminate its potential for causing disease. When used in the context of § 259.30(a) of this part, treatment means either the provision of medical services or the preparation of human or animal remains for interment or cremation.

(b) In addition, when used in this part, the following terms have the meanings given below:

"Biologicals" means preparations made from living organisms and their products, including vaccines, cultures, etc., intended for use in diagnosing, immunizing or treating humans or animals or in research pertaining thereto.

"Blood products" means any product derived from human blood, including but not limited to blood plasma, platelets, red or white blood corpuscles, and other derived licensed products, such as interferon, etc.

"Body fluids" means liquid emanating or derived from humans and limited to blood; cerebrospinal, synovial, pleural, peritoneal and pericardial fluids; and semen and vaginal secretions.

"Central collection point" means a location where a generator consolidates regulated medical waste brought together from original generation points prior to its transport off-site or its treatment on-site (e.g., incineration).

"Covered States" means those States that are participating in the demonstration medical waste tracking program. It includes States identified under Subtitle J of RCRA which have not petitioned out of the program pursuant to § 259.21 of this part and States which have petitioned into the program pursuant to § 259.22. Any other State is a "non-Covered State."

"Decontamination" means the process of reducing or eliminating the presence of harmful substances, such as infectious agents, so as to reduce the likelihood of disease transmission from those substances.

"Destination facility" means the disposal facility, the incineration facility, or the facility that both treats and destroys regulated medical waste, to which a consignment of such is intended to be shipped, specified in Box 8 of the Medical Waste Tracking Form.

"Destroyed regulated medical waste" means regulated medical waste that has been ruined, torn apart, or mutilated through processes such as thermal treatment, melting, shredding, grinding, tearing or breaking, so that it is no longer generally recognizable as medical waste. It does not mean compaction.

"Destruction facility" means a facility that destroys regulated medical waste by ruining or mutilating it, or tearing it apart.

"Infectious agent" means any organism (such as a virus or a bacteria) that is capable of being communicated by invasion and multiplication in body tissues and capable of causing disease or adverse health impacts in humans.

"Intermediate handler" is a facility that either treats regulated medical waste or destroys regulated medical waste but does not do both. The term, as used in this Part, does not include transporters.

"Laboratory" means any research, analytical, or clinical facility that performs health care related analysis or service. This includes medical, pathological, pharmaceutical, and other research, commercial, or industrial laboratories.

"Medical waste" means any solid waste which is generated in the diagnosis, treatment (e.g., provision of medical services), or immunization of human beings or animals, in research pertaining thereto, or in the production or testing of biologicals. The term does not include any hazardous waste identified or listed under Part 261 of this chapter or any household waste as defined in § 261.4(b)(I) of this chapter.

Note to this definition: Mixtures of hazardous waste and medical waste are subject to this part except as provided in § 259.31.

"Original generation point" means the location where regulated medical waste is generated. Waste may be taken from original generation points to a central collection point prior to off-site transport or on-site treatment.

"Oversized regulated medical waste" means medical waste that is too large to be placed in a plastic bag or standard container.

"Regulated medical waste" means those medical wastes that have been listed in § 259.30(a) of this part and that must be managed in accordance with the requirements of this part.

"Tracking form" means the Federal Medical Waste Tracking Form that must accompany all applicable shipments of regulated medical wastes generated within one of the Covered States.

"Treated regulated medical waste" means regulated medical waste that has been treated to substantially reduce or eliminate its potential for causing disease, but has not yet been destroyed.

"Universal biohazard symbol" means the symbol design that conforms to the design shown in 29 CFR 1910.145(f)(8)(ii).

"Untreated regulated medical waste" means regulated medical waste that has not been treated to substantially reduce or eliminate its potential for causing disease.

"Waste category" means either untreated regulated medical waste or treated regulated medical waste.

SUBPART C—COVERED STATES

§ 259.20   States Included in the Demonstration Program.

(a) The regulations of this part apply to all regulated medical waste that is generated in any Covered State. This Subpart further identifies the procedures for States electing to participate or not to participate in the demonstration program.

(b) For purposes of this part, Covered States are the States of Connecticut, Illinois, Indiana, Michigan, Minnesota, New Jersey, New York, Ohio, Pennsylvania, and Wisconsin. Any of these States may elect not to participate in the demonstration program using the procedures in § 259.21 of this subpart. States that the Administrator removes from the demonstration program pursuant to RCRA section 11001(b) are non-Covered States.

(c) Any States not listed in paragraph (b) of this section may petition to participate in the demonstration program pursuant to § 259.22 of this subpart. States that the Administrator has included in the demonstration program pursuant to a State petition are Covered States.

§ 259.21   States Electing Not To Participate.

(a)(1) If Connecticut, New Jersey, or New York elect not to participate in the demonstration program, the Governor of the State must notify the Administrator no later than April 24, 1989, of his decision that the State elects not to participate in the demonstration program. The notification must include:

(i) A statement that the State has implemented a medical waste tracking program that is no less stringent than the demonstration program of this part;

(ii) A copy of the State's regulations implementing that program; and

(iii) A copy of the State statutes authorizing that program, and a copy of the State statutes and regulations governing the State's administrative procedures.

(2) The Administrator will consider the information submitted under paragraph (a)(1) of this section and shall determine whether the State's program is no less stringent than the Federal program under this part. Upon a finding by the Administrator that the State's program is no less stringent than Part 259, the Administrator shall remove the State from the list of Covered States in this subpart.

(b) If Illinois, Indiana, Michigan, Minnesota, Ohio, Pennsylvania, or Wisconsin elect not to participate in the demonstration program, the Governor of the State must provide written notification to the Administrator no later than April 24, 1989.

§ 259.22   States Electing To Participate.

Any State not listed in § 259.20(b) of this subpart may elect to participate in the demonstration program. The Governor of such State must submit a petition to the Administrator no later than April 24, 1989, requesting inclusion in the dem-

Table C–1. Regulated Medical Waste

Waste Class	Description
(1) Cultures and Stocks	Cultures and stocks of infectious agents and associated biologicals, including: cultures from medical and pathological laboratories; cultures and stocks of infectious agents from research and industrial laboratories; wastes from the production of biologicals; discarded live and attenuated vaccines; and culture dishes and devices used to transfer, inoculate, and mix cultures
(2) Pathological Wastes	Human pathological wastes, including tissues, organs, and body parts and body fluids that are removed during surgery or autopsy, or other medical procedures, and specimens of body fluids and their containers
(3) Human Blood and Blood Products	(1) Liquid waste human blood; (2) products of blood; (3) items saturated and/or dripping with human blood; or (4) items that were saturated and/or dripping with human blood that are now caked with dried human blood; including serum, plasma, and other blood components, and their containers, which were used or intended for use in either patient care, testing and laboratory analysis or the development of pharmaceuticals. Intravenous bags are also included in this category
(4) Sharps	Sharps that have been used in animal or human patient care or treatment or in medical, research, or industrial laboratories, including hypodermic needles, syringes (with or without the attached needle), pasteur pipettes, scalpel blades, blood vials, needles with attached tubing, and culture dishes (regardless of presence of infectious agents). Also included are other types of broken or unbroken glassware that were in contact with infectious agents, such as used slides and cover slips
(5) Animal Waste	Contaminated animal carcasses, body parts, and bedding of animals that were known to have been exposed to infectious agents during research (including research in veterinary hospitals), production of biologicals, or testing of pharmaceuticals
(6) Isolation Wastes	Biological waste and discarded materials contaminated with blood, excretion, exudates, or secretions from humans who are isolated to protect others from certain highly communicable diseases, or isolated animals known to be infected with highly communicable disease
(7) Unused Sharps	The following unused, discarded sharps: hypodermic needles, suture needles, syringes, and scalpel blades

onstration program as a Covered State. Upon a determination to accept such a petition, the Administrator shall include the State on the list of Covered States.

§ 259.23 Notice of Participating States.

The Administrator shall publish a notice in the Federal Register listing those States included in the demonstration program after April 24, 1989.

SUBPART D—REGULATED MEDICAL WASTE

§ 259.30 Definition of Regulated Medical Waste.

(a) A regulated medical waste is any solid waste, defined in § 259.10(a) of this part, generated in the diagnosis, treatment (e.g., provision of medical services), or immunization of human beings or animals, in research pertaining thereto, or in the production or testing of biologicals, that is not excluded or exempted under paragraph (b) of this section, and that is listed in the following table:

Note to paragraph (a): The term "solid waste" includes solid, semisolid, or liquid materials, but does not include domestic sewage materials identified in § 261.4(a)(1) of this subchapter.

(b)(1) *Exclusions.* (i) Hazardous waste identified or listed under the regulations in Part 261 of this chapter is not regulated medical waste.

Note to paragraph (b)(1)(i): Mixtures of regulated medical waste and hazardous waste are subject to Part 259, except as provided in § 259.31(b) of this subpart.

(ii) Household waste, as defined in § 261.4(b)(1) of this Chapter, is not regulated medical waste.

(iii) Ash from incineration of regulated medical waste is not regulated medical waste once the incineration process has been completed.

(iv) Residues from treatment and destruction processes are no longer regulated medical waste once the waste has been both treated and destroyed.

(v) Human corpses, remains, and anatomical parts that are intended for interment or cremation are not regulated medical waste.

(2) *Exemptions.* (i) Etiologic agents being transported interstate pursuant to the requirements of the U.S. Department of Transportation, U.S. Department of Health and Human Services, and all other applicable shipping requirements are exempt from the requirements of this part.

(ii) Samples of regulated medical waste transported off-site by EPA- or State-designated enforcement personnel for enforcement purposes are exempt from the requirements of this Part during the enforcement proceeding.

§ 259.31 Mixtures.

(a) Except as provided in paragraph (b) of this section, mixtures of solid waste and regulated medical waste listed in § 259.30(a) of this subpart are a regulated medical waste.

(b) Mixtures of hazardous waste identified or listed in Part 261 of this chapter and regulated medical waste listed in § 259.30(a) of this subpart are subject to the requirements in this part, unless the mixture is subject to the hazardous waste manifest requirements in Part 262 or Part 266 of this chapter.

Note to paragraph (b): Mixtures of regulated medical waste with hazardous waste that is exempt from the hazardous waste manifest requirements (e.g., under 40 CFR 261.5) remain subject to this Part.

SUBPART E—PRE-TRANSPORT REQUIREMENTS

§ 259.39 Applicability.

Generators must comply with the requirements of this subpart prior to shipping waste off-site, and generators must comply with § 259.42 of this Subpart for on-site storage. Transporters, intermediate handlers (e.g., treatment or destruction facilities), and destination facilities must comply with applicable requirements of this subpart, when specified in Subparts H or I of this part.

§ 259.40 Segregation Requirements.

(a)(1) Generators must segregate regulated medical waste intended for transport off-site to the extent practicable prior to placement in containers according to paragraph (a)(2) of this section.

(2) Generators must segregate regulated medical waste into sharps (Classes 4 and 7 of § 259.30(a) of this subpart including sharps containing residual fluid), fluids (quantities greater than 20 cubic centimeters), and other regulated medical waste.

(b) If other waste is placed in the same container(s) as regulated medical waste, then the generator must package, label, and mark the container(s) and its entire contents according to the requirements in §§ 259.41, 259.44, and 259.45 of this part.

§ 259.41   Packaging Requirements.

Generators must ensure that all regulated medical wastes meet the following requirements before transporting or offering for transport such waste off-site. Generators may use one or more containers to meet these requirements.

(a) Generators must ensure that all regulated medical waste is placed in a container or containers that are:

(1) Rigid;

(2) Leak-resistant;

(3) Impervious to moisture;

(4) Has a strength sufficient to prevent tearing or bursting under normal conditions of use and handling; and

(5) Sealed to prevent leakage during transport.

(b)(1) In addition to the requirements of paragraph (a) of this section, generators must package sharps and sharps with residual fluids in packaging that is puncture-resistant.

(2) In addition to the requirements of paragraph (a) of this section, generators must package fluids (quantities greater than 20 cubic centimeters) in packaging that is break-resistant and tightly lidded or stoppered.

(c) Generators need not place oversized regulated medical waste in containers. Generators must note any special handling instructions for these items in Box 14 of the tracking form required under Subpart F and Appendix I of this part.

§ 259.42   Storage of Regulated Medical Waste Prior to Transport, Treatment, Destruction, or Disposal.

Any person who stores regulated medical waste prior to treatment or disposal on-site (e.g., landfill, interment, treatment and destruction, or incineration), or transport off-site, must comply with the following storage requirements:

(a) Store the regulated medical waste in a manner and location that maintains the integrity of the packaging and provides protection from water, rain and wind;

(b) Maintain the regulated medical waste in a nonputrescent state, using refrigeration when necessary;

(c) Lock the outdoor storage areas containing regulated medical waste (e.g., dumpsters, sheds, tractor trailers, or other storage areas) to prevent unauthorized access;

(d) Limit access to on-site storage areas to authorized employees; and

(e) Store the regulated medical waste in a manner that affords protection from animals and does not provide a breeding place or a food source for insects and rodents.

§ 259.43   Decontamination Standards for Reusable Containers.

Generators, transporters, intermediate handlers, and destination facility owners and operators must comply with the following requirements with respect to reusing containers:

(a) All non-rigid packaging and inner liners must be managed as regulated medical waste under this part and must not be reused.

(b) Any container used for the storage and/or transport of regulated medical waste and designated for reuse once emptied, must be decontaminated if the container shows signs of visible contamination.

(c) If any container used for the storage and/or transport of regulated medical waste is for any reason not capable of being rendered free of any visible signs of contamination in accordance with paragraph (b) of this section, the container must be managed (labeled, marked and treated and/or disposed of) as regulated medical waste under this part.

§ 259.44   Labeling Requirements.

Generators must label each package of regulated medical waste according to the following label requirements before transporting or offering for transport off-site:

(a) *Untreated regulated medical waste.* Each package of untreated regulated medical wastes must have a water-resistant label affixed to or printed on the outside of the container. The label must include the words "Medical Waste," or "Infectious Waste," or display the universal biohazard symbol. Red plastic bag(s) used as inner packaging need not display a label.

(b) *Treated regulated medical waste.* Packages containing treated regulated medical wastes are not required to be labeled under this section but are required to be marked according to § 259.45 of this subpart.

§ 259.45   Marking (Identification) Requirements.

Generators (including intermediate handlers) must mark each package of regulated medical waste according to the following marking requirements before the waste is transported or offered for transport off-site:

(a) The outermost surface of each package prepared for shipment must be marked with a water-resistant identification tag of sufficient dimension to contain the following information:

(1) Generator's or intermediate handler's name;

(2) Generator's or intermediate handler's State permit or identification number. If the generator's or intermediate handler's State does not issue permit or identification numbers, then the generator's or intermediate handler's address;

(3) Transporter name;

(4) Transporter State permit or identification number, or if not applicable, then the transporter's address;

(5) Date of shipment; and

(6) Identification of contents as medical waste.

(b) In addition to paragraph (a) of this section, if the generator has used inner containers, including sharps and fluid containers, each inner container must be marked with indelible ink or imprinted with water-resistant tags. The marking must contain the following information:

(1) Generator's or intermediate handler's name;

(2) Generator's or intermediate handler's State permit or identification number. If the generator or intermediate handler's State does not issue permit or identification numbers, then the generator's or intermediate handler's address.

SUBPART F—GENERATOR STANDARDS

§ 259.50   Applicability and General Requirements.

(a) This subpart establishes standards for generators of regulated medical waste.

(b) A person who generates a medical waste, as defined in § 259.10(b) of this part, and who is located in a Covered State, must determine if that waste is a regulated medical waste.

(c) A generator who either treats and destroys or disposes of regulated medical waste on-site (e.g., incineration, burial or sewer disposal covered by section 307(b)–(d), of the Clean Water Act) is not subject to tracking requirements for that waste.

Note to the section: Generators of regulated medical waste with on-site incinerators are subject to the on-site incinerator requirements in Subpart G of this Part. In addition, generators who treat and destroy regulated medical waste are subject to § 259.54(c). Generators who treat or dispose of medical waste on-site may be subject to additional Federal, State or local laws and regulations.

(d) Vessels at port in a Covered State are subject to the requirements of this Part for those regulated medical wastes that are transported ashore in the Covered State. The owner or operator of the vessel and the person(s) removing or accepting waste from the vessel are considered co-generators of the waste.

(e) A generator of regulated medical waste must determine the quantity of regulated medical waste that he generates in a calendar month, and that is transported or offered for transport off-site for treatment, destruction, or disposal.

(1) *Generators of 50 pounds or more per month.* Generators who generate and transport or offer for transport off-site 50 pounds or more of regulated medical waste in a calendar month are subject to the requirements of Subpart E and all of the requirements of this Subpart for each shipment of regulated medical waste.

(2) *Generators of less than 50 pounds per month.* (i) Generators who generate and transport or offer for transport off-site less than 50 pounds of regulated medical waste in a calendar month are subject to the requirements of Subpart E of this Part and § § 259.50, 259.51 and 259.54(b) of this subpart.

(ii) Generators of regulated medical waste who generate less than 50 pounds in a calendar month but who transport or offer for transport off-site more than 50 pounds in any one shipment, are also subject to Subpart E of this part and all of the requirements of this subpart for each shipment of 50 pounds or more.

(f) Generators of regulated medical waste must use transporters who have notified EPA under § 259.72 of this part to transport their regulated medical waste, except as provided in § 259.51 of this subpart.

§ 259.51   Exemptions.

(a) *Generators of less than 50 pounds per month.* Generators who meet the conditions of § 259.50(e)(2) of this subpart are exempt from the requirement to use a transporter who has notified EPA, exempt from the requirement to use the tracking form, and exempt from the requirements of Subpart H of this part provided that the following conditions are met:

(1)(i) The regulated medical waste is transported to a health care facility, an intermediate handler, or a destination facility with which the generator has a written agreement to accept the regulated medical waste; or

(ii) The generator is transporting the regulated medical waste from the original generation point to the generator's place of business; and

(2) The regulated medical waste is transported by the generator (or an authorized employee) in a vehicle owned by the generator or authorized employee; and

Note to the section: Owned vehicle means a vehicle which is owned by or registered to the generator or employee or is under lease by the generator or authorized employee for a minimum of 30 days.

(3) The generator must compile a shipment log and maintain records as required by § 259.54(b)(2).

(b) *Shipments between generator's facilities.* Generators are exempt from the requirement to use a transporter who has notified EPA, exempt from the use of the tracking form, and exempt from the requirements of Subpart H of this part when transporting regulated medical waste from the original generation point to a central collection point, provided they meet all of the following conditions:

(1) The regulated medical waste is transported by the generator (or the generator's authorized employee) in a vehicle owned by the generator or the employee;

(2) The regulated medical waste is brought to a central collection point or treatment facility owned or operated by the generator;

(3) The original generation point and the central collection point or treatment facility are located in the same Covered State; and

(4) The generator compiles and maintains a shipment log at each original generation point and each central collection point as required by § 259.54(a)(2) of this part.

(c) *Shipments of regulated medical waste (Classes 4 and 7) through the U.S. Postal Service.* Generators who meet the conditions of § 259.50(e)(2)(i) of this subpart who transport regulated medical waste (Classes 4 and 7 of § 259.30(a) of this part) by the U.S. Postal Service, are exempt from the requirement to use a transporter who has notified EPA and from the requirement to use the tracking form, provided they meet the following conditions:

(1) The package is sent registered mail, return receipt requested (indicating to whom, signature, date, and address where delivered); and

(2) The generator compiles a shipment log and maintains the original receipt and the returned registered mail receipt as required by § 259.54(b)(3) of this part.

§ 259.52   Use of the Tracking Form.

(a) Except as provided in § § 259.50(e)(2)(i) and 259.51 of this Subpart, a generator who transports or offers for transport regulated medical waste for off-site treatment or disposal, must prepare a tracking form according to this section and the instructions included in Appendix I to this part.

(b) Generators must obtain the tracking form from the following sources:

(1) For generators who transport or offer for transport off-site regulated medical waste to an intermediate handler or a destination facility in a Covered State which prints the tracking form and requires its use, the form from that State; and

Note to paragraph (b)(1): For generators who transport or offer for transport regulated medical waste to another Covered State which prints the tracking form and requires its use, the transporter is required to provide the generator with the receiving State's form.

(2) For all other generators, the tracking form from the State in which the waste was generated,

(3) If the generator's State does not print the tracking form, the generator must use the tracking form in Appendix I of this part.

(c) The generator must prepare at least the number of tracking form copies that will provide the generator, each transporter(s), and each intermediate handler with one copy, and the owner or operator of the destination facility with two copies.

Note to paragraph (c): The destination facility keeps one copy for their records and returns the second copy to the generator.

(d) The generator must also:

(1) Sign the certification statement on the tracking form by hand;

(2) Obtain the handwritten signature of the initial transporter and date of acceptance on the tracking form; and

(3) Retain one copy, in accordance with § 259.54.

(e) For rail shipments of regulated medical waste within the United States that originate at the site of generation, the generator must send at least three (3) copies of the tracking form dated and signed in acccordance with this section to:

(1) The next non-rail transporter, if any; or

(2) The intermediate handler or destination facility if transported solely by rail; or

(3) The last rail transporter to handle the waste in the United States if exported by rail.

§ 259.53   Generators Exporting Regulated Medical Waste.

Generators (including transporters and intermediate handlers that initiate tracking forms) who export regulated medical waste to a foreign country (e.g., Canada) for treatment and destruction, or disposal, must request that the destination facility provide written confirmation that the waste was received. If the generator has not received that confirmation from the destination facility within 45 days from the date of acceptance of the waste by the first transporter, the generator must submit an exception report as required under § 259.55 of this subpart.

§ 259.54   Recordkeeping.

(a) Except as provided in paragraph (b) of this section, each generator must:

(1)(i) Keep a copy of each tracking form signed in accordance with § 259.52 of this part, for at least three (3) years from the date the waste was accepted by the initial transporter; and

(ii) Retain a copy of all exception reports required to be submitted under § 259.55(c) of this subpart.

(2) Generators who meet the conditions of § 259.51(b) of this subpart must meet the following requirements:

(i) A shipment log must be maintained at the original generation point for a period of three (3) years from the date the waste was shipped. The log must contain the following information:

(A) Date of shipment;

(B) Quantity (by weight) of regulated medical waste transported, by waste category (i.e., untreated and treated);

(C) Address or location of central collection points; and

(D) Signature of generator's employee who will transport the waste, indicating acceptance.

(ii) A shipment log must be maintained at each central collection point for a period of three (3) years from the date that regulated medical waste was accepted from each original generation point and must contain the following information:

(A) Date of receipt;

(B) Quantity (by weight) of regulated medical waste accepted, by waste category (i.e., untreated and treated);

(C) Address or location of original generation point; and

(D) Signature of generator or generator's representative who operates the central collection point, indicating acceptance of the waste.

(b) Generators who meet the conditions of § 259.50(e)(2)(i) of this subpart, who do not transport or offer for transport off-site more than 50 pounds of regulated medical waste in a single shipment, and who do not voluntarily comply with the use of the tracking form are subject to the following recordkeeping requirements:

(1) Generators who use a transporter who has notified EPA must maintain a log for a period of three (3) years from the date of shipment that contains the following information for each shipment or pickup:

(i) Transporter's name and address;

(ii) Transporter's State permit or identification number, if one is required by the State;

(iii) Quantity of regulated medical waste transported, by waste category (i.e., untreated and treated);

(iv) Date of shipment; and

(v) The signature of the transporter's representative accepting the regulated medical waste for transport.

(2) Generators who transport regulated medical waste to a health care facility or to a treatment, destruction, or disposal facility as specified in § 259.51(a) of this subpart must compile and maintain a log for a period of three (3) years from the date of the last shipment entered into the log. The log must contain the following information:

(i) Name and address of the intermediate handler, destination facility, or health care facility to which the generator has transported that shipment of regulated medical waste;

(ii) Quantity (by weight) of regulated medical waste transported, by waste category (i.e., untreated and treated);

(iii) Date of shipment; and

(iv) Signature of the generator or his authorized representative who transported the waste.

(3) Generators who transport regulated medical waste by the U.S. Postal Service under § 259.51(c) of this subpart must retain the original U.S. Postal Service receipt and the return mail receipt and maintain a shipment log for a period of three (3) years from the date of shipment. The log must contain the following information:

(i) Quantity (by weight) of regulated medical waste transported, by waste category (i.e., untreated and treated);

(ii) Date of shipment; and

(iii) Name and address of each intermediate handler or destination facility to which the generator has transported the regulated medical waste by the U.S. Postal Service.

(c) Each generator who treats and destroys regulated medical waste on-site by a method or process other than incineration, must maintain the following records:

(1) The approximate quantity by weight, of regulated medical waste that is subject to the treatment and destruction processes;

(2) Approximate percent, by weight, of total waste treated and destroyed that is regulated medical waste;

(3) For regulated medical waste accepted from generators meeting the exemption conditions in § 259.51 (a) or (c), information identifying the generator, the date the waste was accepted, the weight of waste accepted, and the date the waste was treated and destroyed; and

(4) Records must be maintained by the generator for a period of at least three (3) years from the date the waste was treated and destroyed.

§ 259.55 Exception Reporting.

(a) A generator who meets the conditions of § 259.50(e)(1) or (e)(2)(ii) of this subpart must contact the owner or operator of the destination facility, transporter(s), and intermediate handler(s), as appropriate, to determine the status of any tracked waste if he does not receive a copy of the completed tracking form with the handwritten signature of the owner or operator of the destination facility within 35 days of the date the waste was accepted by the initial transporter.

(b) A generator must submit an Exception Report, as described below, to the State and the EPA Regional Administrator for the Region in which the generator is located if he has not received a completed copy of the tracking form signed by the owner or operator of the destination facility within 45 days of the date the waste was accepted by the initial transporter. The Exception Report must be postmarked on or before the 46th day and must include:

(1) A legible copy of the original tracking form for which the generator does not have confirmation of delivery; and

(2) A cover letter signed by the generator or his authorized representative explaining the efforts taken to locate the regulated medical waste and the results of those efforts.

(c) A copy of the exception report must be kept by the generator for a period of at least three (3) years from the due date of the report.

§ 259.56   Additional Reporting.

The Administrator may require generators to furnish additional information concerning the quantities and management methods of medical waste as he deems necessary under RCRA section 11004.

SUBPART G—ON-SITE INCINERATORS

§ 259.60   Applicability.

(a) The regulations in this subpart apply to generators of regulated medical waste who incinerate regulated medical waste on-site.

(b) Generators of regulated medical waste who incinerate such waste on-site and who accept regulated medical waste accompanied by a tracking form are also subject to the requirements of Subpart I of this part.

§ 259.61   Recordkeeping.

(a) Generators must keep an operating log at their incineration facility that includes the following information:

(1)(i) The date each incineration cycle was begun;

(ii) The length of the incineration cycle;

(iii) The total quantity of medical waste incinerated, per incineration cycle; and

(iv) An estimate of the quantity of regulated medical waste incinerated, per incineration cycle.

(2) Generators with on-site incinerators that accept regulated medical waste from generator(s) subject to § 259.51(a) of this Part must maintain the following information for each shipment of regulated medical waste accepted:

(i) The date the waste was accepted;

(ii) The name and State permit or identification number of the generator who originated the shipment. If the State does not issue permit or identification numbers, then the generator's address;

(iii) The total weight of the regulated medical waste accepted from the originating generator; and

(iv) The signature of the individual accepting the waste.

(b)(1) Generators must compile the operating log required by paragraph (a)(1) of this section during the following period: June 22, 1989, to June 22, 1991.

(2) Generators must retain the operating log until at least June 22, 1992.

(c) Generators with on-site incinerators that accept regulated medical waste from generators subject to the tracking form requirements must keep copies of all tracking forms for a period of three years from the date they accepted the waste.

(d) Generators must retain a copy of the on-site incinerator report form required under § 259.62 of this subpart for three (3) years from the date of submission.

§ 259.62   Reporting.

(a) *General.* The owner or operator of an on-site incinerator must prepare and submit two copies of the on-site incinerator report on the form provided in Appendix II of this part to: Chief, Waste Characterization Branch, Office of Solid Waste (OS–332), U.S. Environmental Protection Agency, 401 M Street, SW, Washington, DC 20460. The reports must summarize information collected in the operating log during the first and third six-month period after the effective date of the demonstration program, and must contain the following information in the format provided in Appendix II of this part:

(1) Facility name, mailing address, and location;

(2) Facility type (e.g., hospital, laboratory);

(3) Contact person;

(4) Waste feed information;

(5) The total number of incinerators at the facility that incinerate regulated medical waste and information concerning each incinerator.

(b) Each report must contain the following certification, signed by the facility owner or his authorized representative: I certify that I have personally examined and am familiar with the information submitted in this and all attached documents, and that based on my inquiry of those individuals immediately responsible for obtaining the information, I believe that the submitted information is true, accurate, and complete.

(c)(1) *Dates.* The first report is due February 6, 1990, and must contain information from the first six months of the demonstration program.

(2) The second report is due February 6, 1991, and must contain information from the thirteenth through the eighteenth month of the demonstration program.

SUBPART H—TRANSPORTER REQUIREMENTS

§ 259.70   Applicability.

(a) These requirements apply to transporters, including generators who transport their own waste, and owners and operators of transfer facilities engaged in transporting regulated medical waste generated in a Covered State.

(b) These regulations do not apply to on-site transportation of regulated medical waste, nor to shipments exempted under § 259.51 (a), (b), or (c) of this part.

(c) A transporter of regulated medical waste must also comply with Subpart F of this part when he consolidates two or more shipments of regulated medical waste onto a single tracking form.

(d) Transporters must also comply with Subpart E of this part if they:

(1) Store regulated medical waste in the course of transport; or

(2) Remove regulated medical waste from a reusable container; or

(3) Modify packaging of regulated medical waste.

§ 259.71   Transporter Acceptance of Regulated Medical Waste.

(a) Transporters must not accept for transport any regulated medical waste generated in a Covered State unless the outer surface of the container is labeled and marked in accordance with Subpart E of this part.

(b) Transporters must not accept a shipment of regulated medical waste from a generator unless accompanied by a properly completed tracking form as required under Subpart F of this part, unless the generator is exempt from the use of the tracking form under either § 259.50(e)(2)(i) or § 259.51 of this part.

(c) *Marking (identification).* When regulated medical waste is handled by more than one transporter, each subsequent transporter must attach a water resistant identification tag below the generator's marking on the outer surface of the packaging, that does not obscure the generator's or previous transporter's markings. The transporter taking possession of the shipment must ensure that the tag contains the following information:

(1) Name of transporter taking possession (receiving) of the regulated medical waste;

(2) Transporter State permit or identification number. If the State does not issue permit or identification numbers, then the transporter's address; and

(3) Date of receipt.

§ 259.72   Transporter Notification.

(a)(1)Transporters (including owners or operators of transfer facilities) are prohibited from transporting regulated medical waste generated in a Covered State unless they have notified EPA and the Covered State in writing as provided in this Section.

(2) Transporters who accept regulated medical waste that was generated in a Covered State, or who transport regulated medical waste that was generated in a Covered State, must submit a separate notification form for each Covered State in which the regulated medical waste was generated.

(3)(i) The original and one copy of the transporter notification must be sent to: Chief, Waste Characterization Branch (OS–332), EPA Office of Solid Waste, 401 M Street, SW, Washington, DC, 20460.

(ii) An additional copy must be sent to the Director of the waste management agency in the Covered State for which the transporter is notifying.

(b) Each transporter notification must contain the following information:

(1) Transporter's name, mailing address, and EPA hazardous waste identification number (if any);

(2) Name, address, and telephone number for each transportation or transfer facility (by site) that the transporter will operate from for each Covered State for which the transporter is notifying;

(3) Identifications (State permit or license numbers) required to handle medical or infectious waste; and

(4) The following statement signed by a corporate official or the owner or operator: I certify, under penalty of criminal or civil prosecution for making or submission of false statements, representations, or omissions, that I have read, understand, and will comply with the regulations at 40 CFR Part 259, issued under authority of Subtitle J of the Resource Conservation and Recovery Act.

Note paragraph (b): The Agency has published a suggested form for transporter notification in Appendix IV of this part which may be utilized by transporters notifying EPA.

(c) EPA will issue transporters, who notify under this section, a unique EPA Medical Waste Identification Number for each Covered State for which they have notified. This identification number will apply to all transporter sites identified in paragraph (b)(2) of this section, that relate to each Covered State. Transporters may accept regulated medical waste after notifying under this section. Upon receipt of an EPA Medical Waste Identification Number the transporter must include it on Box 5 of the Medical Waste Tracking Form found in Appendix I of this part.

Note to the section: States may impose or may presently have in place additional licensing, permitting or other requirements that apply to transporters of regulated medical waste.

§ 259.73 Vehicle Requirements.

(a) Transporters must use vehicles to transport regulated medical waste that meet the following requirements:

(1) The vehicle must have a fully enclosed, leak-resistant cargo-carrying body;

(2) The transporter must ensure that the waste is not subject to mechanical stress or compaction during loading and unloading or during transit;

(3) The transporter must maintain the cargo-carrying body in good sanitary condition; and

(4) The cargo-carrying body must be secured if left unattended.

(b) The transporter must use vehicles to transport regulated medical waste that have the following identification on the two sides and back of the cargo-carrying body in letters a minimum of 3 inches in height:

(1) The name of the transporter;

(2) The transporter's State permit or license number, if any; and

(3) A sign or the following words imprinted:

(i) MEDICAL WASTE; or

(ii) REGULATED MEDICAL WASTE.

(c) A transporter must not transport regulated medical waste in the same container with other solid waste unless the transporter manages both as regulated medical waste in compliance with this subpart.

§ 259.74 Tracking Form Requirements.

(a) *General.* A transporter may not accept a shipment of regulated medical waste in excess of 50 pounds from a generator in a Covered State or from a generator in a Covered State who generates more than 50 pounds per month, unless it is accompanied by a tracking form completed in accordance with Appendix I of this part and signed by the generator in accordance with the provisions of § 259.52 of this part. In the case where a transporter intends to deliver regulated medical waste generated in a Covered State to another Covered State, the latter of which supplies its own tracking form and requires its use, the transporter must provide the generator with the form of the Covered State to which the waste is to be sent.

(b) *Acceptance.* Before accepting for transport or transporting any regulated medical waste that is accompanied by a tracking form, the transporter must:

(1) Certify that the tracking form accurately reflects the number and total weight of the packages being transported by signing and dating the tracking form acknowledging acceptance of the regulated medical waste from the generator; and

(2) Return a signed copy of the tracking form to the generator before leaving the generator's site.

(c) *In transit.* The transporter must ensure that the tracking form accompanies the regulated medical waste while in transit.

(d) *Delivery of regulated medical waste in the United States.* A transporter, upon delivery of the regulated medical waste to another transporter (including a transfer facility) or to an intermediate handler or destination facility located in the United States, must:

(1) Obtain the date of delivery and the handwritten signature of the transporter, or the owner or operator of the intermediate handling facility, or destination facility on the tracking form;

(2) Retain one copy of the tracking form in accordance with § 259.77 of this part; and

(3) Give the remaining copies of the tracking form to the accepting transporter, intermediate handler, or destination facility.

(e) *Delivery of regulated medical waste outside the United States.* Any transporter who transports regulated medical waste across an international border, or who delivers regulated medical waste to a transporter or treatment, destruction, or destination facility located in a foreign country (e.g., Canada) must:

(1) Sign the tracking form and verify that the waste has been delivered to the next (foreign) transporter, or treatment, destruction, or destination facility;

(2) Retain one copy of the signed tracking form for his records; and

(3) Return all remaining copies of the tracking form by mail to the generator.

(f) *Rail shipment.* For shipments involving rail transportation, the requirements of § 259.91 of this part apply to rail transporters in lieu of the requirements of paragraphs (b), (c), and (d) of this section.

(g) *Special requirements for waste from generators of less than 50 pounds/month.* A transporter accepting a shipment of less than 50 pounds of regulated medical waste from a generator who generates less than 50 pounds per month need not comply with the requirements of paragraphs (a) through (f) of this section provided that:

(1) The transporter compiles a log, containing the following information for each shipment of regulated medical waste:

(i) The generator's name and State permit or identification number, or, if the generator's State does not issue permit or identification numbers, then the generator's address.

(ii) The quantity of waste accepted (number of packages and total weight by waste category (i.e., "untreated" and "treated")); and

(iii) The date the waste is accepted;

(2) The transporter carries this log in the vehicle while transporting such regulated medical waste to a second transporter;

(3) The transporter dates and signs the generator's log required under § 259.54(b) of this part; and

(4) The transporter complies with § 259.76(a) of this subpart.

§ 259.75   Compliance with the Tracking Form.

(a) Except as provided in paragraph (b) of this section, the transporter must deliver the entire quantity of regulated medical waste that he has accepted from a generator or another transporter to:

(1) The intermediate handler or destination facility listed on the tracking form; or

(2) The next transporter.

(b) If the regulated medical waste cannot be delivered in accordance with paragraph (a) of this section, the transporter must contact the generator for further directions, revise the tracking form according to the generator's instructions, and deliver the entire quantity of regulated medical waste from that generator according to the generator's instructions.

§ 259.76   Consolidating or Remanifesting Waste to a New Tracking Form.

(a) Transporters must complete a tracking form for all regulated medical waste received from generators who meet the conditions of § 259.50(e)(2)(i) of this part (in shipments of less than 50 pounds that are not accompanied by a tracking form).

(b) A transporter may choose to consolidate or remanifest to a single tracking form all shipments of regulated medical waste less than 220 pounds.

Note to paragraph (b): EPA strongly recommends, that, to minimize bookkeeping errors, transporters consolidate or remanifest those shipments from generators who are required to originate the tracking form separately from those shipments by generators who are not required to originate the tracking form.

(c) When the transporter receives the signed tracking form that he initiated from the destination facility, and the regulated medical waste was accompanied by a tracking form originated by a generator, the transporter must:

(1) Attach a copy of the tracking form signed by the destination facility to the generator's original tracking form; and

(2) Retain a copy of each tracking form in accordance with § 259.77 of this subpart; and

(3) Return a copy of each tracking form to the generator within 15 days of receipt of the tracking form from the destination facility.

(4) For each tracking form initiated, either by accepting waste from generators who meet the condition of § 259.50(e)(2)(i) of this part or by consolidating tracking forms onto a new one, the transporter must maintain a consolidation log indicating all shipments consolidated or remanifested on that form. The log must accompany the tracking form and include the following information:

(i) Name of each generator;

(ii) Generator's State permit or identification number. If the generator's State does not issue permit or identification numbers, then the generator's address;

(iii) Date the regulated medical waste was originally shipped by the generator;

(iv) Quantity of regulated medical waste (number of containers and/or weight in pounds) by waste category (i.e., "untreated" or "treated") shipped by each generator; and

(v) The names, State permit or identification numbers of all previous transporters or, if not applicable, the transporters' addresses.

§ 259.77   Recordkeeping.

(a) A transporter of regulated medical waste must keep a copy of the tracking form signed by the generator, himself, the previous transporter (if applicable), and the next party, which may be one of the following: another transporter; or the owner or operator of an intermediate handling facility; or destination facility. The transporter must retain a copy of this form for a period of three (3) years from the date the waste was accepted by the next party.

(b) For regulated medical waste that is not accompanied by a generator-initiated tracking form, the transporter must retain a copy of all transporter-initiated tracking forms and consolidation logs for a period of three (3) years from the date the waste was accepted by the transporter.

(c) For any regulated medical waste that was received by the transporter accompanied by a tracking form and consolidated or remanifested by the transporter to another tracking form, the transporter must:

(1) Retain a copy of the generator-initiated tracking form signed by the transporter for three (3) years from the date the waste was accepted by the transporter; and

(2) Retain a copy of the transporter-initiated tracking form signed by the intermediate handler or destination facility for three (3) years from the date the waste was accepted by the intermediate handler or destination facility.

(d) Retain a copy of each transporter report required by § 259.78 of this subpart for three (3) years after the date of submission.

§ 259.78 Reporting.

(a)(1) A transporter who accepts regulated medical waste generated in a Covered State must submit reports describing the source and disposition of the waste. The reports must be submitted using the form in Appendix III of this part.

(2) Transporters who accept regulated medical waste directly from a generator in a Covered State, or who transport regulated medical waste that was generated in a Covered State, must submit a separate report for each Covered State's waste they have transported.

(b) Each report must be submitted as follows:

(1) One copy must be submitted to: Chief, Waste Characterization Branch (OS–332), Office of Solid Waste, U.S. Environmental Protection Agency, 401 M St., SW, Washington, DC 20460; and

(2) A second copy must be submitted to the Director of the waste management agency in the State for which the transporter has compiled the report.

(c)(1) Each report must contain the following information in the format provided by Appendix III of this part:

(i) The transporter's name, address, and EPA medical waste identification number;

(ii) The name and telephone number of a contact person;

(iii) Total number of generators from whom the transporter accepted regulated medical waste;

(iv) The name, address, and type of each generator from whom the transporter accepted regulated medical waste;

(v) The amount by weight and waste category (untreated or treated) of regulated medical waste accepted from each generator;

(vi) The total, by weight and waste category, of regulated medical waste from all generators in the Covered State that the transporter delivered to an intermediate handler or to a destination facility; and

(vii) The total, by weight and waste category, of regulated medical waste from all generators in the Covered State that the transporter delivered to a second transporter or to a transfer facility.

(viii) The certification signed by the owner or operator, or his authorized representative.

(2) Transporters who transport or deliver regulated medical waste to an intermediate handler or to a destination facility must also provide the following information:

(i) The name and address of each intermediate handler and destination facility to which waste from that Covered State was delivered;

(ii) The amount, by waste category, that was delivered;

(iii) The total number of intermediate handlers and destination facilities to which waste was delivered.

(d) The transporter must submit reports covering the following periods:

(1) A report covering the 180 day period from June 23, 1989, to December 19, 1989.

(2) A report covering the 180 day period from December 20, 1989, to June 17, 1990.

(3) A report covering the 180 day period from June 18, 1990, to December 14, 1990.

(4) A report covering the 180 day period from December 15, 1990, to June 12, 1991.

(e) Transporters must submit the reports required in paragraph (d) of this section on or before the date 45 days after the end of the reporting period.

(f) Each transporter who initiates a tracking form must meet the requirements of § 259.55 of this part, exception reporting, except that the 35 and 45 day periods begin on the day the transporter accepted the waste from the generator.

§ 259.79   Additional Reporting.

The Administrator may require transporters to furnish additional information concerning the quantities and management methods of regulated medical waste as he deems necessary under RCRA section 11004.

SUBPART I—TREATMENT, DESTRUCTION, AND DISPOSAL FACILITIES

§ 259.80   Applicability.

(a) These regulations apply to owners and operators of facilities that receive regulated medical waste generated in a Covered State, including facilities located in non-Covered States that receive regulated medical waste generated in a Covered State. Facilities that are subject to this subpart include:

(1) Destination facilities (i.e., treatment and destruction facilities, a facility that causes the regulated medical waste to meet the conditions of § 259.30(b)(1)(iii) or (iv) of this part including incineration facilities, and disposal facilities); and

(2) Intermediate handlers (i.e., facilities that either treat or destroy the regulated medical waste, but do not cause it to meet the conditions of § 259.30(b)(1)(iii) or (iv) of this part).

(b)(1) Except as provided by paragraph (b)(2) of this section, this subpart does not apply to generators who incinerate regulated medical waste on-site.

(2) This subpart does apply to generators who receive regulated medical waste required to be accompanied by a tracking form.

§ 259.81   Use of the Tracking Form.

(a) *Destination Facility.* When a destination facility receives regulated medical waste accompanied by a tracking form, the owner or operator must:

(1) Sign and date each copy of the tracking form to certify that the regulated medical waste listed on the tracking form was received;

(2) Note any discrepancies as defined in §259.82(a) of this subpart on the tracking form;

(3) Immediately give the transporter at least one copy of the signed tracking form;

(4) Send a copy of the tracking form to the generator (or to the transporter or intermediate handler that initiated the tracking form) within 15 days of the delivery;

(5) Retain a copy of each tracking form in accordance with §259.83 of this subpart.

(b) *Intermediate Handlers.* When an intermediate handler receives regulated medical waste accompanied by a tracking form, the owner or operator must meet the following requirements:

(1) The owner or operator must meet all the requirements for generators under both subparts E and F of this part including signing the tracking form accepting the waste as specified in Box 20 and entering the new tracking form number in Box 21 when initiating a new tracking form for each shipment of regulated medical waste that has either been treated or destroyed.

(2) The owner or operator must maintain a log matching the original generator's tracking forms to the tracking form that he initiates. This log must include:

(i) Name(s) of generator(s);

(ii) Generator's State permit or identification number. If the State does not issue permit or identification numbers, then the generator's address;

(iii) The date the regulated medical waste was originally shipped by the generator or the generator's unique tracking form number;

(iv) The new tracking form number to which the waste is assigned;

(3) Within 15 days of receipt of the tracking form that he initiated and that was signed by the destination facility, the intermediate handler must:

(i) Attach a copy of the tracking form signed by the destination facility to the original tracking form initiated by the generator identified in §259.81(b)(2)(i) above;

(ii) Send a copy of each tracking form to the generator who initiated the tracking form; and

(iii) Retain a copy of each tracking form in accordance with the requirements of §259.83 of this subpart.

(c) *Rail shipments.* If a destination facility or intermediate handler receives from a rail transporter regulated medical waste that is accompanied by shipping papers containing the information required on the medical waste tracking form, with the exception of the generator's certification and chain of custody signatures, the owner or operator or his agent, must:

(1) Sign and date each copy of the tracking form or the shipping papers (if the tracking form has not been received);

(2) Note any discrepancies as defined in §259.82(a) of this subpart on each copy of the tracking form or shipping papers (if the tracking form has not been received);

(3) Immediately give the rail transporter at least one copy of the tracking form or shipping papers (if the tracking form has not been received);

(4)(i) If the facility is a destination facility, send a copy of the signed and dated tracking form to the generator within 15 days after the delivery. If the owner or operator has not received the tracking form within 15 days of delivery, he must send a copy of the signed and dated shipping papers to the party initiating the tracking form;

(ii) If the facility is an intermediate handler, retain a copy of the tracking form (or the shipping papers if the tracking form has not been received), until he receives a copy of the tracking form signed by the owner or operator of the destination facility. He then must:

(A) Attach a copy of the tracking form signed by the destination facility to the original tracking form (or the shipping papers if the tracking form has not been received) initiated by another party;

(B) Send a copy of each tracking form (or each set of shipping papers) to the party who initiated the tracking form; and

(C) Retain a copy of each tracking form in accordance with the requirements of § 259.83 of this subpart.

(5) The destination facility and intermediate handlers must retain a copy of the tracking form (or shipping papers if signed in lieu of the tracking form) for at least three (3) years from the date of acceptance of the regulated medical waste.

Note to paragraph (c): Destination facilities and intermediate handlers receiving shipments by rail should expect to receive the tracking form from the generator, or the preceding non-rail transporter who will have sent the tracking form to the facility by some other means (e.g., by mail).

§ 259.82   Tracking Form Discrepancies.

(a) Tracking form discrepancies are:

(1) For containers, any variation in piece count such as a discrepancy of one box, pail, or drum in a truckload;

(2) For waste by categories (i.e., untreated or treated) discrepancies in number of containers for each category of regulated medical waste as described on the label imprinted or affixed to the outer surface of the package;

(3) Packaging that is broken, torn, or leaking; and

(4) Regulated medical waste that arrives at an intermediate handler or a destination facility unaccompanied by a tracking form, where the owner or operator knows such form is required, or for which the tracking form is incomplete or not signed.

(b) Upon discovering a discrepancy, the owner or operator must attempt to resolve (e.g., with telephone conversations) the discrepancy with the waste generator, the transporter and/or the intermediate handler. If the discrepancy is not resolved, the owner or operator must submit a letter, within 15 days of receiving the waste, to the EPA Regional Administrator(s) for both the State of generation and the State in which the facility is located as well as to the appropriate State agency for the Covered State in which the generator is located. The letter must describe the nature of the discrepancy and the attempts the owner or operator has undertaken to reconcile it. The owner or operator must include with the letter a legible copy of the tracking form or shipping papers in question. If the discrepancy is the type specified in paragraph (a)(4) of this section, the report must specify the quantity of waste received, the transporter, and the generator(s).

§ 259.83   Recordkeeping.

(a) The owner or operator of a destination facility or an intermediate handler receiving regulated medical waste generated in a Covered State must maintain records for a minimum of three (3) years from the date the waste was accepted. These records must contain the following information:

(1) Copies of all tracking forms required by the following paragraphs of this subpart: § 259.81(a)(5); (b)(3)(iii); and (c)(4)(ii)(C); and the logs required by § 259.81(b)(2) of this subpart;

(2) The name and State permit or identification number of each generator who delivered waste to the destination facility or intermediate handler under § 259.51(a) of this part, if the State does not issue permit or identification numbers then the generator's address; and

(3) Copies of all discrepancy reports required by § 259.82(b) of this subpart.

(b) The owner or operator of a destination facility or an intermediate handler that accepts regulated medical waste from generator(s) subject to § 259.51(a) of this part must maintain the following information for each shipment of regulated medical waste accepted:

(1) The date the waste was accepted;

(2) The name and State permit or identification number of the generator who originated shipment. If the State does not issue permit or identification numbers, then the generator's address;

(3) The total weight of the regulated medical waste accepted from the originating generator; and

(4) The signature of the individual accepting the waste.

§ 259.84   Additional Reporting.

The Administrator may require owners or operators of destination facilities and intermediate handlers to furnish additional information concerning the quantities and management methods of medical waste as he deems necessary under RCRA section 11004.

SUBPART J—RAIL SHIPMENTS OF REGULATED MEDICAL WASTE

§ 259.90   Applicability.

(a) These requirements apply to persons engaged in rail transportation of regulated medical waste generated in a Covered State.

(b) Rail transporters of regulated medical waste must also comply with Subpart H of this part, Transporter Requirements, except as otherwise provided in § 259.74(f) of this part.

§ 259.91   Rail Shipment Tracking Form Requirements.

(a) The following requirements apply to all shipments of regulated medical waste involving rail transport:

(1) When accepting regulated medical waste generated in a Covered State from a non-rail transporter, the initial rail transporter must:

(i) Sign and date the tracking form acknowledging acceptance of the regulated medical waste;

(ii) Return a copy of the tracking form to the non-rail transporter;

(iii) Forward at least three copies of the tracking form to:

(A) The next non-rail transporter, if any; or

(B) The intermediate handler or destination facility, if the shipment is delivered to that facility by rail; or

(C) The last rail transporter designated to handle the waste in the United States; and

(iv) Retain one copy of the tracking form and rail shipping paper in accordance with § 259.77 of this part.

(2) Rail transporters must ensure that a shipping paper containing all the information required on the tracking form (excluding permitting or licensing numbers, generator certification, and signatures) accompanies the shipment at all times. Intermediate rail transporters are not required to sign either the tracking form(s) or shipping paper(s).

(3) When delivering regulated medical waste to an intermediate handler or destination facility, a rail transporter must:

(i) Obtain the date of delivery and handwritten signature of the owner or operator of the facility on the tracking form or the shipping papers (if the tracking form has not been received by the facility); and

(ii) Retain a copy of the tracking form or signed shipping paper in accordance with § 259.77 of this part.

(4) When delivering regulated medical waste to a non-rail transporter, a rail transporter must:

(i) Obtain the date of delivery and the handwritten signature of the next non-rail transporter on the tracking form; and

(ii) Retain a copy of the tracking form in accordance with § 259.77 of this part.

(5) Upon accepting regulated medical waste generated in a Covered State from a rail transporter, a non-rail transporter must sign and date the tracking form (or the shipping papers if the tracking form has not been received by the transporter) and provide a copy to the rail transporter.

From Environmental Protection Agency: Standards for the tracking and management of medical waste; Interim final rule and request for comments. Fed. Reg., 54:12371–12382, 1989.

Appendix D

Needlestick Protocol

1. Significant Exposures
   A. Contaminated needlestick
   B. Puncture wound from a contaminated, sharp dental instrument
   C. Contamination of any obviously open wound or the mucous membranes by saliva, blood, or a mixture of both saliva and blood
2. Exposure to the patient's blood or saliva on the unbroken skin is not considered significant
3. Protocol
   A. Immediately cleanse the wound thoroughly with soap and water
   B. Obtain the patient's and exposure recipient's permission for blood testing and arrange for pretest counseling
   C. Have a sample of the patient's blood drawn the same day as the exposure. The blood should be tested for HBsAg and anti-HIV
   D. The person who was exposed should also have blood drawn to test for anti-HBs and anti-HIV the same day as the exposure. If the exposure recipient received hepatitis B vaccine and was post-tested to prove seroconversion and immunity, hepatitis testing is not required
   E. The exposure recipient should be notified of the signs and symptoms associated with anti-HIV seroconversion and given the opportunity for clinical evaluation
   F. Hepatitis Blood Test Results and Treatment Recommendations

Patient's Antigen Status	*Recipient of Exposure*
1. HBsAg negative	1a. Hepatitis B vaccine if not already received
2. HBsAg positive	2a. Anti-HBs positive recipient: *No treatment*
	2b. Hepatitis B vaccine recipient with laboratory proven seroconversion: *No treatment necessary*
	2c. Hepatitis B vaccine recipient without laboratory proven seroconversion: *One additional dose of vaccine and one dose of HBIG if anti-HBs negative on testing*
	2d. Anti-HBs negative recipient: *HBIG starting within 48 hours after exposure (0.06 ml/kg intramuscularly) and hepatitis B vaccination series started within 7 days*

G. HIV Blood Test Results and Treatment Recommendations

Patient's Antigen Status *Recipient of Exposure*

1. Diagnosed AIDS, anti-HIV positive, refuses testing, or unknown source

   1a. Anti-HIV positive: *Post-test counseling and medical evaluation*

   1b. Anti-HIV negative: *Post-test counseling and repeat testing at 6, 12 and 24 weeks*

2. Anti-HIV negative

   2a. Anti-HIV positive: *Post-test counseling and medical evaluation*

   2b. Anti-HIV negative: *Post-test counseling and optional followup at 12 weeks*

HBsAg refers to the hepatitis B surface antigen
Anti-HBs refers to the antibody to the hepatitis B surface antigen
HBIG refers to hepatitis B immune globulin
Anti-HIV refers to the antibody to the human immunodeficiency virus
Adapted from Centers for Disease Control (ACIP): Protection against viral hepatitis. MMWR, *39*(RR-2):19–21, 1990; and Centers for Disease Control: Public Health Service statement on management of occupational exposure to human immunodeficiency virus, including considerations regarding zidovudine postexposure use. MMWR, *39*(RR-1):1–14, 1990.

Appendix E

Guide to Chemical Agents for Disinfection and/or Sterilization

Office Sterilization and Asepsis Procedures (OSAP) Research Foundation

GUIDE TO CHEMICAL AGENTS FOR DISINFECTION AND/OR STERILIZATION

January, 1992

IMMERSION ONLY

PRODUCTS (EPA Reg #)	CHEMICAL CLASSIFICATION	TB DIRECTIONS (TEST)**	ADA ACCEPTED	STERILANT	STERILANT REUSE (DAYS)
Multicide Plus (1043-36)	1% phenylphenol, 5% benzyl chlorophenol, soap	1:32, 20 min, 20C (AOAC)	No	No	None
CoeSteril ColdSpor (55195-2)	Glutaraldehyde 10%, 0.5% phenylphenol, 0.1% amylphenol	1:20, 10 min, 20C (AOAC)	Yes	1:5, 10 hrs, 20C	30
Glutarex (7182-4)	Glutaraldehyde 2% neutral	FS, 10 min 20C (AOAC)	Yes	FS*, 10 hrs, 20C	None
Banicide (15136-1) Sterall, Wavicide 01	Glutaraldehyde 2% acidic	20 min (FS), 30 min (1:4), 20C (Quant)	Yes	FS, 5 hrs, 40C FS, 10 hrs, 21C	None 30
Cidex Plus (7078-14)	Glutaraldehyde 3.2% alkaline	FS, 20 min, 25C (Quant)	Yes	FS, 10 hrs, 20C	28
CoeCide XL Plus (46781-4) Maxicide Plus Metricide Plus 30 Aristocrat Plus 30	"	FS, 20 min, 20C (AOAC)	Yes	FS, 10 hrs, 20C	30
Cidex 7 (7078-1)	Glutaraldehyde 2% alkaline	FS, 90 min, 25C (Quant)	Yes	FS, 10 hrs, 20C	28
Germ-X (10352-29)	"	FS, 10 min, 20C (AOAC)	Yes	FS, 10 hrs, 20C	None
Baxter/Omnicide Omnicide ProCide (46851-2)	"	FS, 45 min, 20C (AOAC)	Yes	FS, 10 hrs, 20 C	28
CoeCide XL Healthco 30 Maxicide Metricide Protec-Top Vitacide (46781-2)	"	FS, 20 min, 20C (AOAC)	Yes	FS, 10 hrs, 20C	30

SURFACE ONLY

Product	Active Ingredient	Dilution / Time			
Alcide LD (45631-15) Exspor (45631-03)	Chlorine Compounds	10:1:1, 3 min, 20C (AOAC) 4:1:1, 3 min, 20C	Yes	No 4:1:1, 6 hrs, 20C	None None
Bleach (5.25%)		1:10, 10 min, 20C	No	No	None
Lysol Spray (777-53)	0.1% phenylphenol, 79% ethanol	10 min, 20C (AOAC)	Yes	No	None
Coe Spray-The Pump (334-417)	0.216% phenylphenol, 0.054% tert amylphenol, 66% ethanol	10 min, 20C (AOAC)	Yes	No	None
ProCide Spray (46851-5)	0.28% phenylphenol 0.03% benzyl chlorophenol	10 min, 20C (AOAC)	Yes	No	None
Sterall Spray (15136-6)	0.25% glutaraldehyde	30 min, RT (AOAC)	No	No	None

SURFACE/IMMERSION

Product	Active Ingredient	Dilution / Time			
Biocide, Surf-A-Cide (4959-16)	Iodophor (1.75% titrable iodine)	1:213, 10–25 min, 20C (AOAC)	Yes	No	None
Iodofive (1677-22)	Iodophor (1.75% titrable iodine)	1:213, 5 min, 20C (AOAC) (10 min hydrophilic viruses)	Yes	No	None
Omni II, Vitaphene (46851-1)	9.0% phenylphenol 1% benzyl chlorophenol	1:32, 10 min, 20C (AOAC)	Yes	No	None
Asepti-phene 128 (303-87) Cidaldent	4.28% phenylphenol 3.49% benzyl chlorophenol 1.92% tert amylphenol	1:128, - (AOAC)	No	No	None

*   Full Strength.
** Test used for TB label claim: AOAC = Association of Official Analytical Chemists; Quant = Quantitative TB Test

Adapted from ADA Accepted Products of 10/1/90. Other products available. Listing does not imply endorsement, recommendation or warranty. 20C = 68F, 25C = 77F. Purchasers are legally required to consult the package insert for changes in formulation and recommended product uses. Check materials compatibility before use on dental equipment. Updated tables are available from the OSAP Research Foundation 800/243-1233.

Appendix F

Office Sterilization and Asepsis Procedures (OSAP) Research Foundation

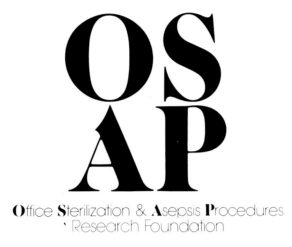

THE CONCEPT

The Office Sterilization and Asepsis Procedures (OSAP) Research Foundation evolved from the combined concerns of academicians, practitioners, distributors, and manufacturers dedicated to finding solutions to the constant problem of the microbiologic assault facing the office practitioner. Providing standards for protection of the office personnel and practitioner is the goal.

MISSION STATEMENT

The Office Sterilization and Asepsis Procedures (OSAP) Research Foundation is dedicated to the establishment, implementation, and maintenance of standards in aseptic techniques and providing the professions with leading information critical to the practitioner to develop a formalized infection control program.

OBJECTIVES

1. Achieve factual advertising
2. Provide educational forums for the professions and industry
3. Provide and monitor practical guidelines in infection control
4. Promote quality research relating to infection control
5. Interface with other regulatory agencies and organizations (i.e., ADA, EPA, FDA, CDC, AMA, AHA, OSHA, and AAMI)

THE FUNDING

Portions of the OSAP budget are supported by educational grants from the following industry members as of January, 1992.

A-dec, Inc.
American Dental Corp, Inc.
Ash/Dentsply
Block Drug Corp.
* Cottrell, Ltd
Cox Sterile Products, Inc.
DW Technology
Forest Medical Products, Inc.
GC America/Coe
* Health-Sonics Corp.
Hu-Friedy
Hygenic Corp.
Johnson & Johnson Medical Inc.
Midwest Dental Products Corp.
Pelton & Crane/Siemens
Pinnacle Products, Inc.
Porter Instrument Co., Inc.
* Henry Schein Company
Semantodontics/SmartPractice
Silverman's Dental Supply
Young Dental Manufacturing

* Founding Members

MEMBERSHIP CATEGORIES

Health Care Professional
Individual: Persons with an interest in infection control and office asepsis
Student: Full-time students enrolled in a health care education program
Health Care Institution
Institutional: Institutions with an interest in infection control and office asepsis
Industry Membership
Full Industry: Manufacturers and distributors with an interest in infection control and office asepsis
Associate Industry: Health care professional with commercial affiliation
Associate Distributor: Distributors of infection control products who are not full industry members with no voting privileges

CODE OF ETHICS

As members of this Foundation, representatives shall observe the highest standards of integrity, frankness, and responsibility in dealing with others:

1. by encouraging the use of only those products and techniques that are safe and effective.
2. by making, in all advertising, packaging, and printed material, only those statements which are accurate and free of the capacity to mislead or deceive the consumer.
3. by requiring all members and representatives to be accurate in their descriptions of products, techniques, and services.

4. by complying with all Federal, state and local laws, standards and regulatory agencies as they apply to the industry and profession.
5. by complying with all national, state, and local health care association guidelines and standards.

ACADEMIC ADVISORY PANEL

A panel of academicians and clinicians, recognized in their field, contribute information instrumental in the organizational and educational efforts for OSAP. As part of their contributions to this Research Foundation, this panel reviews advertising materials and product literature for accuracy in descriptions of products, techniques, and services. The panel is available to answer questions regarding infection control from the membership. Of the authors and contributors, Drs. Cottone, Crawford, Miller, Molinari, Runnells, and Young are members of this panel.

For additional information and membership forms, write or call:

Office Sterilization and Asepsis Procedures (OSAP) Research Foundation
2150 West 29th Ave., Suite 500
Denver, CO 80211
(800)-243-1233

Index

Page numbers in *italics* indicate figures; those followed by t indicate tables.

in homosexual and bisexual men, 53
in intravenous drug users, 53-55
manifestations of, *58-59,* 58-64
 dermatologic, 65
 gastrointestinal, 65
 hematologic, 67, 67t
 neurologic, 62, 66-67
 ophthalmologic, 66
 oral, 65, 66t
 nonopportunistic infections in, 64
 opportunistic infections in, 62-64, 63t
 organ systems in, 64-67
 pediatric, 57
 classification of, 61t
 persistent generalized lymphadenopathy due
  to, 62
 prevalence of, among blood donors, 49
 response to hepatitis B vaccine and, 44
 serologic testing for, 48-49
Human T-cell lymphotrophic virus type III
  (HTLV-III). *See* Human immunodeficiency
  virus
Hutchinson's triad, 12
Hypertension, 86-87
Hyperthyroidism
 symptoms and signs of, 88
Hypochlorite solution(s). *See* Sodium
  hypochlorite
Hypothyroidism
 symptoms and signs of, 88

Immune deficiency
 history suggestive of, 83
Immunity
 active, 32t, 33
 passive, 32t, 32-33
Immunization
 recommendations for oral health care workers,
  93-97
Impression(s)
 cleaning and disinfection of, 165, 190, 191t
 American Dental Association
  recommendations for, 221t, 225
 in laboratory, 193, *194*
 dental office procedures for handling, 189-192
Impression tray(s)
 plastic
  sterilization of, 164
Indigestion
 causes of, 87
Infection control
 checklist for, 217t
 "commandments" of, 209-213, 212t
 cost-effectiveness of, 213
 in laboratory, 189-198
 in radiology, 167-175
 rationale for, 71-79
 recommendations for
  American Dental Association, 215-228
  chronology of, 78t
Infectious disease(s), 3-17. *See also* particular
  diseases
 childhood, 5-6
 history of concern about, in dentistry, 3-4
 respiratory, 4-5
 sexually transmitted, 6-13
Infectious hepatitis. *See* Hepatitis A
Infectious mononucleosis, 13
 pharyngitis due to, 4

Infective endocarditis
 antibiotic prophylaxis for, 86, 87t
Influenza
 immunization recommendations for, 96
Instrument(s)
 in radiology
  sterilization of, 170
 recirculation of, 112-113, *159,* 159-165
  facility for. *See* Instrument Recirculation
   Center
 sharp. *See* Sharp(s)
 sterilization of, 107-112, 108t-111t, 114t-115t.
  See also Sterilization
  American Dental Association
   recommendations for, 221-224, 222t-223t
 storage of, 163-164
Instrument Recirculation Center (IRC), *178-179,*
  184-188, *186*
 processing counter in, 186-188
 special considerations in design of, 185-186
Interstitial keratitis
 in congenital syphilis, 12
Intravenous drug user(s)
 human immunodeficiency virus infection in,
  53-55
Iodine, 123-124
Iodophor(s), 123-124, 124t
 for prosthesis disinfection, 190t
Isopropyl alcohol, 122-123, 123t

Jaundice
 causes of, 88
Joint(s)
 swollen, painful
  causes of, 84
Joint replacement
 infection after, 84

Kaposi's sarcoma, 64
 intraoral, 65
 of eyelid and conjunctiva in acquired
  immunodeficiency syndrome, 66
Keratitis
 interstitial, in congenital syphilis, 12
Keratoconjunctivitis
 herpetic, 8
Koplik's spot(s), 6

Label(s)
 Alert, 191-192, *192*
 biohazard, 237-238
Laboratory
 aseptic techniques for use in, 193-196, *194-195*
 barrier techniques for use in, 193
 infection control in, 189-198, *197*
  American Dental Association
   recommendations for, 226
  checklist for, 221t
 office procedures for material to be sent to,
  189-192
LAV (lymphadenopathy-associated virus). *See*
  Human immunodeficiency virus
Lung disease
 chronic obstructive
  oxygen use in, 86
Lymphadenopathy
 persistent generalized (PGL), 62

Pumice
  management of, 194
    American Dental Association
      recommendations on, 226

Quaternary ammonium preparation(s), 121-122,
    122t

Radiology
  design of unit for, 183
  extent of contamination in, 141, 143, 167-169,
    168
  infection control in, 167-175
    preventive measures for, 141-143, 170-173
  recommended cleanup procedures for, 170,
    224
  two-person technique for, 171-172, 172
Recombivax HB, 35-38, 36t, 37, 38t
  contraindication for, 36
Renewal
  in instrument recirculation, 162-163
Respiratory infection(s), 4-5
Respiratory system
  evaluation of, 85-86
Retinal detachment
  symptoms of, 85
Reuse life
  defined, 127
Rhagade(s), 12
Rheumatic heart disease
  infective endocarditis risk and, 86, 87t
Rhinitis
  causes of, 85
  syphilitic, 12
Rubber dam(s), 102
Rubber prophylaxis cup(s), 164
Rubella, 5-6
  immunization recommendations for, 93-94
Rubeola, 6
  immunization recommendations for, 94
Rust
  prevention of, with autoclave sterilization, 108

Saber skin, 12
Saddle nose, 12
Saliva
  areas contaminated by, during dental
    procedures, 71-75, 73, 76-77
  demonstration of spread of, 145
  human immunodeficiency virus transmission
    by, 50, 68
Scaphoid scapula(e), 12
Seborrheic dermatitis
  in acquired immunodeficiency syndrome, 65
Seizure(s), 89
Sensitivity
  of diagnostic tests, 48
Serum hepatitis. *See* Hepatitis B
Sexually transmitted disease(s), 6-13. *See also*
    particular diseases
Shade verification, 195, 196
Sharp(s)
  disposal of, 155, 160, 160, 164
    proposed OSHA standard on, 234
  handling of
    American Dental Association
      recommendations on, 220

Shelf life
  defined, 127
Sink(s)
  design of, 143, 143, 180, 182-183
  for Instrument Recirculation Center
    design of, 185-186
Sinusitis
  acute, 4
  chronic, 4
Skin
  evaluation of, 84
  irritations to, with glove use, 100, 100t
  resident flora of, 98
  transient flora of, 98
Soap(s), 121
  for handwashing, 99
Sodium hypochlorite (bleach), 124-125, 125t
  for environmental surface disinfection
    American Dental Association
      recommendations for, 224
  for prosthesis disinfection, 190, 190t
Spaulding classification, 119, 119t-120t, 173-174
Specificity
  of diagnostic tests, 48
Spore testing device(s)
  for sterilization monitoring, 116, 163
Staphylococcus(-i)
  pneumonia due to, 4
Sterilization, 107-117, 114t-115t
  chemical agents for, 219t, 272t-273t
  classification of objects for, 119t, 173-174
  cold, 120, 127
  defined, 75, 107
  disinfection vs., 107
  dry heat, 109t, 109-110
  ethylene oxide, 111t, 111-112
  glutaraldehyde, 126-127
  monitoring of, 113-116, 163
  of handpieces, 113
    American Dental Association
      recommendations for, 224
    preparation for, 145
  packaging for, 113, 162-163
    materials for, 162
  physical methods of, 107-112
  recommendations for, 162-163
    American Dental Association, 220-224, 222t-
      223t
  sources of error in, 115
  steam, 107-108, 108t
  unsaturated chemical vapor, 110t, 110-111
Storage
  of sterilized instruments, 163-164
Substantivity
  defined, 99
Suction system, 144
Suction tip(s)
  plastic
    sterilization of, 164
Surface(s). *See* Environmental surface(s)
Swallowing
  causes of difficulty in, 87
Syphilis, 10-12
  congenital, 11-12
  late, 11
  primary, 10
  secondary, 11